Cell Biology Research Progress

Cytoskeleton:
Cell Movement, Cytokinesis and Organelles Organization

CELL BIOLOGY RESEARCH PROGRESS

Additional books in this series can be found on Nova's website at:

https://www.novapublishers.com/catalog/index.php?cPath=23_29&seriesp=
Cell+Biology+Research+Progress

Additional e-books in this series can be found on Nova's website at:

https://www.novapublishers.com/catalog/index.php?cPath=23_29&seriespe=
Cell+Biology+Research+Progress

CELL BIOLOGY RESEARCH PROGRESS

CYTOSKELETON: CELL MOVEMENT, CYTOKINESIS AND ORGANELLES ORGANIZATION

SÉBASTIEN LANSING
AND
TRISTAN ROUSSEAU
EDITORS

Nova Biomedical Press, Inc.
New York

Copyright © 2010 by Nova Science Publishers, Inc.

All rights reserved. No part of this book may be reproduced, stored in a retrieval system or transmitted in any form or by any means: electronic, electrostatic, magnetic, tape, mechanical photocopying, recording or otherwise without the written permission of the Publisher.

For permission to use material from this book please contact us:
Telephone 631-231-7269; Fax 631-231-8175
Web Site: http://www.novapublishers.com

NOTICE TO THE READER

The Publisher has taken reasonable care in the preparation of this book, but makes no expressed or implied warranty of any kind and assumes no responsibility for any errors or omissions. No liability is assumed for incidental or consequential damages in connection with or arising out of information contained in this book. The Publisher shall not be liable for any special, consequential, or exemplary damages resulting, in whole or in part, from the readers' use of, or reliance upon, this material.

Independent verification should be sought for any data, advice or recommendations contained in this book. In addition, no responsibility is assumed by the publisher for any injury and/or damage to persons or property arising from any methods, products, instructions, ideas or otherwise contained in this publication.

This publication is designed to provide accurate and authoritative information with regard to the subject matter covered herein. It is sold with the clear understanding that the Publisher is not engaged in rendering legal or any other professional services. If legal or any other expert assistance is required, the services of a competent person should be sought. FROM A DECLARATION OF PARTICIPANTS JOINTLY ADOPTED BY A COMMITTEE OF THE AMERICAN BAR ASSOCIATION AND A COMMITTEE OF PUBLISHERS.

Library of Congress Cataloging-in-Publication Data

Cytoskeleton : cell movement, cytokinesis, and organelles organization / editors, Sébastien Lansing and Tristan Rousseau.
   p. cm.
Includes index.
ISBN 978-1-60876-559-1 (hardcover)
1. Cytoskeleton. 2. Cell receptors. I. Lansing, Sébastien. II. Rousseau, Tristan.
QH603.C96C973 2009
571.6'54--dc22
                    2009044357

Published by Nova Science Publishers, Inc. ✢ *New York*

Contents

Preface		vii
Chapter I	Follow the Leader: When the Urokinase Receptor Coordinates Cell Adhesion, Motility and Proliferation with Cytoskeleton Organization *Marco Archinti, Gabriele Eden, Ronan Murphy and Bernard Degryse*	1
Chapter II	LIMK1, The Key Enzyme of Actin Remodeling Bridges Spatial Organization of Nucleus and Neural Transmission: From Heterochromatin via Non-Coding RNAs to Complex Behavior *Anna V. Medvedeva, Alexander V. Zhuravlev and Elena V. Savvateeva-Popova*	37
Chapter III	Common Tasks of Cytoskeleton and Dystrophin in Muscular and Neurological Functions: Perpectives in Gene Therapy *Joel Cerna Cortés, Dominique Mornet, Doris Cerecedo, Francisco García-Sierra, Janet Hummel, Eliud Alfredo García Montalvo, Olga Lidia Valenzuela Limón, Valery Melnikov, Sergio Adrián Montero Cruz, Juan Alberto Osuna Castro, Alejandra Mancilla, Rafael Rodríguez-Muñoz and Bulmaro Cisneros*	69
Chapter IV	Measuring Reciprocal Regulation of Mesenchymal Stem Cell and Tumor Cell Motility in Two and Three Dimensions In Vitro *Vilma Sardão, Teresa Rose-Hellekant, Ed Perkins, Amy Greene and Jon Holy*	101
Chapter V	Centriole Duplication or DNA Replication - What Starts Earlier? *R. E. Uzbekov and I. B. Alieva*	127
Chapter VI	The Myosin Light Chain-IQGAP Interaction: What is its Function? *David J. Timson*	139

Chapter VII	Migrating Plant Cell: F-Actin Asymmetry Directed by Phosphoinositide Signaling *Koji Mikami*	149
Chapter VIII	Membrane Microdomains and Neural Impulse Propagation: Field Effects in Cytoskeleton Corrals *Ron Wallace*	161
Chapter IX	Scaffolding Proteins that Regulate the Actin Cytoskeleton in Cell Movement *S. J. Annesley and P. R. Fisher*	179
Chapter Sources		309
Index		228

Preface

In this book, the authors review the effects of uPAR on the actin, intermediate filaments and microtubules that constitute the cell cytoskeleton, and the mechanisms used by uPAR to modulate intracellular signalling and temporally fine tune cytoskeletal dynamics. The effects of cytoskeletal components of uPAR expression and cellular distribution are examined as well. In addition, Duchenne Muscular Dystrophy (DMD) is an inherited disorder characterized by progressive muscular degeneration and cognitive impairment due to mutations in the DMD gene. Elucidation of the molecular basis for this illness has determined that cytoskeleton and the product of the DMD gene called dystrophin work in a coordinated way to maintain fibre muscle integrity. The authors describe the scientific path that allows elucidation of the molecular basis of DMD. Furthermore, cell motility is central to many aspects of cell, tissue, and organ function in both health and disease. Some of the more popular published experimental approaches to study cell motility are discussed. Also examined are the IQGAP family of proteins, which are now known to act at the interface between cellular signalling pathways and the actin cytoskeleton.

Chapter I - Since the cloning of the urokinase receptor (uPAR) in 1985, challenging data on the structure and the roles of this receptor have been reported. Originally described as a protease receptor that binds the urokinase-type plasminogen activator (uPA) and thus a central element of the plasminogen activation cascade, uPAR is now also recognized as an anchorage (by binding to the extracellular matrix protein, vitronectin) and a signalling receptor. uPAR is a glycosylphosphatidylinositol (GPI)-anchored protein that does not possess an intracellular domain, but uPAR is nonetheless a full signalling receptor with major functions in cell adhesion, migration, and proliferation. This receptor successfully achieves these functions through its lateral relationships with a wide array of other membrane receptors such as seven-transmembrane domain receptors, integrins and growth-factor receptors. The regulation of these fundamental biological functions implies that uPAR also finely controls the state of organization of the cell cytoskeleton. Indeed, either cell spreading, motility or cytokinesis cannot be correctly executed without the appropriate cytoskeleton reorganization. In this chapter, the authors review the effects of uPAR on the actin, intermediate filaments and microtubules that constitute the cell cytoskeleton, and the mechanisms used by uPAR to modulate intracellular signalling and temporally fine tune cytoskeletal dynamics. In addition, the authors also discuss the effects of cytoskeletal components on uPAR expression and cellular distribution.

Chapter II - According to present knowledge, systemic realization of genetic activity in the dynamic spatial organization of the genome in the nucleus provides such a level of plasticity of complex biological systems that allows them to adequately respond to environmental stimuli or signals during the development, modulate and shift the balance of contacting components and dimensions of their interactions, resulting in structural rearrangements. The chromosome positions within the nucleus determine both normal development and progression of genomic diseases, i.e., changes according to the environmental requirements, current needs of the organism, and its individual experience. At the same time, the striking output of the evolution of higher organisms, largely ignored to date, is that only 1.2% of the mammalian genome encodes proteins and the vast majority of the expressed information is in RNA. There are hundreds of thousands of non-coding (nc) RNAs, as well as many other yet-to-be-discovered small regulatory RNAs . A new paradigm envisions the interactions between these two worlds, the one of protein and the other of RNA, as providing a dynamic link between the transcriptome and the environment and, therefore, the progressive maturation and functional plasticity of the nervous system in health and disease. Also, a wide repertoire of ncRNAs plays an important role in chromatin organization, gene expression, and disease etiology via a signal cascade of actin remodeling (LIMK1, cofilin, actin). The activity of the protein kinase LIMK1 that controls spine development, local dendritic translation at postsynaptic sites and ionotropic glutamate receptor trafficking is regulated by a brain-specific miRNA miR-134. This miRNA is localized to the synapto-dendritic compartment of rat hippocampal neurons and negatively regulates the size of dendritic spines--postsynaptic sites of excitatory synaptic transmission. Moreover, LIMK1 hemizygosity is considered to cause cognitive defects in a genome disorder Williams syndrome. Drosophila is a helpful model organism to determine the sequence of events in this system of hierarchical relationships. Drosophila LIMK1 gene (*agnostic*) with a specific chromosome architecture around the gene capable of generating miRNAs, recapitulates many features both of Williams syndrome and of neurodegenerative disorders. Mutants in the gene have increased expression of LIMK1 and cofilin, modified chromosome packaging and homologous and nonhomologous pairing, implemented in different rates of unequal recombination. Also, they display congofilic inclusions both in the adult brain and larval tissues presumably leading to severe defects in learning and memory during courtship conditioning.

Chapter III - Duchenne Muscular Dystrophy (DMD) is an inherited disorder characterized by progressive muscular degeneration and cognitive impairment due to mutations in the DMD gene. This disease seriously affects the quality of life of DMD patients causing death due to cardiac and respiratory complications before 30 years of age. Elucidation of the molecular basis for this illness has determined that cytoskeleton and the product of the DMD gene called dystrophin works in a coordinated way to maintain fibre muscle integrity. It is known that cytoskeleton via its association with the integrin complexes modulates migration of stem cells during embryogenesis to give rise to diverse tissues and organs. This association is also important in performing basic neurological processes such as synaptogenesis. Recent findings have shown that the DMD gene is also manifested in the central nervous system where it has different functions from that seen in muscle. Among the most clearly defined tasks of DMD gene in neurons is its involvement in modulating the formation of beta 1-integrin complexes. This chapter describes the scientific path that allowed elucidation of the molecular basis for Duchenne Muscular Dystrophy. The up dated knowledge to explain the role of the DMD gene in neurological functions is also described together with the advances in the design of therapeutic strategies focused on restoration of the DMD gene function in patients.

Chapter IV - Cell motility is central to many aspects of cell, tissue, and organ function in both health and disease. Examples include the morphogenetic events of embryogenesis, the functioning of the immune system, wound healing, angiogenesis, and the metastatic spread of cancer. Consequently, numerous methods have been developed to study cell motility. One rapidly growing area of interest in the cell motility field involves the interactions between tumor cells, surrounding stromal cells, and mesenchymal stem cells (MesSCs), which can be recruited to tumor sites. Important motility-related questions include how MesSCs are able to home to tumor sites, and, once present at a tumor site, how they affect the metastatic potential of the tumor cells. This chapter discusses and compares some of the more popular published experimental approaches to study cell motility, with an emphasis on assays that are suitable for studies of MesSC-tumor cell interactions *in vitro*. Both two-dimensional and three-dimensional cell motility assays are described, along with the specific strengths and weaknesses of each assay for interrogating specific subcomponents of the motility process. The authors also describe a novel murine breast cancer-MesSC model system that is well suited for *in vitro*, as well as *in vivo* studies of the motility events associated with tumor cell-MesSC interactions.

Chapter V - Animal centrosome an organelle consists of centrioles and associated structures surrounded by pericentriolar material, is the major microtubule organizing center in interphase cell and spindle pole component in mitosis and indispensable organelle for cilia and flagella formation.

In diploid cells, the centrosome usually includes not more then two centrioles and since the number of centrosomes in the cell is determined by the number of centrioles, cells have developed effective mechanisms to control centriole formation and to tightly coordinate this process with DNA replication. Duplication of this organelle and chromosomes redoubling during DNA replication are two principal events of cell cycle in the course of cell division progression. The principal question is what starts earlier, the duplication of centrioles or DNA replication? During last five years, some proteins, which participate in the process of procentriole formation, were found, but temporal sequences of cell cycle events are not still fully investigated. Traditionally the time of centriole replication beginning denote like G_1/S or even S, although precise analysis was not ever undertaken.

In present study, the ultrastructural analysis of centrosomes from cells that were previously in one's lifetime observed after mitosis was used in combination with autoradiography of the same cells. PE cells were individually monitored after mitosis and procentriole appearance was detected by electron microscopy as soon as 5–6 h after mitosis. This period was 1–2 h shorter than minimal duration of G_1-phase in PE cell line. Ultrastructural serial sections analysis of centrosomes in the cells with known "cell cycle age" in combination with ^{3}H-thimidine autoradiography study of the same cells directly confirmed that centrioles duplication started earlier than cells entered in S-phase of cell cycle, i.e., preceded the DNA replication. The data were obtained showed that centriole duplication started before the beginning of DNA replication.

Chapter VI - The first members of the IQGAP family of proteins were characterised over 15 years ago. It is now known that these molecules act at the interface between cellular signalling pathways and the actin cytoskeleton. They bind to a diverse range of signalling molecules – including those involved in calcium, GTPase, kinase and growth factor signalling. One intriguing interaction is that between mammalian IQGAP1 and the myosin essential light chain isoform, Mlc1sa. Although this has been demonstrated *in vitro*, its *in vivo* role is not known. Indeed, it would be tempting to dismiss it as an experimental artefact, except for the existence of a parallel interaction in the budding yeast, *Saccharomyces cerevisae*. In this organism, the IQGAP-like protein (Iqg1p) interacts with a myosin essential light chain (Mlc1p). This interaction is critical for the correct execution of cytokinesis. IQGAP-like proteins also play key roles in cytokinesis in other fungi. Recent work implicating mammalian IQGAP1 in cytokinesis may help explain the role of the interaction in higher eukarytotes.

Chapter VII - Polarity is a fundamental cell property essential for differentiation, proliferation and morphogenesis in unicellular and multicellular organisms. It is well known that polarized distribution of F-actin is important in providing the driving force for directional migration in mammalian leukocytes and *Dictyostelium* cells. Phosphoinositide (PI) signaling, including phosphatidylinositol kinases and phospholipases, is also critical for the formation of cell polarity in these cells. A monospore from the marine red alga *Porphyra yezoensis* is well known as a migrating plant cell and thus is a unique and useful material for investigating polarity determination in plant cells. As in leukocytes and *Dictyostelium* cells, monospore migration requires asymmetrical distribution of F-actin, whose establishment is regulated by the phosphatidylinositol 3-kinase and phospholipase C, whereas phospholipase D is involved in the maintenance of F-actin distribution. These findings indicate that the regulation of F-actin asymmetry by PI signaling cascades is evolutionarily conserved in terms of the establishment of cell polarity in migrating eukaryotic cells.

Chapter VIII - The possibility that an ensemble of neural-membrane lipids could regulate the duration of the ion-channel "open" conformation may have direct implications for local gating of the action potential (AP). The control of channel dynamics is equivalent to controlling the transmembrane ion conductances responsible for neural depolarization and hyperpolarization. Accordingly, if a membrane region in an axon were to contain (for example) clusters of Na^+ channels with relatively longer open states, such a structure would be conducive to a local depolarization (spike) and the continuing propagation of the neural impulse. By contrast, if the Na^+ channels had brief open states, the structure would be conducive to impulse propagation failure. Modulation of the membrane state through other channel types would of course also be possible. A good example is the A-current delayed-rectifier K^+ channel (K_A), currently the object of intensive research because of its possible role in conduction failure. The K_A channel is gated by membrane hyperpolarization, which it increases and prolongs by rapidly conducting potassium ions out of the cytosol. A prolonged open time for this channel could hypothetically strengthen the delayed-rectifier effect and significantly increase the probability of conduction block.

This chapter examines the possible role of neural membrane microdomains in regulating the propagation of the action potential. These data are particularly important because they appear consistent with the concept that "local switches" regulate AP propagation (Scott, 1995). The chapter begins with an overview of the experimental evidence for AP conduction failure. It then examines the two major alternative models: one emphasizing the role of impedance mismatch due to neuron branching geometry; the other emphasizing the role of prolonged hyperpolarization due to the A-current potassium channel (K_A). A model emphasizing the possible interaction of a microdomain-cytoskeleton system with neuron branching geometry will then be presented (Wallace, 2004).. Because of the large number of studies bearing on the subject, the K_A channel will be used as the basic example, although the possible contributions of other channel types will be briefly discussed. The chapter concludes with a discussion of how microdomain regulation of AP propagation may explain a number of neuron features that strikingly depart from cable properties.

Chapter IX - Actin is the main component of the microfilament system in all eukaryotic cells and is essential for most intra- and inter-cellular movement including muscle contraction, cell movement, cytokinesis, cytoplasmic organisation and intracellular transport. The polymerisation and depolymerisation of actin filaments in nonmuscle cells is highly regulated and the reorganisation of the actin cytoskeleton can occur within seconds after chemotactic stimulation. There are many proteins which are involved in the regulation of the actin cytoskeleton. These include receptors which receive chemotactic stimuli, G proteins, second messengers, signalling molecules, kinases, phosphatases and transcription factors. These proteins are varied and numerous and are involved in multiple pathways. Despite the large number of proteins, there are not enough to coordinate the various responses of the cytoskeleton. An additional level of regulation is conferred by scaffolding proteins.

Due to the presence of numerous protein interaction domains, scaffolding proteins can tether various proteins to a certain location within the cell to facilitate the rapid transfer of signals from one protein to the next. This colocalisation of the components of a particular pathway also helps to prevent unwanted crosstalk with components of other pathways. Tethering receptors, kinases, phosphatases and cytoskeletal components to a particular location within a cell helps ensure efficient relaying and feedback inhibition of signals to enable rapid activation and inactivation of responses. Scaffolding proteins are also thought to stabilise the otherwise weak interactions between particular proteins in a cascade and to catalyse the activation of the pathway components. There are numerous scaffolding proteins involved in the regulation of the cytoskeleton and this chapter has focussed on examples from several groups of scaffolding proteins including the MAPK scaffolds, the AKAPs, scaffolds of the post synaptic density and actin binding scaffolding proteins.

Chapter I

Follow the Leader: When the Urokinase Receptor Coordinates Cell Adhesion, Motility and Proliferation with Cytoskeleton Organization

Marco Archinti[1], Gabriele Eden[2], Ronan Murphy[3] and Bernard Degryse**

[1]Institute for Research in Biomedicine, Parc Cientific de Barcelona, Baldiri Reixac 10, 08028 Barcelona, Spain.
[2]Division of Nephrology, Hannover Medical School, Hannover, Germany.
[3]School of Health and Human Performance, Faculty of Science and Health, Dublin City University, Glasnevin, Dublin 9, Ireland.

Abstract

Since the cloning of the urokinase receptor (uPAR) in 1985, challenging data on the structure and the roles of this receptor have been reported. Originally described as a protease receptor that binds the urokinase-type plasminogen activator (uPA) and thus a central element of the plasminogen activation cascade, uPAR is now also recognized as an anchorage (by binding to the extracellular matrix protein, vitronectin) and a signalling receptor. uPAR is a glycosylphosphatidylinositol (GPI)-anchored protein that does not possess an intracellular domain, but uPAR is nonetheless a full signalling receptor with major functions in cell adhesion, migration, and proliferation. This receptor successfully achieves these functions through its lateral relationships with a wide array of other membrane receptors such as seven-transmembrane domain receptors, integrins and growth-factor receptors. The regulation of these fundamental biological functions implies that uPAR also finely controls the state of organization of the cell cytoskeleton. Indeed, either cell spreading, motility or cytokinesis cannot be correctly executed without the appropriate cytoskeleton reorganization. In this chapter, we review the effects of uPAR

---

* Corresponding author: E-mail: degryse.bernard@hsr.it

on the actin, intermediate filaments and microtubules that constitute the cell cytoskeleton, and the mechanisms used by uPAR to modulate intracellular signalling and temporally fine tune cytoskeletal dynamics. In addition, we also discuss the effects of cytoskeletal components on uPAR expression and cellular distribution.

Introduction

Glycosylphosphatidylinositol (GPI)-anchored proteins form a unique class of proteins that are bound to the outside leaflet of the plasma membrane. This family of receptors includes functionally diverse proteins such as enzymes, adhesion molecules, surface antigens, others active proteins and receptors [for reviews see Paulick and Bertozzi, 2008; Orlean and Menon, 2007].

The urokinase receptor (uPAR) belongs to the latter sub-family of GPI-anchored proteins. uPAR is a multi-ligand and multi-functional receptor that regulates pericellular proteolysis and protease activation, gene expression, cell proliferation, adhesion and migration. These roles are reflected at the molecular level by the functioning of uPAR which is known as a protease (that binds urokinase), anchorage (that binds vitronectin), and as a signalling receptor. The latter is certainly the most surprising characteristic because uPAR being a GPI-anchored protein has no intracellular domain. However, this receptor successfully mediates signals to the cell through its lateral relationships with a wide array of other receptors namely seven-transmembrane domain receptors such as FPRL1; endocytic receptors such as LRP-1 (low density lipoprotein receptor-related protein-1), VLDL-R (Very Low-Density Lipoprotein Receptor), the mannose 6-phosphate/IGF-II receptor (CD222, CIMPR), or uPARAP (Endo180); caveolin; the gp130 cytokine receptor; tyrosine kinase receptors such as the EGF receptor (EGFR), the PDGF receptor (PDGFR) or the IGF-1 receptor (IGF-1R); and integrins [for reviews see Blasi and Carmeliet, 2002; Degryse, 2003, 2008; Ragno, 2006].

The partners of uPAR are structurally different and exert various molecular functions. This diversity certainly explains how uPAR manages basic but essential physiological processes for instance cell adhesion, migration and proliferation. At the first glance, these processes are divergent and have rather contrasting goals i.e. immobility vs. motion vs. growth respectively. However, the least common denominator of all these processes is the cell cytoskeleton. Without a tight and timely control of the cytoskeleton organization, all these fundamental processes would fail or would not even start. It is remarkable that uPAR succeeds in regulating the specific organization of the cytoskeleton during such divergent cellular processes.

In this chapter, we focus on the relationship between uPAR and the cell cytoskeleton summarizing our current knowledge. We also discuss the influence of the cytoskeleton on uPAR.

Structure of a Leader

The Extracellular Domains of uPAR

In humans, the gene of uPAR is located on chromosome 19 (19q13.1-q13.2), which is then transcribed into a 1.4 kb mRNA and later translated into a 335-residue precursor. At the N-terminal, the removal of a signal peptide of 22 amino acids leads to a 313-residue single polypeptide chain presenting five potential glycosylation sites. uPAR is modified post-translationally at the C-terminal by the cleavage of a 30-residue GPI anchor sequence signal and the attachment of the GPI anchor. Full-length uPAR consists of a 283-residue single-chain protein. The molecular weight of the non-glycosylated polypeptide is approximately 35,000 while the one of the glycoprotein is about 55,000-60,000 [Nielsen et al., 1988; Roldan et al., 1990; Blasi and Carmeliet, 2002].

uPAR is a cysteine-rich molecule, and disulphide bonds give a structure comprised of 3 homologous domains. Domain I is located at the N-terminus while the GPI anchor added post-translationally is placed at the C-terminus of domain III [for reviews on uPAR see Blasi and Camerliet, 2002; Degryse, 2003, 2008; Ragno, 2006]. Domain II contains the D2A sequence (residues $_{130}$IQEGEEGRPKDDR$_{142}$ of human uPAR) that was the first identified region of uPAR involved in uPAR-integrin interactions [Degryse et al., 2005]. The minimum active sequence composed by the four residues GEEG was also reported [Degryse et al., 2005]. D2A-derived synthetic peptide binds at least to integrins αvβ3 and α5β1 inducing integrin- but not uPAR-dependent signalling thereby stimulating cell migration. Moreover, our most recent experimental data demonstrated that D2A is also mitogenic and represents the first identified mitogenic sequence of uPAR [Eden et al., in preparation]. So far, the D2A sequence is the only region of uPAR that has been described to have intrinsic signalling activities inducing cell migration and growth [Degryse et al., 2005]. Changing the two glutamic acids into two alanines in the D2A motif generated two inhibitors of cell migration, the D2A-Ala and GAAG peptides [Degryse et al., 2005]. Interestingly, D2A-Ala and GAAG are also inhibitors of cell proliferation and tumour growth in vivo [Eden et al., in preparation]. Other sites of uPAR-integrin interactions have been identified in the domain III of uPAR [Chaurasia et al., 2006; Wei et al., 2007]. The synthetic peptide corresponding to sequence $_{240}$GCATASMCQ$_{248}$ of human uPAR disrupts suPAR-α5β1 integrin complex [Chaurasia et al., 2006]. In addition, mutants of uPAR bearing single point mutation S245A or H249A, and D262A fail to associate to integrins α5β1 and α3β1 respectively [Chaurasia, 2006; Wei, 2007].

Linker regions are present in between domain I and II, and domain II and III. The DI-DII linker region is highly sensitive to proteolytic cleavage and harbors the first identified chemotactically active sequence SRSRY (human sequence) that is involved in the interactions with seven-transmembrane domain receptors such as FPRL1 [Resnati et al., 1996, 2002; Fazioli et al., 1997; Degryse et al., 1999; de Paulis et al., 2004; Gargiulo et al., 2005; Seleri et al., 2005]. The SRSRY motif is not always exposed on the uPAR surface. By binding to uPAR, urokinase (uPA) induces a crucial change of conformation that results in the exposition of the SRSRY chemotactic epitope. This conformational change permits uPAR-seven-transmembrane domain receptor interaction by metamorphosing uPAR into a ligand of FPRL1 which in its turn mediates signalling and promotes cell migration (Figure 1A).

uPAR exists under different forms. Soluble uPAR (suPAR) is generated by the degradation of the GPI anchor. Moreover, high levels of the soluble forms of uPAR are markers of cancers and correlate with poor clinical prognosis [Stephens et al., 1999; Mustjoki et al., 1999; Sier et al., 1999]. Proteolytic cleavage in the DI-DII linker region of both membrane-bound uPAR and suPAR by a variety of proteases including uPA produces DI fragment and DIIDIII-uPAR [Ploug and Ellis, 1994]. Interestingly, DIIDIII-uPAR is chemotactically active mimicking the effects of uPA. This fact suggests that the proteolytic cleavage has led to the exposition of the SRSRY motif and that DIIDIII-uPAR can bind to FPRL1 [Fazioli et al., 1997]. However, the proteolytic cleavage can occur at other sites in the DI-DII linker region generating two kinds of DIIDIII-uPAR possessing or not the intact SRSRY sequence. Therefore, only full-length uPAR and suPAR, SRSRY-DIIDIII-uPAR and SRSRY-DIIDIII-suPAR can stimulate cell migration. Furthermore, all forms of DIIDIII-uPAR cannot bind to uPA or vitronectin (VN). In contrast, the two-chain kinin-free high molecular weight kininogen (HKa) is capable of binding domains II and III of both DIIDIII-uPAR and full-length uPAR in a Zn^{2+}-dependent manner [Colman et al., 1997; Chavakis et al., 2000]. HKa and VN are competitive binding partners providing uPAR with interesting anti-adhesive and adhesive properties.

The three-dimensional structure of uPAR has been resolved recently [Llinas et al., 2005; Huang et al., 2005; Barinka et al., 2006; Huai et al., 2006]. The three external domains form a globular-like structure in the form of a "croissant" creating a central pocket where uPA the main ligand of uPAR can bind. The crystal data are coherent with previous biochemical studies showing that all three domains are involved in the binding of uPA but with domain I being predominant. The crystal structure also revealed that the whole external part of uPAR constitutes a very large surface useful for the binding of the other soluble ligands (Table 1) and lateral partners of uPAR (Table 2).

The Lipid Anchor of uPAR

The GPI anchor is certainly the most original and important characteristic of uPAR. Due to this lipid anchor, uPAR is entirely located on the outer side of the plasma membrane. uPAR has neither transmembrane nor intracellular domains.

In many reviews on uPAR the fact that GPI anchoring is a very complicated and metabolically expensive process is too often simply not mentioned [for reviews see Orlean and Menon, 2007; Paulick and Bertozzi, 2008]. GPI anchors are widely present among eukaryotic organisms including protozoa, yeasts, fungi, plants, insects, and mammals. GPI anchoring is extremely important in the embryonic development of mammals as the deficiency of GPI biosynthesis results in fetal lethality [Orlean and Menon, 2007; Paulick and Bertozzi, 2008]. About >20 genes are involved in the synthesis of the anchor that take place in the endoplasmic reticulum. It is only when completed that the whole GPI anchor will be assembled to the protein bearing a GPI anchor sequence signal at the C-terminus. The common structure of the GPI anchor consists of three domains: a phosphoethanolamine linker (that is bound to the C-terminus of the protein), a conserved glycan core, and a phospholipid tail. The glycan core is the subject of variability meaning that the GPI anchors from diverse GPI-anchored proteins are not identical [Orlean and Menon, 2007; Paulick and Bertozzi, 2008]. In the literature, examples of the influence of the nature of the GPI anchor on the functions of the proteins can be found [Nicholson and Stanners, 2006]. However, so far no correlation has been reported between the structure and the function of the GPI anchors. The exact functions of the complex GPI anchors are still being discussed [Paulick and Bertozzi, 2008].

The same uncertainty can be extended to the functions of the GPI anchor of uPAR. Very little knowledge can be claimed beside the fact that the GPI anchor provides uPAR with a convenient and efficient link to the cell surface. However, a few interesting statements can reasonably be made based on the published literature. First, the GPI anchor seems to influence the conformation of uPAR. It is indeed well known that soluble and GPI-bound uPAR have different conformations [Høyer-Hansen et al., 2001; Andolfo et al., 2002]. A similar change of conformation has also been reported for Thy-1 another GPI-anchored protein [Barboni et al., 1995].

The presence of the GPI anchor may represent a convenient signal to address a protein in particular domains of the plasma membrane, the lipid rafts [Varma and Mayor, 1998; Friedrichson and Kurzchalia, 1998; Nicholson and Stanners, 2006]. This is also true for uPAR that was reported to be present in lipid rafts and caveolae [Okada et al., 1995; Stahl and Mueller, 1995; Koshelnick et al., 1997; Wei et al., 1999; Schwab et al., 2001; Cunningham et al., 2003; Sitrin et al., 2004; Sahores et al., 2008]. In addition, uPA enhances uPAR redistribution into lipid rafts [Sahores et al., 2008]. The effect of uPA suggests that the conformation of the receptor may exert an influence on uPAR localization into lipid rafts [Sahores et al., 2008]. Dimerization of uPAR was also suggested to redirect uPAR into lipid rafts and to be required for VN binding [Sidenius et al., 2002; Cunningham et al., 2003].

The influence of the GPI anchor on uPAR has not been thoroughly studied. In one study, the presence or the absence of the GPI anchor does not appear to interfere with uPAR functioning [Li et al., 1994]. The comparison of uPAR with a chimeric uPAR built using the extracellular domains attached to the transmembrane and intracellular domains of the α chain of the IL-2 receptor, showed that the kinetics of binding, internalization and degradation of the uPA/Plasminogen activator inhibitor-1 (PAI-1) complex were identical [Li et al., 1994]. These data are consistent with the fact that cleaved suPAR (that exposes the SRSRY epitope) can mimic the effects of uPAR [Resnati et al., 1996].

A more recent study employed a reverse strategy. The GPI anchor of uPAR was associated with different external domains [Madsen et al., 2007]. In that report, a chimeric receptor composed of the GPI anchor of uPAR and PAI-1 was compared to uPAR. PAI-1 was chosen because this serpin binds to VN in a similar region [Okumura et al., 2002]. The chimeric receptor mimicked the effects of uPAR on cell morphology suggesting that the external domains of uPAR play a minor role [Madsen et al., 2007].

The Functioning of uPAR or How to be a Top Dog

Classically, it is a well accepted paradigm that uPAR exerts both protease-dependent and protease-independent functions. On the one hand, by binding uPA, uPAR regulates pericellular proteolysis and protease activation. On the other hand, by binding its soluble ligands (Table 1) and interacting with its membrane-bound partners (Table 2), uPAR serves as a signalling receptor.

The first identified function of uPAR was to be the receptor of uPA. Thus, uPAR is a major player in the regulation of pericellular proteolysis. uPAR enhances the rate of activation of pro-uPA into uPA, initiating and/or increasing the activation of plasminogen into active plasmin [Ellis et al., 1989]. At the same time, uPAR masters the localization of uPA activity at discrete points of the cell surface. The perfect control of pericellular proteolysis is of particular relevance in the context of cell movement such as cell migration or proliferation. The adherent cell has to sever its links with its surrounding cells before starting migrating or dividing. The degradation of extracellular matrix (ECM) and of basement membrane proteins, intravasation and extravasation represent key steps in tumour invasion and/or metastastic dissemination. Concerning cell proliferation uPAR exerts an additional role by ruling growth factors activation. Indeed, uPA activates growth factors such as basic fibroblast growth factor (bFGF), pro-transforming growth factor-β (pro-TGF-β), and pro-hepatocyte growth factor (pro-HGF) [Odekon et al., 1992, 1994; Naldini et al., 1992, 1995].

Table 1. The external ligands of uPAR

Nature	Roles	Name
Inactive zymogen	Precursor of uPA Induces cell adhesion, migration and proliferation	Pro-urokinase (pro-uPA)
Serine protease	Activates plasminogen into plasmin Induces cell adhesion, migration and proliferation	High molecular weight form urokinase (HMW-uPA)
Complex of uPA and its physiological inhibitor PAI-1	No proteolytic activity Blocks uPA-dependent cell migration Promotes uPAR and integrin internalization	PAI-1/uPA complex
Extracellular matrix and plasma protein	Induces cell adhesion and migration Cofactor of PAI-1	Vitronectin (VN)
Plasma protein	Pro-inflammatory activity Inhibits VN-dependent cell adhesion and migration	Two chain high molecular weight kininogen (HKa)
Secreted protein	Development of brain speech areas	SRPX2 [Royer-Zeimmour et al., 2008]
Anchor-less microbial surface protein from *Streptococcus Pyogenes*	Glycolytic enzyme Induces bacterial adherence to host cells	Streptococcal surface deshydrogenase (SDH) [Jin et al., 2005]

Table 2. The lateral ligands of uPAR

Nature	Roles	Name
GPI-linked protein	Plasminogen activation Pericellular proteolysis Cell adhesion, migration and proliferation	Urokinase receptor (uPAR)
Seven-transmembrane domain receptors	Cell migration	FPRL1, FPRL2, FPR
Integrins	Cell adhesion and migration	α3β1, α4β1, α5β1, α6β1, α9β1, αvβ3, αvβ5, αvβ6, αMβ2, αLβ2, αXβ2
Receptor tyrosine kinases	Cell proliferation and migration	EGFR, PDGFR, IGF-1R
Endocytic receptors	uPAR internalization (LRP-1 induces both uPAR and integrin internalization)	LRP-1, LRP1B, VLDL-R, mannose 6-phosphate-R, endo180
Scaffolding/ structural protein	Intracellular signalling	Caveolin
Cytokine receptor	Cell migration	gp130
Complement receptor	Complement activation	gC1qR
Adhesion receptor	Cell adhesion	L-selectin
Serine protease	Pericellular proteolysis	Seprase

However, beside its permissive functions as a protease receptor, uPAR also exerts important inducing functions as a signalling receptor. uPAR mediates various signals including proliferative and migratory signals. The SRSRY sequence is responsible for the migratory properties of uPAR through seven-transmembrane domain receptors implicating uPAR as a cell surface chemokine [Blasi, 1999; Fazioli et al., 1997; Degryse et al., 1999] or MACKINE (Membrane-Anchored ChemoKINE-like proteins) [Degryse, 2003]. Furthermore, the D2A region via direct interactions with the integrins induces integrin-dependent signalling and cell migration [Degryse et al., 2005]. The D2A motif can also initiate a mitogenic signal resulting in EGFR activation and cell growth [Eden et al., in preparation]. Here, it appears clearly that standing on the top of a long list of membrane-bound partners such as seven transmembrane domain receptors, receptor tyrosine kinases and integrins, provides an ultimate advantage. Being in pole position, uPAR can rule diverse receptors and signalling pathways. Recent experimental data further support that idea. uPAR controls the activity of a variety of receptors including integrins and EGFR. uPAR expression boosts integrin-dependent cell migration [Degryse et al., 2005]. While in the absence of uPAR or when uPAR activity is blocked, the EGFR does not function [Jo et al., 2007; D'Alessio et al., 2008; Eden et al., in preparation].

Interestingly, uPAR may also control its own activity through the formation of uPAR dimers. Dimerization has been suggested to be crucial for the binding of VN but also for the redistribution of uPAR into the lipid rafts [Sidenius et al., 2002; Cunningham et al., 2003]. It is quite tempting to assume that dimerization represents a mechanism of uPAR activation as suggested [Sitrin et al., 2000; Cunningham et al., 2003]. Furthermore, dimerization is the common activation mechanism of many receptors and signalling proteins including the ErbB family and Janus kinases [for reviews see Wieduwilt and Moasser, 2008; Aaronson and Horvath, 2002], and lipid rafts are viewed as convenient signalling platforms [for a review see Lajoie et al., 2009].

However, it may not just be that simple, and dimerization may be as well considered an inactivation mechanism. VN-bound uPAR i.e. the uPAR dimer does not seem to induce signalling. We previously reported that VN binding to uPAR did not initiate signalling and failed to promote cell migration [Degryse et al., 2001a]. In addition, both full-length VN and VN_{40-459} fragment lacking the SMB domain (which cannot bind to uPAR) have similar chemotactic activity supporting the idea that VN-induced migratory signal does not depend on VN binding to uPAR [Degryse et al., 2005]. Furthermore, VN binding to uPAR provided cell anchorage but failed to induce cell spreading [Stahl and Mueller, 1997; Sidenius and Blasi, 2000]. A more recent study revealed that uPAR monomers are engaged in signalling complexes as shown by the measurement of diffusion coefficients of monomers and dimers suggesting that uPAR monomers rather than dimers are the active form of uPAR [Malengo et al., 2008].

uPAR mobility onto the plasma membrane may be correlated with its functions. It is the change of conformation of the receptor induced by uPA leading to the exposition of the SRSRY motif (i.e. the activation of uPAR) that controls the cellular distribution of uPAR. uPA-bound uPAR redistributes to particular areas of the cell surface [Resnati et al., 1996; Degryse et al., 1999]. For instance, in rat smooth muscle cells challenged with uPA, uPAR accumulates at the leading edge of the migrating cell [Degryse et al., 1999]. It is the same mechanism (the conformational change that results in the exposition of the SRSRY epitope) that promotes lateral interactions with other membrane receptors such as FPRL1 and integrins resulting in the formation of large signalling complexes [Bohuslav et al., 1995]. In perfect agreement, uPA-induced chemotaxis is inhibited by both anti-uPAR and anti-$\alpha v \beta 3$ antibodies [Degryse et al., 1999]. The reverse relationship is also true, both anti-uPAR and anti-$\alpha v \beta 3$ antibodies efficiently block VN-induced cell migration [Degryse et al., 2001a]. Moreover, uPA binding to uPAR (thus, again the activation of uPAR) increases the relocalization of uPAR into lipid rafts [Sahores et al., 2008]. Lipids rafts and caveolae constitutes microdomains of the plasma membrane forming convenient signalling platforms where uPAR interacts with its membrane-bound ligands and regulates downstream signalling molecules such as c-Src and FAK (Focal Adhesion Kinase) [for a review see Lajoie et al., 2009]. The presence of uPAR in these micro-domains appears connected to signalling as uPAR was reported to associate to and stabilize integrin-caveolin-β_1 complex [Wei et al., 1999; Chapman et al., 1999]. In addition, uPAR clustering initiates uPA-dependent signalling [Sitrin et al., 2000, 2004].

The internalization of uPAR is thought to be an essential mechanism that maintains the uPAR system running. Thanks to the internalization process, free uPAR is recycled back at special locations on the cell surface such a new focal adhesions assembled at the leading edge of the migrating cell [Prager et al., 2004]. The internalization of uPAR via the clathrin-coated pathway is initiated by PAI-1, the physiological inhibitor of uPA. The formation of PAI-1/uPA complex allows the interactions with the low density lipoprotein receptor-related protein (LRP-1), and then direct interactions between LRP-1 and uPAR [Nykjaer et al., 1992, 1994; Conese et al., 1995; Czekay et al., 2001]. The whole LRP-1/PAI-1/uPA/uPAR complex is internalized, then the PAI-1/uPA complex is degraded while uPAR is recycled back to the cell surface from the early endosomes [Nykjaer et al., 1997]. It is easy to understand that for the efficient PAI-1-induced internalization of uPAR, the presence of a whole intact uPAR (for its uPA binding capacity) is required on the cell membrane. In fact, DIIDIII-uPAR is poorly internalized. uPA, uPA/PAI-1 and LRP-1 do not bind to DIIDIII-uPAR, and consequently this shorter form of uPAR is not efficiently internalized [Høyer-Hansen et al., 1992; Nykjaer et al., 1998; Ragno et al., 1998].

The cellular importance of regenerating ligand-free uPAR on the cell surface is further illustrated by the recent discovery of a new mechanism of internalization and recycling of uPAR [Cortese et al., 2008]. Beside the classical clathrin-mediated LRP-1-dependent internalization of uPAR, a micropinocytic-like route that is PAI-1/uPA- and lipid rafts-independent provides the cell with endocytosis and rapid recycling of uPAR [Cortese et al., 2008].

A third mechanism of uPAR internalization involves the mannose 6-phosphate/insulin-like growth factor-II receptor (Cation-Independent Mannose 6-Phosphate Receptor, CIMPR). Here again, this internalization receptor negatively regulates uPAR functions [Leksa et al., 2002]. Interestingly, the CIMPR-dependent mechanism is the only route described so far leading to the internalization of both the full-length and the shorter form of uPAR. Indeed, the CIMPR binds and internalizes both uPAR and DIIDIII-uPAR in an uPA-independent manner [Nykjaer et al., 1998]. Tumour cells exhibit more copies of DIIDIII-uPAR than of full-length uPAR on their cell surface [Ragno et al., 1998].

Evidence supports the idea that the regeneration of ligand-free uPAR on the plasma membrane is crucial for the functioning of the uPAR system. In that way, new interactions with uPA or VN are possible, and the localization of uPAR is under control [Prager et al., 2004]. Thus, uPAR internalization is a convenient and powerful mechanism for the regulation of both uPAR activity and location. In the absence of uPAR regeneration on the cell membrane, cells stop migrating [Degryse et al., 2001b]. By promoting the LRP-1-dependent internalization of uPAR and also of integrins, PAI-1 blocks uPA-induced cell migration and promotes cell detachment [Degryse et al., 2001b; Czekay et al., 2003]. Indeed, uPAR internalization can also regulate the activity and the number of integrins present on the cell surface [Czekay et al., 2003]. A mechanism that is valid for different integrins [Czekay et al, 2003]. Thus, uPAR internalization is a fast and convenient mechanism of integrin regulation that once again highlights the importance of the uPAR-integrin interactions.

Conversely, blocking the internalization of uPA/uPAR results in increased production and expression of uPA/uPAR on the cell surface, subsequently enhancing plasminogen activation, cell motility and tumoural cell invasion [Weaver et al., 1997; Webb et al., 1999, 2000; Sid et al., 2006].

The formation of uPAR-integrin complex is certainly the main step of the functioning of uPAR and lays the foundation stone of the uPAR signalosome or chameleon signalosome [Degryse, 2008]. The uPAR-integrin constitute a convenient and adaptable signalling complex better defined as chameleon signalosome that consents to build up larger signalling complexes and to adjust their compositions in order to meet the evolving cellular requirements as the cell adhere, migrate or proliferate. The impressive figure of the 156 components of the integrin adhesome i.e. the molecules that interact with and constitute the integrin network makes clear that the benefits of combining the uPAR system with the integrin system are great [Zaidel-Bar et al., 2007]. The large family of integrin receptors mediates bi-directional signalling and is connected to the cell cytoskeleton. Integrins are multi-ligands receptors and possess numerous membrane-bound partners [Porter and Hogg, 1998]. Integrins are for instance indispensable partners of growth factor and cytokine receptors. However, further studies will be necessary to completely determine uPAR-integrin interactions and the mechanism(s) these receptors use to regulate each other. Yet, three different models can be proposed (Figure 1).

The interactions of uPAR with the integrins play a primary role in the regulation of uPAR activity. The formation of uPAR-integrin complex is required and seems to precede the interactions of uPAR with FPRL1 (Figure 1A) [for a review see Degryse, 2008]. Furthermore, by regulating integrin activity uPAR is in perfect position to regulate important biological processes. The integrins control essential functions in embryonic development and in adult tissue homeostasis, inflammation, cell differentiation, adhesion, migration, cell cycle progression, angiogenesis and tumour metastasis. In particular, by mediating cell attachment integrins promote cell survival and resistance to genotoxic injury i.e. adhesion-mediated radioresistance/drug resistance of tumour cells. Thus, considering the vital roles of both uPAR and integrin systems, it is no surprise that they are widely used and abused in disease states such as cancers.

uPAR Connections with the Cell Cytoskeleton

The paradigm that uPAR is a signalling receptor without intracellular domain that cannot directly interact with intracellular signalling effectors is highly challenging. However, it is not uncommon that GPI-anchored proteins succeed in inducing signalling. Other examples have been reported in the literature that we briefly illustrate here.

Thy-1 is a GPI-anchored protein that shares by many aspects the properties of uPAR. Thy-1 induces complex signalling through integrins, cellular tyrosine kinases, cytokines and growth factors [for a review see Rege and Hagood, 2006]. Like uPAR, Thy-1 regulates FAK and the Src family of kinases and is localized in lipid rafts [Rege et al., 2006; Rege and Hagood, 2006]. Thy-1 is also involved in apoptosis, and cell adhesion, migration and proliferation [Rege and Hagood, 2006].

The erythropoietin-producing hepatocellular carcinoma (Eph) receptors constitute the largest family of receptor tyrosine kinases (RTKs). This family of receptors plays a key role in attraction/repulsion, migration, and adhesion of the axons, and synapse formation during the development of the central nervous system [for a review see Aoto and Chen, 2007]. The A-ephrin ligands of the EphA receptors are GPI-linked to the cell membrane. Similarities with uPAR include the regulation of integrin activity via FAK and other kinases, and clustering into lipid rafts [Bourgin et al., 2007; Aoto and Chen, 2007]. But most strikingly,

A-ephrin-EphA receptor interactions are involved in cell-cell contacts by forming trans-interactions [Aoto and Chen, 2007]. A similar situation has been reported for uPAR [Tarui et al., 2001]. uPAR can engage into trans-interaction with the integrins, thereby mediating cell-cell interactions [Tarui et al., 2001].

uPAR is involved in major basic biological processes such cell adhesion, migration, and proliferation that require the reorganization of the cell cytoskeleton.

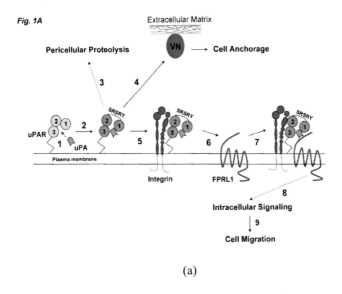

(a)

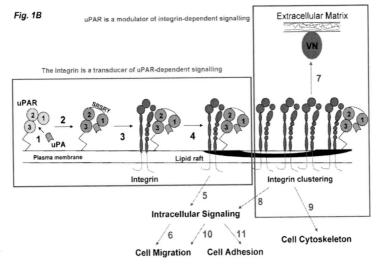

(b)

Figure 1. (Continued)

Fig. 1C

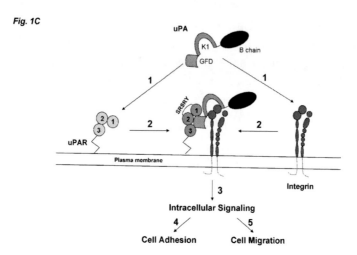

(c)

A) The classical model. The conformational change of uPAR is induced by the binding of its ligand uPA (1), resulting in the exposure of SRSRY, the chemotactic epitope situated in the DI-DII linker region of uPAR (2). The binding of uPA to uPAR also serves regulating pericellular proteolysis by locating uPA activity at discrete points of the cell surface (3), and increase the affinity of uPAR for VN (4). Lateral interactions with the integrins are favored, and the uPAR-integrin signalling complex is formed (5). For a simplified representation, this complex is represented as a single integrin and a single uPAR. However, larger complex including other signalling proteins such as FAK or c-Src are more likely to exist. uPAR is now metamorphosed into a ligand of seven-transmembrane domain receptors such as FPRL1 (6). The binding of uPAR to FPRL1 (7) promotes cell signalling (8) and finally cell migration (9).

B) The recruiting officer model. It is a powerful model in which uPAR is either an activator (red square) or a modulator (blue square) of integrin-dependent signalling. The binding of uPA to uPAR (1) induces the conformational change of uPAR and the exposition of the SRSRY motif (2). uPAR associates to the integrins (3) via direct interactions of the sequence D2A located in domain II that allows secondary interactions with other sequences present in domain III (4). Acting as an activator, the D2A sequence activates integrin-dependent signalling (5), thereby stimulating cell migration (6). Acting as a recruiting officer, uPAR localizes the integrins into the lipid rafts and promotes integrin clustering (4). Once activated and aggregated, integrins bind to VN (7) initiating intracellular signalling (8), and connect to the actin cytoskeleton (9) promoting cell migration (10) or adhesion (11).

C) The uPA bridge model. By binding concurrently to both uPAR and integrin (1), one single molecule of uPA serves as a molecular bridge bringing together uPAR and the integrin (2). uPA binds to uPAR through its growth factor domain (GFD) and to the integrin via its kringle domain (K1) as shown here. Binding of uPA to integrin through its catalytic chain (B chain) has also been reported. The association of uPAR with the integrin generates an active uPAR-integrin complex, which activates cell signalling (3), and cell adhesion (4) or migration (5).

This figure was created modifying an artwork originally published in: The Cancer Degradome - Proteases in Cancer Biology, 2008, pp 451-474, chapter 23, The urokinase receptor (uPAR) and integrins constitute a cell migration signalosome, by Bernard Degryse, figure 23.2. © 2008 Springer Science + Business Media, LLC. With kind permission of Springer Science and Business Media.

Figure 1. Three models explaining uPAR-integrin interactions.

uPAR and Cell Adhesion

There is no doubt that cell adhesion is a crucial biological process for the morphogenesis of organs and later for the maintenance of tissues [for reviews see Gumbiner, 1996; Arnaout et al., 2007]. For instance, the thyroid gland does not function without the correct three-dimensional structure of the follicle that permits iodine uptake, thyroglobulin storage and thyroid hormones synthesis. Diverse mechanisms of cellular adhesion are known such as cadherins, adherens and occluding junctions, desmosomes, hemidesmosomes, and of course the integrins. The latter are particularly involved in the connections with other cells, the extracellular matrix, and the basement membrane. Integrins provide a network rich of 24 receptors that are conveniently activated through affinity and avidity mechanisms [for a review see Harburger and Calderwood, 2009]. Deactivation of the integrins occurs through disengagement from the ligand, and disassembly of integrin clusters that see the integrin disconnection from the cytoskeleton. For example, the tetraspanin CD151 plays a regulatory function in integrin deactivation [Zijlstra et al., 2008]. Internalization is also implicated in the redistribution of the integrins at the right cellular place. In addition to their role as adhesion receptor i.e. mechanical receptor, integrins play also the role of signalling receptor mediating signals to the cells via intracellular signalling molecules such as FAK, Src family of kinases, and Integrin-linked kinase (ILK). Moreover, integrins can initiate bidirectional signalling, which represents a major difference between uPAR- and integrin-dependent signalling. Inside-out signalling regulates the extracellular binding activity of integrins, whereas outside-in signalling induced by binding of ligands such as ECM proteins, generates signals that are transmitted into the cell.

uPAR is both directly and indirectly involved in cell adhesion. By binding VN, uPAR can directly influence cell adhesion by providing at least one of the first steps of cellular adhesion i.e. cell anchorage. VN binding to uPAR does not induce cell spreading and signalling [Stahl and Mueller, 1997; Sidenius and Blasi, 2000; Degryse et al., 2001a]. However, the fact that the same receptor provides cell anchorage and proteolytic activity gives to the cell the possibility to cut cell-cell or cell-substrate contacts while avoiding detachment and its negative consequences i.e. anoikis.

uPAR can indirectly regulate cell adhesion via the integrins. uPAR interacts directly with 11 of the 24 receptors of the integrin family (Table 2) [for a recent review see Degryse, 2008]. However, this number will certainly increase because uPAR have been reported to interact with the $\beta1$, $\beta2$, $\beta3$ and $\beta5$ integrin subfamilies. By regulating integrin activity, uPAR can potentially influence the 156 components of the adhesome [Zaidel-Bar et al., 2007]. The models explaining uPAR-integrin interactions have been presented above (see Figure 1). uPAR can use the integrins as adaptors that mediate uPAR-induced signals to the cell (Figure 1B). As a recruiting officer, uPAR can also be the architect of the building of the focal adhesions (Figure 1B). The exclusion of uPAR from focal adhesions leads to their disruption [Wickstrom et al., 2001]. Others links between uPAR and integrins have been reported. The level of expression of uPA/uPAR appears to be controlled by the integrins and vice-versa [Nip et al., 1995; Bianchi et al., 1996; Wang et al., 1998; Ghosh et al., 2000; Khatib et al., 2001; Adachi et al., 2001; Hapke et al., 2001a,b; Besta et al., 2002]. Furthermore, the activation state of the integrins and the level of expression of uPAR are correlated [Chintala et al., 1997; Aguirre-Ghiso et al., 1999]. Last, uPAR-integrin interactions seems to govern uPAR and integrins co-localization [Ciambrone and McKeown-Longo, 1992; Degryse et al., 1999; Ghosh et al., 2000, 2006].

In vitro, cell adhesion can be separated in several steps that lead from round cell to flat cell that is from a floating/detached cell to the firm attachment to the substrate and adoption of the final typical cellular morphology. These steps include electrostatic contact with the substrate, anchorage, attachment, and spreading. Because of the requirement of force transmission across the cell, the key players are integrins and the actin cytoskeleton. The early focal complexes which later mature into focal adhesions are clusters of integrins that due to the connections with the actin cytoskeleton serve as foundation points for the actin stress fibers that will shape the morphology of the cell [Arnaout et al., 2007]. Other members of the cell cytoskeleton involved in focal contacts are for instance the proteins connecting integrins and actin such as Arp2/3 complex, α-actinin, talin, and vinculin. However, many other proteins will bind to tail of the integrins and become involved as the cluster of integrins mature. These proteins can be adaptor protein such as paxillin or signalling kinases such as FAK or ILK. Of course, uPAR itself is a component of the focal adhesion and as stated above it may be regarded as the architect of this structure [Arnaout et al., 2007].

Experimental studies support the idea that uPAR can directly and indirectly influence cell adhesion by controlling cell anchorage and integrin activity respectively. uPAR was identified as an adhesion receptor that binds to VN promoting adhesion of non-adherent human pro-myeloid U937 cells [Waltz and Chapman, 1994]. In human HEK 293 cells (which are devoid of uPAR) expression of uPAR increased cell adhesion to VN, and resulted in a radical change in morphology. Parental cells formed circular-like aggregates while uPAR-transfected cells looked more elongated and less aggregated [Wei et al., 1994]. However, in these HEK 293 cells adhesion to VN is mainly uPAR- and non-integrin-dependent. In melanoma cells, uPAR promoted attachment on VN but failed to stimulate cell spreading [Stahl and Mueller, 1997]. Similarly, expression of uPAR in 32D cells led to cell anchorage but not to cell spreading supporting anyway a direct role uPAR in cell adhesion [Sidenius and Blasi, 2000]. Thanks to uPAR binding to VN, the 32D cells bound to the substrate but remained rounded [Sidenius and Blasi, 2000].

Interestingly, upregulation or downregulation of uPAR has an impact on cell morphology and cytoskeleton organization that is believed to be exerted through the integrins. On the one hand, increase in cell size and shape was correlated with the overexpression of uPAR and two integrins [Hill et al., 2004]. Overexpression of uPAR in murine fibroblasts dramatically changed cell morphology and cytoskeletal organization [Kjøller and Hall, 2001]. Cells exhibited a decrease of actin stress fiber content and the formation of spectacular protrusions looking like the leading edge of a motile cell. An observation further strengthened by the fact that the protrusion formation was Rac-dependent. Rac is a small GTPase modulating membrane ruffling and lamellipodia formation involved in cell motility [Kjøller and Hall, 2001]. These data were recently reproduced and extended [Madsen et al., 2007; Hillig et al., 2008]. The underlying questions are: does VN induce signalling and cellular effects via its binding to uPAR? Are the lateral interactions of uPAR with the integrins required? The discussion is always open and complicated because VN is a ligand of both uPAR and integrins. There is no a priori reason for VN to not induce effects through binding to uPAR.

However, a clear demonstration is still lacking. In an adhesion assay performed on VN matrix in the presence of a cyclic-RGD peptide (which inhibits integrin-VN interactions) cells expressing wt-uPAR showed a rounded-shape with less protrusions suggesting that VN exerts its effects through the integrins [Hillig et al., 2008]. In a further attempt to solve that question Madsen et al. used a chimeric receptor composed of the GPI anchor of uPAR attached to the serpin domain of PAI-1. The authors reported that the chimeric GPI-PAI-1 receptor fully reproduced the effects of uPAR on cell morphology precluding lateral interactions with the integrins. However, the authors might as well have re-created lateral interactions with the integrins. PAI-1 is indeed a known ligand of LRP-1 (which is both a scavenger and a signalling receptor) capable of inducing cell migration through binding to this receptor [Degryse et al., 2004], and LRP-1 has been reported to bind to the integrins [Czekay et al., 2003; Salicioni et al., 2004; Gonias et al., 2004; Akkawi et al., 2006; Hu et al., 2007]. Thus, the formation of VN/GPI-PAI-1/LRP-1/integrin complex is plausible and might have substituted the VN/uPAR/integrin complex.

On the other hand, downregulation of uPAR has also impressive effects on cell morphology and actin cytoskeleton [Chintala et al., 1997]. The authors used the human glioma cells SNB19 transfected with antisense uPAR. In contrast to parental cells which were spindle shaped, antisense-transfected cells displayed a round shape with an actin cytoskeleton reflecting this shape. In addition, cells were larger and failed to spread correctly [Chintala et al., 2007].

Other reports underline the role of uPAR as a regulator of the actin cell cytoskeleton, and uPAR connection with the integrins. uPAR can mediate mechanical force across the cell which appears similar to that of integrins suggesting a physical link of uPAR with the cytoskeleton [Wang et al., 1995]. Indeed, uPAR is connected to the actin cytoskeleton via the integrins [Margheri et al., 2006]. The stiffness and the stiffening response are dependent on the actin cytoskeleton and the responses drop off upon actin stress fibers disruption [Wang et al., 1995].

In the skeletal muscle, uPAR seems to be involved in the regulation of cell adhesion and spreading through a new mechanism requiring its proteolytic-dependent activity. uPA is capable to cleave the integrin $\alpha 7$, and the resulting cleaved $\alpha 7$ increases cell adhesion and spreading on laminin ($\alpha 7\beta 1$ is a laminin-binding integrin) suggesting a new mechanism of integrin regulation involved in myogenic differentiation [Liu et al., 2008]. A similar effect of uPA has been reported for integrin $\alpha 6$ which again may represent another mechanism of regulation of cell adhesion [Demetriou et al., 2004; Demetriou and Cress, 2004].

Our present knowledge on the influence of uPAR on intermediate filaments is to say the least minimal. uPA/uPAR were suggested to activate desmosomes (cell-cell contacts) and hemidesmosomes (cell-substrate contacts) turnover [Kitajima et al., 1999]. The adhesion structures desmosomes and hemidesmosomes are molecular complexes that connect the plasma membrane to intermediate filaments of the keratin family.

Therefore, taken altogether all these studies show that disturbing uPAR has dramatic consequences on cell spreading, cell morphology, and actin cytoskeleton.

uPAR and the Cytoskeleton in the Migrating Cell

Cell migration during embryonic development leads to the formation of organs greatly facilitating to the elaboration of the organism [for reviews see Horwitz and Webb, 2003; Ridley et al., 2003; Bagorda et al., 2006; Gerthoffer, 2008; Bretscher, 2008]. Later, cell migration is implicated in the immune responses and wound healing. In a few words, cell migration shapes and defends the life. Unfortunately, the back of the medal is less glorious. In western societies, cell migration is involved in the most lethal diseases that are cancers and vascular diseases.

The influence of uPAR on cell migration is well described both in vitro and in vivo. Again, the reasons for such a broad impact have their roots in the duality of uPAR functions. uPAR, the protease receptor clears the path of the migrating cell while uPAR, the signalling receptor starts the race. It is some kind of surprising that uPAR is capable of governing the migration of both adherent and non-adherent cells. In both, it is an integrated process requiring the concomitant and continuous regulation of signalling, receptors availability (internalization and recycling), cell polarity, pericellular proteolysis, cell extension, cell adhesion and de-adhesion, cytoskeleton organization, mechanical forces and energy. However, just after the reception of the migratory signal, the responses will be slightly different, the adherent cell will cut its cell-cell contacts that otherwise will prevent cell migration, whereas the non-adherent cell will create cell-substratum contacts in order to be able to migrate. This fact is amazing and further supports the idea that uPAR is a part of a highly adaptable signalosome, the chameleon signalosome.

uPAR signalling is really complex which in some way can be expected just because uPAR interacts with many partners that are signalling receptors (Table 2). The first identified adaptor of uPAR was the seven-transmembrane domain receptor FPRL1 [Resnati et al., 2002]. Other have been reported since then including other seven-transmembrane domain receptors, integrins, EGFR, PDGFR, the cytokine receptor gp130 [de Paulis et al., 2004; Gargiulo et al., 2005; Seleri et al., 2005; Degryse et al., 2005; Liu et al., 2002; Kiyan et al., 2005; Koshelnick et al., 1997; for reviews see Blasi and Carmeliet, 2002; Ragno, 2006; Binder et al., 2007; Degryse, 2003, 2008]. The best characterized signalling pathways that are downstream of uPAR are the MAP kinase pathway and the Jak/Stat pathway [Simon et al., 1996; Yu et al., 1997; Aguirre Ghiso et al., 1999, 2001, 2003; Liu et al., 2002; Degryse et al., 2001a; Dumler et al., 1998, 1999a,b; Kusch et al., 2000; Patecki et al., 2007]. Other membrane and downstream signalling molecules can also be mentioned such as LRP-1; Endo180 (uPARAP); FAK; phosphatidylinositol-3 kinase (PI-3K); Src kinases family; $G_{i/o}$ proteins; DOCK180; adaptor proteins p130Cas, CrkII; small GTPases RhoA, Cdc42 and Rac; phosphatase SHP-2 [Nykjaer et al., 1992, 1994; Conese et al., 1995; Czekay et al., 2001; Behrendt et al., 2000; Engelholm et al., 2001; Sturge et al., 2003; Tang et al., 1998; Degryse et al., 1999, 2001a,b; Bohuslav et al., 1995; Smith et al., 2008; Kunigal et al., 2006; Furmaniak-Kazmierczak et al., 2007; Carlin et al., 2005; Kiyan et al., 2009].

The effects of uPAR on the actin cytoskeleton of migrating cells are rapid and transient. In the rat smooth muscle cells challenged with pro-uPA, changes were observed within 5 minutes [Degryse et al., 1999]. The first signs of cell movement were showed by the appearance of membrane ruffling but all cell-cell contacts were not yet disrupted. The actin stress fibers that were evenly distributed in the unstimulated cells started to disappear (Figure 2A,C), while vinculin was being relocated at the periphery of the cell (Figure 2B,D). Subsequently, the cells formed a leading edge by the accumulation of actin on one side indicating that the polarization of the cells was well engaged. After 30 minutes, the cell exhibited the classical elongated and polarized hand-mirror shape typical of motile cells. A semi-ring of actin was observed at the leading edge of the cell in between a double row of vinculin. Vinculin distribution was not uniform, higher in the leading part of the cell and lower in the trail. Membrane ruffling was still displayed at the top of the leading edge. In Figure 2O, one cell revealed an impressive network of actin around the cell nucleus. This particular network could likely have been formed to pull the nucleus while the cell is moving forward. However, regulation of the shape of the nucleus by mechanotransduction is also involved in gene regulation [Wang et al., 2009]. After 120 minutes, as the cells stopped migrating, cells displayed characteristics of shape and cytoskeleton organization which were closed to those of unstimulated cells. Cell morphology was unpolarized and actin reformed the evenly distributed stress fiber network. Only vinculin were subtly localized at the periphery of the cells (Figure 2T) [Degryse et al., 1999]. In the same paper using the rat smooth muscle cells, we showed that uPAR, integrins αvβ3 and β1, and c-Src were all present at the leading of the cell after 30 minutes of stimulation with pro-uPA [Degryse et al., 1999]. Thus, the spatial and temporal changes observed in a motile cell are not limited to cell morphology and actin cytoskeleton but also include adhesion receptors and signalling molecules [Horwitz and Webb, 2003; Ridley et al., 2003; Bagorda et al., 2006; Gerthoffer, 2008; Bretscher, 2008]. Modeling the migrating cell suggested that the creation of a positive gradient i.e. the redistribution of receptors at the leading edge required a short time of residence within the membrane [Bretscher, 2008]. The existence of the three-known mechanisms of internalization of uPAR is thus fully justified.

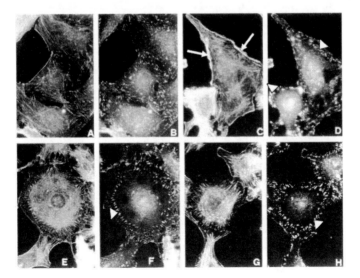

Part 1

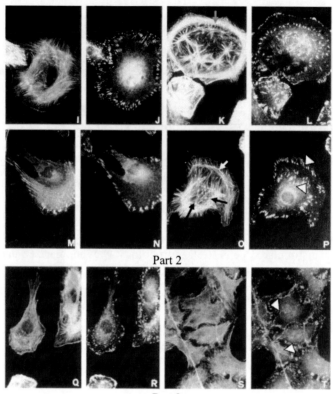

Part 2

Part 3

The sequential pictures reveal the effects of uPAR-dependent signalling on actin cytoskeleton (A, C, E, G, I, K, M, O, Q, S), and vinculin (B, D, F, H, J, L, N, P, R, T). Unstimulated rat smooth muscle cells (A, B) and cells stimulated with pro-uPA (1 nM) for 5 minutes (C, D), 10-15 minutes (E, F, G, H, I, J), 30 minutes (K, L, M, N, O, P, Q, R), and 120 minutes (S, T) are shown. The effects of uPAR on the actin cytoskeleton are rapid and transient [Degryse et al., 1999]. After 5 minutes, membrane ruffles (large arrows in Figure 2C) were visible but all cell-cell contacts were not yet disrupted. The actin stress fibers that were evenly distributed in the unstimulated cells started to disappear (compare Figure 2A and Figure 2C), and vinculin was redistributed at the periphery of the cell (arrowheads in Figure 2D, F, H). Subsequently, a leading edge was formed by the accumulation of actin on one side of the cell (grey arrow in Figure 2K) indicating the on-going polarization of the cells. After 30 minutes, the cell exhibited the classical elongated and polarized hand-mirror shape typical of motile cell. A semi-ring of actin was observed at the leading edge of the cell (white arrow in Figure 2O) in between a double row of vinculin (arrowheads in Figure 2P). Vinculin distribution was not uniform, higher in the leading part of the cell and lower in the trail. Membrane ruffling was still showing at the top of the leading edge. In Figure 2O, one cell revealed an impressive network of actin around the cell nucleus (black arrows). This particular network would likely serve to pull the nucleus while the cell is moving forward. After 120 minutes, cells stopped migrating, and displayed characteristics of shape and cytoskeleton organization which were closed to those of unstimulated cells i.e. unpolarized morphology, and stress fibers that were equally distributed. Only vinculin was localized at the periphery of the cells (arrowheads in Figure 2T) [Degryse et al., 1999].

This research was originally published in *Blood*. Degryse, B; Resnati, M; Rabbani, SA; Villa, A; Fazioli, F; Blasi, F. Src-dependence and pertussis-toxin sensitivity of urokinase receptor-dependent chemotaxis and cytoskeleton reorganization in rat smooth muscle cells. *Blood*, 1999 Jul 15, 94(2), 649-662. © 1999 The American Society of Hematology.

Figure 2. uPAR controls the actin cytoskeleton during cell migration.

The sequence of events just described illustrates very well that the reorganization of actin cytoskeleton mirrors the changes in cell morphology and focal adhesions (as reported by vinculin). uPAR is a component of focal adhesions that disassemble upon uPAR removal correlating with actin stress fibers disorganization [Wickstrom et al., 2001; Ghosh et al., 2006]. Focal adhesions are clusters of integrins whose activity relies on uPAR. These data provide a molecular explanation for the huge impact of uPAR on cell migration. uPAR down-regulation alters the actin cytoskeleton, and inhibits cell migration [Chintala et al., 1997; Degryse et al., 2001b]. Whereas up-regulating uPAR results in increased protrusion formation, cell migration and invasion [Weaver et al., 1997; Webb et al., 1999, 2000; Kjøller and Hall, 2001; Sid et al., 2006; Madsen et al., 2007; Hillig et al., 2008].

Focal adhesions are essential for the dynamic regulation of cell migration. However, other cell-matrix adhesion structures lamellipodia, filopodia, podosome and invadopodia are involved in cell migration. These structures are important for cell motility. Cellular protrusions acting as sticky fingers probe the ECM during cell migration [Galbraith et al., 2007]. Interestingly, the members of the uPAR system: uPA, PAI-1 and VN under their free and complex forms can determine the fate of these protrusions by providing "Stop" and "Go" signals [Degryse, 2008]. Lamellipodia, filopodia, podosome and invadopodia are by some aspects similar to focal adhesions [Block et al., 2008]. Thus, it not a surprise to find uPAR in membrane ruffles and pseudopodia [Bastholm et al., 1994]. uPAR is indeed present in lamellipodia where it associates with integrins and other molecules including RTKs and downstream signalling factors [Kindzelskii et al., 1996, 1997; Wilson and Gibson, 1997]. uPAR-integrin interactions are dynamic and are not the outcome of a diffusion-regulated process [Weinand et al., 1999]. uPAR is believed to drive cell motility via the activation of the MAP kinases ERKs, Rac, and then lamellipodia formation [Vial et al., 2003]. The catalytic-dependent influence of uPAR may be also involved. The uPA/uPAR proteolytic activity is important for lamellipodia and the podosome-like structure invadopodia where uPAR associates with the gelatinase, seprase in a cytoskeleton- and integrin-dependent manner [Artym et al., 2002; Kindzelskii et al., 2004]. In addition, the metalloproteases MM9, MT1-MMP (MMP14) localized together with uPA/uPAR in the invadopodia [Furmaniak-Kazmierczak et al., 2007]. Last, the down-regulation of uPAR provokes the reduction of podosomes, cell rounding and EGFR exocytosis [Abu-Ali et al., 2008]. Similarly, uPAR-deficient osteoclasts display a delayed podosome belt formation that supports a function of uPAR in podosome maturation [Furlan et al., 2007].

The available information regarding uPAR and its relationship with the microtubules is unfortunately minimalist. Using the same cellular model, the rat smooth muscle cells, we also questioned the effects of uPAR on microtubules organization [Degryse et al., 2001a]. In unstimulated cells, microtubules distribution was uniform reflecting the unpolarized morphology of the cells (Figure 3). Within 30 minutes, pro-uPA induced the formation of the hand-mirror shape indicating that the cells are polarized. The microtubules network was reorganized and polarized (Figure 3). In the leading part, the microtubules radiated to reach and follow the leading edge of the migrating cell [Degryse et al., 2001a]. The literature on the microtubules during cell migration indicates the crucial function of the small GTPase Cdc42 in organizing cell polarity and the localization of the centrosome or main microtubule-organizing centre (MTOC) in front or behind the nucleus depending on cell type along with the Golgi apparatus [Ridley et al., 2003]. In the smooth muscle cells, the MTOC is located in front of the nucleus [Gerthoffer, 2008]. The function of the microtubules may be to facilitate the redistribution of uPAR at the leading of the migrating cell where it can be connected to the integrins, vinculin, and thus the actin cytoskeleton [Washington and Dore-Duffy, 1994]. Microtubules are also thought to be involved in the disassembly of focal contacts in the trailing part of the cells [Gerthoffer, 2008].

In summary, by driving cell migration uPAR coordinates a complicated integrated process. Motile cells exhibit many differences with respect to resting cells, for instance: a polarized morphology, a reverse gradient of intracellular calcium, the organization of cell-adhesion structures such as focal adhesion that are clusters of integrins, and filipodia or lamellipodia that constitute the leading edge of the cell, the reorganization of the cytoskeleton including actin, microtubules and intermediate filaments, and the localization at the leading edge of the cell of molecules capable of mediating the migratory signal.

uPAR in the Mitotic Cell

Cell growth or cell proliferation sees a cell population increases in size. In vitro cell growth is exponential and commonly expressed in doubling time i.e. the period of time required to obtain a number of cells twice bigger than the starting value. Cell division also known as cell cycle is the basic physiological process of cell proliferation. It is the process where a pre-existing cell gives two daughter cells. The cell cycle is separated in several step namely the G_0, G_1, S, G_2 (the interphase), and M (the mitosis) phases. It is during the M phase that takes place the actual division of the mother cell that will give two daughter cells. This cycle will end with the separation of these two cells by the process of cytokinesis. It is also cell division that produces all the cells of one individual during fetal development, and childhood growth. Later, in the adulthood cell division will maintain the correct cell number of the organs. Unfortunately, pathologies involving cell proliferation are known such as cancers but others such as the thyroid goitres do not necessarily require cell transformation.

Unlike in cell migration, the role of uPAR in the regulation of cell proliferation is not well documented [for a review see Hildenbrand et al., 2008]. uPA was first identified as a mitogen, and then uPAR was implicated as well [Kirchheimer et al., 1987a,b, 1988; Rabbani et al., 1990; Kanse et al., 1997; Fischer et al., 1998]. Induction of cell proliferation does not seem to be a protease-dependent effect of uPAR because the amino-terminal fragment (ATF) of uPA devoid of catalytic activity reproduces the effects of full-length uPA [Rabbani et al., 1990; Fischer et al., 1998]. The main signalling pathway that appears activated is the MAP kinase pathway [Simon et al., 1996; Tang et al., 1998; Nguyen et al., 1999, 2000; Webb et al., 2000; Degryse et al., 2001a; Juretic et al., 2001; Hildenbrand et al., 2008]. The Ossowski's group have carried out in depth studies on the relationship between uPAR expression, the MAP kinase pathway activation and tumour dormancy giving a vivid illustration of the role of uPAR in cell proliferation [Yu et al., 1997; Aguirre Ghiso et al., 1999, 2001, 2003; Estrada et al., 2009]. Another step forward has been made with the identification that the sequence D2A located in the domain II was the mitogenic epitope of uPAR [Degryse et al., 2007]. The mechanism of action has been characterized and the publication of this research is currently underway [Eden et al., in preparation].

Regrettably, there are no studies in the literature that described the influence of uPAR on the cell cytoskeleton during cell division. The only alternative is to speculate and discuss briefly potential functions. The integrins are recognized players in the control of cell cytoskeleton throughout mitosis. The integrins are involved in centrosome functioning, assembly of the mitotic spindle and cytokinesis [Reverte et al., 2006]. In particular, is seems clear that integrins control the spindle axis i.e. the orientation of the mitotic spindle [for a review see Toyoshima and Nishida, 2007]. Thus, it is reasonable to hypothesize that as a co-factor of the integrins, uPAR may be involved in similar functions.

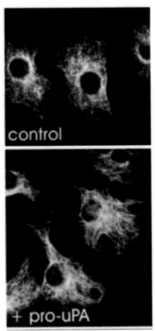

The pictures display the organization of the microtubules in unstimulated rat smooth muscle cells (control), and in cells stimulated with pro-uPA (10 nM) for 30 minutes (+ pro-uPA).
This research was originally published in *Oncogene*. Degryse, B; Orlando, S; Resnati, M; Rabbani, SA; Blasi, F. Urokinase/urokinase receptor and vitronectin/αvβ3 integrin induce chemotaxis and cytoskeleton reorganization through different signaling pathways. *Oncogene*, 2001 Apr 12, 20(16), 2032-2043. © 2001 Nature Publishing Group.

Figure 3. uPAR modulates the organization of the microtubule network.

uPAR, A Mechanosensor?

Mechanotransduction is the cellular transformation of mechanical stimuli into biochemical signals. Force or biomechanical stimulus can influence the activity of receptors, cell-cell and cell-matrix contacts and gene expression [for reviews see Silver and Siperko, 2003; Katsumi et al., 2004; Katoh et al., 2008; Chen, 2008; Gieni and Hendzel, 2008]. Integrins which form cell-matrix adhesion structures are extracellularly connected to the

ECM and intracellularly associated to the actin cytoskeleton. Thus, integrins serve as biomechanical sensors and mediators of biomechanical forces, translating them into biochemical signals [Katsumi et al., 2004]. External force promotes the formation of focal complexes that mature into focal adhesions. Thereby, external force gets in touch with actin cytoskeletal tension [Katsumi et al., 2004, 2005]. The signalling that is activated by mechanotransduction via the integrins appears to be the classical pathways involving c-Src, FAK, or small GTPases [Katsumi et al., 2004].

uPAR may also be a sensor and mediator of biomechanical forces. In fact, uPAR can transmit external forces to the actin cytoskeleton and thus to the cell in a manner similar to that of the integrins suggesting a direct connection with the cytoskeleton [Wang et al., 1995]. These somewhat unexpected data can have a rational molecular explanation. uPAR interacts with the integrins and is a constituent of the cell-matrix adhesion structures such as focal adhesions formed by the integrins.

The Cell Cytoskeleton Regulates uPAR Functions

If uPAR has a net impact on cytoskeleton organization, the reverse relationship is also true. The cell cytoskeleton has been showed to regulate uPAR functions. However, the information is somewhat limited. Presently, only uPAR gene expression, distribution, and interactions have been studied.

The drug-induced disruption of the actin filaments or microtubules enhances uPA and uPAR gene expression [Irigoyen et al., 1997; Bayraktutan and Jones, 1995]. These results may be correlated with the rapid disappearance of the stress fibers at beginning of cell migration (see Figure 2C), and has been supposed to increase cell migration [Bayraktutan and Jones, 1995].

Both microtubules and actin filaments affect the cellular distribution of uPAR. The localization of uPAR on the cell surface is dependent on the microtubules, and the disruption of microtubules with colchicine inhibits both the cell membrane and cytoplasmic location of uPAR. On the cell surface, uPAR associates with actin stress fibers at focal contact via the integrins. The disruption of the actin filaments with cytochalasin also alters uPAR distribution [Washington and Dore-Duffy, 1994].

In the migrating cell, uPAR is localized at the leading edge in the lamellipodia where it interacts with seprase, another protease. The disruption of the microtubule network with colchicine or the disorganization of the actin cytoskeleton with cytochalasin dissociates the uPAR-seprase complex suggesting that the cytoskeleton is an active inducer of uPAR-seprase interactions. The dissociating effect of the drugs was reproduced using an anti-β1 integrin antibody enlightening once again the importance of the functional relationship between uPAR and the integrins [Artym et al., 2002].

Conclusion

uPAR is a multi-ligand (both soluble and membrane-bound ligands), and a multi-functional receptor that can serve as molecular switch activating/deactivating other receptors, and downstream signalling pathways. Integrins are essential partners of uPAR. By combining the soluble and membrane-bound ligands of uPAR with the components of the integrin adhesome, the formation of uPAR-integrin complex set up the foundation stone of the uPAR signalosome or chameleon signalosome that permits to assemble larger signaling complexes and to adjust their compositions in order to adapt and survive the diverse environments and situations as the cells adhere, migrate or grow [Degryse, 2008].

Beside its essential functions as a signalling receptor, uPAR has a notable influence on the cell cytoskeletal dynamics and turnover. Again the interactions of uPAR with the integrins appear to be crucial. However, most but not all the effects of uPAR on the cell cytoskeleton are exerted through the association of this receptor with the integrins. uPAR controls cell morphology, the formation of cellular protrusions, and the organization of the actin filaments and the microtubules. uPAR also seals the fate of focal adhesions and other adhesion structures. However, many key issues are still unresolved. For example, the influence of uPAR on the intermediate filaments or on the cell cytoskeleton during cell division is still covered by the shadow of ignorance.

References

Aaronson, DS; Horvath, CM. A road map for those who don't know JAK-STAT. *Science*, 2002 May 31, 296(5573), 1653-1655.

Abu-Ali, S; Fotovati, A; Shirasuna, K. Tyrosine-kinase inhibition results in EGFR clustering at focal adhesions and consequent exocytosis in uPAR down-regulated cells of head and neck cancers. *Mol Cancer*, 2008 Jun 3, 7, 47.

Adachi, Y; Lakka, SS; Chandrasekar, N; Yanamandra, N; Gondi, CS; Mohanam, S; Dinh, DH; Olivero, WC; Gujrati, M; Tamiya, T; Ohmoto, T; Kouraklis, G; Aggarwal, B; Rao, JS. Down-regulation of integrin alpha(v)beta(3) expression and integrin-mediated signalling in glioma cells by adenovirus-mediated transfer of antisense urokinase-type plasminogen activator receptor (uPAR) and sense p16 genes. *J Biol Chem*, 2001 Dec 14, 276(50), 47171-47177.

Aguirre Ghiso, JA; Kovalski, K; Ossowski, L. Tumor dormancy induced by downregulation of urokinase receptor in human carcinoma involves integrin and MAPK signalling. *J Cell Biol*, 1999 Oct 4, 147(1), 89-104.

Aguirre-Ghiso, JA; Estrada, Y; Liu, D; Ossowski, L. ERK(MAPK) activity as a determinant of tumor growth and dormancy; regulation by p38(SAPK). *Cancer Res*, 2003 Apr 1, 63(7), 1684-1695.

Aguirre-Ghiso, JA; Liu, D; Mignatti, A; Kovalski, K; Ossowski, L. Urokinase receptor and fibronectin regulate the ERK(MAPK) to p38(MAPK) activity ratios that determine carcinoma cell proliferation or dormancy in vivo. *Mol Biol Cell*, 2001 Apr, 12(4), 863-879.

Akkawi, S; Nassar, T; Tarshis, M; Cines, DB; Higazi, AA. LRP and alphavbeta3 mediate tPA activation of smooth muscle cells. *Am J Physiol Heart Circ Physiol*, 2006 Sep, 291(3), H1351-H1359.

Andolfo, A; English, WR; Resnati, M; Murphy, G; Blasi, F; Sidenius, N. Metalloproteases cleave the urokinase-type plasminogen activator receptor in the D1-D2 linker region and expose epitopes not present in the intact soluble receptor. *Thromb Haemost*, 2002 Aug, 88(2), 298-306.

Aoto, J; Chen, L. Bidirectional ephrin/Eph signalling in synaptic functions. *Brain Res.*, 2007 Dec 12, 1184, 72-80.

Arnaout, MA; Goodman, SL; Xiong, JP. Structure and mechanics of integrin-based cell adhesion. *Curr Opin Cell Biol*, 2007 Oct, 19(5), 495-507.

Artym, VV; Kindzelskii, AL; Chen, WT; Petty, HR. Molecular proximity of seprase and the urokinase-type plasminogen activator receptor on malignant melanoma cell membranes: dependence on beta1 integrins and the cytoskeleton. *Carcinogenesis*, 2002 Oct, 23(10), 1593-1601.

Bagorda, A; Mihaylov, VA; Parent, CA. Chemotaxis: moving forward and holding on to the past. *Thromb Haemost*, 2006 Jan, 95(1), 12-21.

Barboni, E; Rivero, BP; George, AJ; Martin, SR; Renoup, DV; Hounsell, EF; Barber, PC; Morris, RJ. The glycophosphatidylinositol anchor affects the conformation of Thy-1 protein. *J Cell Sci*, 1995 Feb, 108(Pt 2), 487-497.

Barinka, C; Parry, G; Callahan, J; Shaw, DE; Kuo, A; Bdeir, K; Cines, DB; Mazar, A; Lubkowski, J. Structural basis of interaction between urokinase-type plasminogen activator and its receptor. *J Mol Biol*, 2006 Oct 20, 363(2), 482-495.

Bastholm, L; Nielsen, MH; De Mey, J; Danø, K; Brünner, N; Høyer-Hansen, G; Rønne, E; Elling, F. Confocal fluorescence microscopy of urokinase plasminogen activator receptor and cathepsin D in human MDA-MB-231 breast cancer cells migrating in reconstituted basement membrane. *Biotech Histochem*, 1994 Mar, 69(2), 61-67.

Bayraktutan, U; Jones, P. Expression of the human gene encoding urokinase plasminogen activator receptor is activated by disruption of the cytoskeleton. *Exp Cell Res*, 1995 Dec, 221(2), 486-495.

Behrendt, N; Jensen, ON; Engelholm, LH; Mørtz, E; Mann, M; Danø, K. A urokinase receptor-associated protein with specific collagen binding properties. *J Biol Chem*, 2000 Jan 21, 275(3), 1993-2002.

Besta, F; Massberg, S; Brand, K; Müller, E; Page, S; Grüner, S; Lorenz, M; Sadoul, K; Kolanus, W; Lengyel, E; Gawaz, M. Role of beta(3)-endonexin in the regulation of NF-kappaB-dependent expression of urokinase-type plasminogen activator receptor. *J Cell Sci*, 2002 Oct 15, 115(Pt20), 3879-3888.

Bianchi, E; Ferrero, E; Fazioli, F; Mangili, F; Wang, J; Bender, JR; Blasi, F; Pardi, R. Integrin-dependent induction of functional urokinase receptors in primary T lymphocytes. *J Clin Invest*, 1996 Sep 1, 98(5), 1133-1141.

Binder, BR; Mihaly, J; Prager, GW. uPAR-uPA-PAI-1 interactions and signalling: a vascular biologist's view. *Thromb Haemost*, 2007 Mar, 97(3), 336-342.

Blasi, F. The urokinase receptor. A cell surface, regulated chemokine. *APMIS*, 1999 Jan, 107(1), 96-101.

Blasi, F; Carmeliet P. uPAR: a versatile signalling orchestrator. *Nat Rev Mol Cell Biol*, 2002 Dec, 3(12), 932-943.

Block, MR; Badowski, C; Millon-Fremillon, A; Bouvard, D; Bouin, AP; Faurobert, E; Gerber-Scokaert, D; Planus, E; Albiges-Rizo, C. Podosome-type adhesions and focal adhesions, so alike yet so different. *Eur J Cell Biol*, 2008 Sep, 87(8-9), 491-506.

Bohuslav, J; Horejsí, V; Hansmann, C; Stöckl, J; Weidle, UH; Majdic, O; Bartke, I; Knapp, W; Stockinger, H. Urokinase plasminogen activator receptor, beta 2-integrins, and Src-kinases within a single receptor complex of human monocytes. *J Exp Med*, 1995 Apr 1, 181(4), 1381-1390.

Bourgin, C; Murai, KK; Richter, M; Pasquale, EB. The EphA4 receptor regulates dendritic spine remodeling by affecting beta1-integrin signalling pathways. *J Cell Biol*, 2007 Sep 24, 178(7), 1295-1307.

Bretscher, MS. On the shape of migrating cells--a 'front-to-back' model. *J Cell Sci*, 2008 Aug 15, 121(Pt16), 2625-2628.

Carlin, SM; Resink, TJ; Tamm, M; Roth, M. Urokinase signal transduction and its role in cell migration. *FASEB J*, 2005 Feb, 19(2), 195-202.

Chapman, HA; Wei, Y; Simon, DI; Waltz, DA. Role of urokinase receptor and caveolin in regulation of integrin signalling. *Thromb Haemost*, 1999 Aug, 82(2), 291-297.

Chaurasia, P; Aguirre-Ghiso, JA; Liang, OD; Gardsvoll, H; Ploug, M; Ossowski, L. A region in urokinase plasminogen receptor domain III controlling a functional association with alpha5beta1 integrin and tumor growth. *J Biol Chem*, 2006 May 26, 281(21), 14852-14863.

Chavakis, T; Kanse, SM; Lupu, F; Hammes, HP; Müller-Esterl, W; Pixley, RA; Colman, RW; Preissner, KT. Different mechanisms define the antiadhesive function of high molecular weight kininogen in integrin- and urokinase receptor-dependent interactions. *Blood*, 2000 Jul 15, 96(2), 514-522.

Chen, CS. Mechanotransduction - a field pulling together? *J Cell Sci*, 2008 Oct 15, 121(Pt20), 3285-3292.

Chintala, SK; Mohanam, S; Go, Y; Venkaiah, B; Sawaya, R; Gokaslan, ZL; Rao, JS. Altered in vitro spreading and cytoskeletal organization in human glioma cells by downregulation of urokinase receptor. *Mol Carcinog*, 1997 Dec, 20(4), 355-365.

Ciambrone, GJ; McKeown-Longo, PJ. Vitronectin regulates the synthesis and localization of urokinase-type plasminogen activator in HT-1080 cells. *J Biol Chem*, 1992 Jul 5, 267(19), 13617-13622.

Colman, RW; Pixley, RA; Najamunnisa, S; Yan, W; Wang, J; Mazar, A; McCrae, KR. Binding of high molecular weight kininogen to human endothelial cells is mediated via a site within domains 2 and 3 of the urokinase receptor. *J Clin Invest*, 1997 Sep 15, 100(6), 1481-1487.

Conese, M; Nykjaer, A; Petersen, CM; Cremona, O; Pardi, R; Andreasen, PA; Gliemann, J; Christensen, EI; Blasi, F. alpha-2 Macroglobulin receptor/Ldl receptor-related protein(Lrp)-dependent internalization of the urokinase receptor. *J Cell Biol*, 1995 Dec, 131(6Pt1), 1609-1622.

Cortese, K; Sahores, M; Madsen, CD; Tacchetti, C; Blasi, F. Clathrin and LRP-1-independent constitutive endocytosis and recycling of uPAR. PLoS ONE. 2008, 3(11), e3730.

Cunningham, O; Andolfo, A; Santovito, ML; Iuzzolino, L; Blasi, F; Sidenius, N. Dimerization controls the lipid rafts partitioning of uPAR/CD87 and regulates its biological functions. *EMBO J*, 2003 Nov 17, 22(22), 5994-6003.

Czekay, RP; Aertgeerts, K; Curriden, SA; Loskutoff, DJ. Plasminogen activator inhibitor-1 detaches cells from extracellular matrices by inactivating integrins. *J Cell Biol*, 2003 Mar 3, 160(5), 781-791.

Czekay, RP; Kuemmel, TA; Orlando, RA; Farquhar, MG. Direct binding of occupied urokinase receptor (uPAR) to LDL receptor-related protein is required for endocytosis of uPAR and regulation of cell surface urokinase activity. *Mol Biol Cell*, 2001 May, 12(5), 1467-1479.

D'Alessio S, Gerasi L, Blasi F. uPAR-deficient mouse keratinocytes fail to produce EGFR-dependent laminin-5, affecting migration in vivo and in vitro. *J Cell Sci*, 2008 Dec 1, 121(Pt 23), 3922-32.

de Paulis, A; Montuori, N; Prevete, N; Fiorentino, I; Rossi, FW; Visconte, V; Rossi, G; Marone, G; Ragno, P. Urokinase induces basophil chemotaxis through a urokinase receptor epitope that is an endogenous ligand for formyl peptide receptor-like 1 and -like 2. *J Immunol*, 2004 Nov 1, 173(9), 5739-5748.

Degryse, B. Is uPAR the centre of a sensing system involved in the regulation of inflammation? *Curr Med Chem-Anti-Inflammatory & Anti-Allergy Agents*, 2003, 2(3), 237-259.

Degryse, B. The urokinase receptor (uPAR) and integrins constitute a cell migration signalosome. In: Dylan Edwards, Gunilla Høyer-Hansen, Francesco Blasi, Bonnie F. Sloane editors. *The Cancer Degradome: Proteases in Cancer Biology*. New-York: Springer; 2008, 451-474.

Degryse, B; Eden, G; Arnaudova, R; Furlan, F; Blasi, F. Identification of a Mitotic Epitope in the Domain 2 of the Urokinase Receptor (uPAR). *In: 11th International Workshop on Molecular and Cellular Biology of Plasminogen Activation*. Vår Gård Saltsjöbaden, Sweden, 16-20th June 2007. Abstract 068.

Degryse, B; Neels, JG; Czekay, RP; Aertgeerts, K; Kamikubo, Y; Loskutoff, DJ. The low density lipoprotein receptor-related protein is a motogenic receptor for plasminogen activator inhibitor-1. *J Biol Chem*, 2004 May 21, 279(21), 22595-22604.

Degryse, B; Orlando, S; Resnati, M; Rabbani, SA; Blasi, F. Urokinase/urokinase receptor and vitronectin/αvβ3 integrin induce chemotaxis and cytoskeleton reorganization through different signalling pathways. *Oncogene*, 2001a Apr 12, 20(16), 2032-2043.

Degryse, B; Resnati, M; Czekay, RP; Loskutoff, DJ; Blasi, F. Domain 2 of the urokinase receptor contains an integrin-interacting epitope with intrinsic signalling activity: generation of a new integrin inhibitor. *J Biol Chem*, 2005 Jul 1, 280(26), 24792-24803.

Degryse, B; Resnati, M; Rabbani, SA; Villa, A; Fazioli, F; Blasi, F. Src-dependence and pertussis-toxin sensitivity of urokinase receptor-dependent chemotaxis and cytoskeleton reorganization in rat smooth muscle cells. *Blood*, 1999 Jul 15, 94(2), 649-662.

Degryse, B; Sier, CF; Resnati, M; Conese, M; Blasi, F. PAI-1 inhibits urokinase-induced chemotaxis by internalizing the urokinase receptor. *FEBS Lett*, 2001b Sep 14, 505(2), 249-254.

Demetriou, MC; Cress, AE. Integrin clipping: a novel adhesion switch? *J Cell Biochem*, 2004 Jan 1, 91(1), 26-35.

Demetriou, MC; Pennington, ME; Nagle, RB; Cress, AE. Extracellular alpha 6 integrin cleavage by urokinase-type plasminogen activator in human prostate cancer. *Exp Cell Res*, 2004 Apr 1, 294(2), 550-558.

Dumler, I; Kopmann, A; Wagner, K; Mayboroda, OA; Jerke, U; Dietz, R; Haller, H; Gulba, DC. Urokinase induces activation and formation of Stat4 and Stat1-Stat2 complexes in human vascular smooth muscle cells. *J Biol Chem*, 1999b Aug 20, 274(34), 24059-24065.

Dumler, I; Kopmann, A; Weis, A; Mayboroda, OA; Wagner, K; Gulba, DC; Haller, H. Urokinase activates the Jak/Stat signal transduction pathway in human vascular endothelial cells. *Arterioscler Thromb Vasc Biol*, 1999a Feb, 19(2), 290-297.

Dumler, I; Weis, A; Mayboroda, OA; Maasch, C; Jerke, U; Haller, H; Gulba, DC. The Jak/Stat pathway and urokinase receptor signalling in human aortic vascular smooth muscle cells. *J Biol Chem*, 1998 Jan 2, 273(1), 315-321.

Ellis, V; Scully, MF; Kakkar, VV. Plasminogen activation initiated by single-chain urokinase-type plasminogen activator. Potentiation by U937 monocytes. *J Biol Chem*, 1989 Feb 5, 264(4), 2185-2188.

Engelholm, LH; Nielsen, BS; Netzel-Arnett, S; Solberg, H; Chen, XD; Lopez Garcia, JM; Lopez-Otin, C; Young, MF; Birkedal-Hansen, H; Danø, K; Lund, LR; Behrendt, N; Bugge, TH. The urokinase plasminogen activator receptor-associated protein/endo180 is coexpressed with its interaction partners urokinase plasminogen activator receptor and matrix metalloprotease-13 during osteogenesis. *Lab Invest*, 2001 Oct, 81(10), 1403-1414.

Estrada, Y; Dong, J; Ossowski, L. Positive crosstalk between ERK and p38 in melanoma stimulates migration and in vivo proliferation. *Pigment Cell Melanoma Res*, 2009 Feb, 22(1), 66-76.

Fazioli, F; Resnati, M; Sidenius, N; Higashimoto, Y; Appella, E; Blasi, F.A urokinase-sensitive region of the human urokinase receptor is responsible for its chemotactic activity. *EMBO J*, 1997 Dec 15, 16(24), 7279-7286.

Fischer, K; Lutz, V; Wilhelm, O; Schmitt, M; Graeff, H; Heiss, P; Nishiguchi, T; Harbeck, N; Kessler, H; Luther, T; Magdolen, V; Reuning, U. Urokinase induces proliferation of human ovarian cancer cells: characterization of structural elements required for growth factor function. *FEBS Lett*, 1998 Oct 30, 438(1-2), 101-105.

Friedrichson, T; Kurzchalia, TV.Microdomains of GPI-anchored proteins in living cells revealed by crosslinking. *Nature*, 1998 Aug 20, 394(6695), 802-805.

Furlan, F; Galbiati, C; Jorgensen, NR; Jensen, JE; Mrak, E; Rubinacci, A; Talotta, F; Verde, P; Blasi, F. Urokinase plasminogen activator receptor affects bone homeostasis by regulating osteoblast and osteoclast function. *J Bone Miner Res*, 2007 Sep, 22(9), 1387-1396.

Furmaniak-Kazmierczak, E; Crawley, SW; Carter, RL; Maurice, DH; Côté, GP. Formation of extracellular matrix-digesting invadopodia by primary aortic smooth muscle cells. *Circ Res*, 2007 May 11, 100(9), 1328-1336.

Galbraith, CG; Yamada, KM; Galbraith, JA. Polymerizing actin fibers position integrins primed to probe for adhesion sites. *Science*, 2007 Feb 16, 315(5814), 992-995.

Gargiulo, L; Longanesi-Cattani, I; Bifulco, K; Franco, P; Raiola, R; Campiglia, P; Grieco, P; Peluso, G; Stoppelli, MP; Carriero, MV. Cross-talk between fMLP and vitronectin receptors triggered by urokinase receptor-derived SRSRY peptide. *J Biol Chem*, 2005 Jul 1, 280(26), 25225-32.

Gerthoffer, WT. Migration of airway smooth muscle cells. *Proc Am Thorac Soc*, 2008 Jan 1, 5(1), 97-105.

Ghosh, S; Brown, R; Jones, JC; Ellerbroek, SM; Stack, MS. Urinary-type plasminogen activator (uPA) expression and uPA receptor localization are regulated by alpha 3beta 1 integrin in oral keratinocytes. *J Biol Chem*, 2000 Aug 4, 275(31), 23869-23876.

Ghosh, S; Johnson, JJ; Sen, R; Mukhopadhyay, S; Liu, Y; Zhang, F; Wei, Y; Chapman, HA; Stack, MS. Functional relevance of urinary-type plasminogen activator receptor-alpha3beta1 integrin association in proteinase regulatory pathways. *J Biol Chem*, 2006 May 12, 281(19), 13021-13029.

Gieni, RS; Hendzel, MJ. Mechanotransduction from the ECM to the genome: are the pieces now in place? *J Cell Biochem*, 2008 Aug 15, 104(6), 1964-1987.

Gonias, SL; Wu, L; Salicioni, AM. Low density lipoprotein receptor-related protein: regulation of the plasma membrane proteome. *Thromb Haemost*, 2004 Jun, 91(6), 1056-1064.

Gumbiner, BM. Cell adhesion: the molecular basis of tissue architecture and morphogenesis. *Cell*, 1996 Feb 9, 84(3), 345-357.

Hapke, S; Gawaz, M; Dehne, K; Köhler, J; Marshall, JF; Graeff, H; Schmitt, M; Reuning, U; Lengyel, E. Beta(3)A-integrin downregulates the urokinase-type plasminogen activator receptor (u-PAR) through a PEA3/ets transcriptional silencing element in the u-PAR promoter. *Mol Cell Biol*, 2001a Mar, 21(6), 2118-21132.

Hapke, S; Kessler, H; Arroyo de Prada, N; Benge, A; Schmitt, M; Lengyel, E; Reuning, U. Integrin alpha(v)beta(3)/vitronectin interaction affects expression of the urokinase system in human ovarian cancer cells. *J Biol Chem*, 2001b Jul 13, 276(28), 26340-26348.

Harburger, DS; Calderwood, DA. Integrin signalling at a glance. *J Cell Sci*, 2009 Jan 15, 122(Pt2), 159-163.

Hildenbrand, R; Gandhari, M; Stroebel, P; Marx, A; Allgayer, H; Arens, N. The urokinase-system--role of cell proliferation and apoptosis. *Histol Histopathol*, 2008 Feb, 23(2), 227-236.

Hill, DA; Chiosea, S; Jamaluddin, S; Roy, K; Fischer, AH; Boyd, DD; Nickerson, JA; Imbalzano, AN. Inducible changes in cell size and attachment area due to expression of a mutant SWI/SNF chromatin remodeling enzyme. *J Cell Sci*, 2004 Nov 15, 117(Pt24), 5847-5854.

Hillig, T; Engelholm, LH; Ingvarsen, S; Madsen, DH; Gårdsvoll, H; Larsen, JK; Ploug, M; Danø, K; Kjøller, L; Behrendt, N. A composite role of vitronectin and urokinase in the modulation of cell morphology upon expression of the urokinase receptor. *J Biol Chem*, 2008 May 30, 283(22), 15217-15223.

Horwitz, R; Webb, D. Cell migration. *Curr Biol*, 2003 Sep 30, 13(19), R756-R759.

Høyer-Hansen, G; Pessara, U; Holm, A; Pass, J; Weidle, U; Danø, K; Behrendt, N. Urokinase-catalysed cleavage of the urokinase receptor requires an intact glycolipid anchor. *Biochem J*, 2001 Sep 15, 358(Pt 3), 673-679.

Høyer-Hansen, G; Rønne, E; Solberg, H; Behrendt, N; Ploug, M; Lund, LR; Ellis, V; Danø, K. Urokinase plasminogen activator cleaves its cell surface receptor releasing the ligand-binding domain. *J Biol Chem*, 1992 Sep 5, 267(25), 18224-18229.

Hu, K; Wu, C; Mars, WM; Liu, Y. Tissue-type plasminogen activator promotes murine myofibroblast activation through LDL receptor-related protein 1-mediated integrin signalling. *J Clin Invest*, 2007 Dec, 117(12), 3821-3832.

Huai, Q; Mazar, AP; Kuo, A; Parry, GC; Shaw, DE; Callahan, J; Li, Y; Yuan, C; Bian, C; Chen, L; Furie, B; Furie, BC; Cines, DB; Huang, M. Structure of human urokinase plasminogen activator in complex with its receptor. *Science*, 2006 Feb 3, 311(5761), 656-659.

Huang, M; Mazar, AP; Parry, G; Higazi, AA; Kuo, A; Cines, DB. Crystallization of soluble urokinase receptor (suPAR) in complex with urokinase amino-terminal fragment (1-143). *Acta Crystallogr D Biol Crystallogr*, 2005 Jun, 61(Pt 6), 697-700.

Irigoyen, JP; Besser, D; Nagamine, Y. Cytoskeleton reorganization induces the urokinase-type plasminogen activator gene via the Ras/extracellular signal-regulated kinase (ERK) signalling pathway. *J Biol Chem*, 1997 Jan 17, 272(3), 1904-1909.

Jin, H; Song, YP; Boel, G; Kochar, J; Pancholi, V. Group A streptococcal surface GAPDH, SDH, recognizes uPAR/CD87 as its receptor on the human pharyngeal cell and mediates bacterial adherence to host cells. *J Mol Biol*, 2005 Jul 1, 350(1), 27-41.

Jo, M; Thomas, KS; Takimoto, S; Gaultier, A; Hsieh, EH; Lester, RD; Gonias, SL. Urokinase receptor primes cells to proliferate in response to epidermal growth factor. *Oncogene*, 2007 Apr 19, 26(18), 2585-2594.

Juretic, N; Santibáñez, JF; Hurtado, C; Martínez, J. ERK 1,2 and p38 pathways are involved in the proliferative stimuli mediated by urokinase in osteoblastic SaOS-2 cell line. *J Cell Biochem*, 2001 Jun 26-Jul 25, 83(1), 92-98.

Kanse, SM; Benzakour, O; Kanthou, C; Kost, C; Lijnen, HR; Preissner, KT. Induction of vascular SMC proliferation by urokinase indicates a novel mechanism of action in vasoproliferative disorders. *Arterioscler Thromb Vasc Biol*, 1997 Nov, 17(11), 2848-2854.

Katoh, K; Kano, Y; Ookawara, S. Role of stress fibers and focal adhesions as a mediator for mechano-signal transduction in endothelial cells in situ. *Vasc Health Risk Manag*, 2008, 4(6), 1273-1282.

Katsumi, A; Naoe, T; Matsushita, T; Kaibuchi, K; Schwartz, MA. Integrin activation and matrix binding mediate cellular responses to mechanical stretch. *J Biol Chem*, 2005 Apr 29, 280(17), 16546-16549.

Katsumi, A; Orr, AW; Tzima, E; Schwartz, MA. Integrins in mechanotransduction. *J Biol Chem*, 2004 Mar 26, 279(13), 12001-12004.

Khatib, AM; Nip, J; Fallavollita, L; Lehmann, M; Jensen, G; Brodt, P. Regulation of urokinase plasminogen activator/plasmin-mediated invasion of melanoma cells by the integrin vitronectin receptor alphaVbeta3. *Int J Cancer*, 2001 Feb 1, 91(3), 300-308.

Kindzelskii, AL; Amhad, I; Keller, D; Zhou, MJ; Haugland, RP; Garni-Wagner, BA; Gyetko, MR; Todd, RF 3rd; Petty, HR. Pericellular proteolysis by leukocytes and tumor cells on substrates: focal activation and the role of urokinase-type plasminogen activator. *Histochem Cell Biol*, 2004 Apr, 121(4), 299-310.

Kindzelskii, AL; Eszes, MM; Todd, RF 3rd; Petty, HR. Proximity oscillations of complement type 4 (alphaX beta2) and urokinase receptors on migrating neutrophils. *Biophys J*, 1997 Oct, 73(4), 1777-1784.

Kindzelskii, AL; Laska, ZO; Todd, RF 3rd; Petty, HR. Urokinase-type plasminogen activator receptor reversibly dissociates from complement receptor type 3 (alpha M beta 2' CD11b/CD18) during neutrophil polarization. *J Immunol*, 1996 Jan 1, 156(1), 297-309.

Kirchheimer, JC; Wojta, J; Christ, G; Binder, BR. Proliferation of a human epidermal tumor cell line stimulated by urokinase. *FASEB J*, 1987a Aug, 1(2), 125-128.

Kirchheimer, JC; Wojta, J; Christ, G; Hienert, G; Binder, BR. Mitogenic effect of urokinase on malignant and unaffected adjacent human renal cells. *Carcinogenesis*, 1988 Nov, 9(11), 2121-2123.

Kirchheimer, JC; Wojta, J; Hienert, G; Christ, G; Heger, ME; Pflüger, H; Binder, BR. Effect of urokinase on the proliferation of primary cultures of human prostatic cells. *Thromb Res*, 1987b Nov 1, 48(3), 291-298.

Kitajima, Y; Aoyama, Y; Seishima, M. Transmembrane signalling for adhesive regulation of desmosomes and hemidesmosomes, and for cell-cell datachment induced by pemphigus IgG in cultured keratinocytes: involvement of protein kinase C. *J Investig Dermatol Symp Proc*, 1999 Sep, 4(2), 137-144.

Kiyan, J; Haller, H; Dumler, I. The tyrosine phosphatase SHP-2 controls urokinase-dependent signalling and functions in human vascular smooth muscle cells. *Exp Cell Res*, 2009 Apr 1, 315(6), 1029-1039.

Kiyan, J; Kiyan, R; Haller, H; Dumler, I. Urokinase-induced signalling in human vascular smooth muscle cells is mediated by PDGFR-beta. *EMBO J*, 2005 May 18, 24(10), 1787-1797.

Kjøller, L; Hall, A. Rac mediates cytoskeletal rearrangements and increased cell motility induced by urokinase-type plasminogen activator receptor binding to vitronectin. *J Cell Biol*, 2001 Mar 19, 152(6), 1145-1157.

Koshelnick, Y; Ehart, M; Hufnagl, P; Heinrich, PC; Binder, BR. Urokinase receptor is associated with the components of the JAK1/STAT1 signalling pathway and leads to activation of this pathway upon receptor clustering in the human kidney epithelial tumor cell line TCL-598. *J Biol Chem*, 1997 Nov 7, 272(45), 28563-28567.

Kunigal, S; Gondi, CS; Gujrati, M; Lakka, SS; Dinh, DH; Olivero, WC; Rao, JS. SPARC-induced migration of glioblastoma cell lines via uPA-uPAR signalling and activation of small GTPase RhoA. *Int J Oncol*, 2006 Dec, 29(6), 1349-57.

Kusch, A; Tkachuk, S; Haller, H; Dietz, R; Gulba, DC; Lipp, M; Dumler, I. Urokinase stimulates human vascular smooth muscle cell migration via a phosphatidylinositol 3-kinase-Tyk2 interaction. *J Biol Chem*, 2000 Dec 15, 275(50), 39466-39473.

Lajoie, P; Goetz, JG; Dennis, JW; Nabi, IR. Lattices, rafts, and scaffolds: domain regulation of receptor signalling at the plasma membrane. *J Cell Biol*, 2009 May 4, 185(3), 381-385.

Leksa, V; Godár, S; Cebecauer, M; Hilgert, I; Breuss, J; Weidle, UH; Horejsí, V; Binder, BR; Stockinger, H. The N terminus of mannose 6-phosphate/insulin-like growth factor 2 receptor in regulation of fibrinolysis and cell migration. *J Biol Chem*, 2002 Oct 25, 277(43), 40575-40582.

Li, H; Kuo, A; Kochan, J; Strickland, D; Kariko, K; Barnathan, ES; Cines, DB. Endocytosis of urokinase-plasminogen activator inhibitor type 1 complexes bound to a chimeric transmembrane urokinase receptor. *J Biol Chem*, 1994 Mar 18, 269(11), 8153-8158.

Liu, D; Aguirre Ghiso, J; Estrada, Y; Ossowski, L. EGFR is a transducer of the urokinase receptor initiated signal that is required for in vivo growth of a human carcinoma. *Cancer Cell*, 2002 Jun, 1(5), 445-457.

Liu, J; Gurpur, PB; Kaufman, SJ. Genetically determined proteolytic cleavage modulates alpha7beta1 integrin function. *J Biol Chem*, 2008 Dec 19, 283(51), 35668-35678.

Llinas, P; Le Du, MH; Gårdsvoll, H; Danø, K; Ploug, M; Gilquin, B; Stura, EA; Ménez, A. Crystal structure of the human urokinase plasminogen activator receptor bound to an antagonist peptide. *EMBO J*, 2005 May 4, 24(9), 1655-1663.

Madsen, CD; Ferraris, GM; Andolfo, A; Cunningham, O; Sidenius, N. uPAR-induced cell adhesion and migration: vitronectin provides the key. *J Cell Biol*, 2007 Jun 4, 177(5), 927-939.

Malengo, G; Andolfo, A; Sidenius, N; Gratton, E; Zamai, M; Caiolfa, VR. Fluorescence correlation spectroscopy and photon counting histogram on membrane proteins: functional dynamics of the glycosyl-phosphatidylinositol-anchored urokinase plasminogen activator receptor. *J Biomed Opt*, 2008 May-Jun, 13(3), 031215.

Margheri, F; Manetti, M; Serratì, S; Nosi, D; Pucci, M; Matucci-Cerinic, M; Kahaleh, B; Bazzichi L; Fibbi, G; Ibba-Manneschi, L; Del Rosso, M. Domain 1 of the urokinase-type plasminogen activator receptor is required for its morphologic and functional, beta2 integrin-mediated connection with actin cytoskeleton in human microvascular endothelial cells: failure of association in systemic sclerosis endothelial cells. *Arthritis Rheum*, 2006 Dec, 54(12), 3926-3938.

Mustjoki, S; Alitalo, R; Stephens, RW; Vaheri, A. Blast cell-surface and plasma soluble urokinase receptor in acute leukemia patients: relationship to classification and response to therapy. *Thromb Haemost*, 1999 May, 81(5), 705-710.

Naldini, L; Tamagnone, L; Vigna, E; Sachs, M; Hartmann, G; Birchmeier, W; Daikuhara, Y; Tsubouchi, H; Blasi, F; Comoglio, PM. Extracellular proteolytic cleavage by urokinase is required for activation of hepatocyte growth factor/scatter factor. *EMBO J*, 1992 Dec, 11(13), 4825-4833.

Naldini, L; Vigna, E; Bardelli, A; Follenzi, A; Galimi, F; Comoglio, PM. Biological activation of pro-HGF (hepatocyte growth factor) by urokinase is controlled by a stoichiometric reaction. *J Biol Chem*, 1995 Jan 13, 270(2), 603-611.

Nguyen, DH; Catling, AD; Webb, DJ; Sankovic, M; Walker, LA; Somlyo, AV; Weber, MJ; Gonias, SL. Myosin light chain kinase functions downstream of Ras/ERK to promote migration of urokinase-type plasminogen activator-stimulated cells in an integrin-selective manner. *J Cell Biol*, 1999 Jul 12, 146(1), 149-164.

Nguyen, DH; Webb, DJ; Catling, AD; Song, Q; Dhakephalkar, A; Weber, MJ; Ravichandran, KS; Gonias, SL. Urokinase-type plasminogen activator stimulates the Ras/Extracellular signal-regulated kinase (ERK) signalling pathway and MCF-7 cell migration by a mechanism that requires focal adhesion kinase, Src, and Shc. Rapid dissociation of GRB2/Sps-Shc complex is associated with the transient phosphorylation of ERK in urokinase-treated cells. *J Biol Chem*, 2000 Jun 23, 275(25), 19382-19388.

Nicholson, TB; Stanners, CP. Specific inhibition of GPI-anchored protein function by homing and self-association of specific GPI anchors. *J Cell Biol*, 2006 Nov 20, 175(4), 647-659.

Nielsen, LS; Kellerman, GM; Behrendt, N; Picone, R; Danø, K; Blasi, F. A 55,000-60,000 Mr receptor protein for urokinase-type plasminogen activator. Identification in human tumor cell lines and partial purification. *J Biol Chem*, 1988 Feb 15, 263(5), 2358-2363.

Nip, J; Rabbani, SA; Shibata, HR; Brodt, P. Coordinated expression of the vitronectin receptor and the urokinase-type plasminogen activator receptor in metastatic melanoma cells. *J Clin Invest*, 1995 May, 95(5), 2096-103.

Nykjaer, A; Christensen, EI; Vorum, H; Hager, H; Petersen, CM; Røigaard, H; Min, HY; Vilhardt, F; Møller, LB; Kornfeld, S; Gliemann, J. Mannose 6-phosphate/insulin-like growth factor-II receptor targets the urokinase receptor to lysosomes via a novel binding interaction. *J Cell Biol*, 1998 May 4, 141(3), 815-828.

Nykjaer, A; Conese, M; Christensen, EI; Olson, D; Cremona, O; Gliemann, J; Blasi, F. Recycling of the urokinase receptor upon internalization of the uPA:serpin complexes. *EMBO J*, 1997 May 15, 16(10), 2610-2620.

Nykjaer, A; Kjøller, L; Cohen, RL; Lawrence, DA; Garni-Wagner, BA; Todd, RF 3rd; van Zonneveld, AJ; Gliemann, J; Andreasen, PA. Regions involved in binding of urokinase-type-1 inhibitor complex and pro-urokinase to the endocytic alpha 2-macroglobulin receptor/low density lipoprotein receptor-related protein. Evidence that the urokinase receptor protects pro-urokinase against binding to the endocytic receptor. *J Biol Chem*, 1994 Oct 14, 269(41), 25668-25676.

Nykjaer, A; Petersen, CM; Møller, B; Jensen, PH; Moestrup, SK; Holtet, TL; Etzerodt, M; Thøgersen, HC; Munch, M; Andreasen, PA; Gliemann, J. Purified alpha 2-macroglobulin receptor/LDL receptor-related protein binds urokinase.plasminogen activator inhibitor type-1 complex. Evidence that the alpha 2-macroglobulin receptor mediates cellular degradation of urokinase receptor-bound complexes. *J Biol Chem*, 1992 Jul 25, 267(21), 14543-14546.

Odekon, LE; Sato, Y; Rifkin, DB. Urokinase-type plasminogen activator mediates basic fibroblast growth factor-induced bovine endothelial cell migration independent of its proteolytic activity. *J Cell Physiol*, 1992 Feb, 150(2), 258-263.

Odekon, LE; Blasi, F; Rifkin, DB. Requirement for receptor-bound urokinase in plasmin-dependent cellular conversion of latent TGF-beta to TGF-beta. *J Cell Physiol*, 1994 Mar, 158(3), 398-407.

Okada, SS; Tomaszewski, JE; Barnathan, ES. Migrating vascular smooth muscle cells polarize cell surface urokinase receptors after injury in vitro. *Exp Cell Res*, 1995 Mar, 217(1), 180-187.

Okumura, Y; Kamikubo, Y; Curriden, SA; Wang, J; Kiwada, T; Futaki, S; Kitagawa, K; Loskutoff, DJ. Kinetic analysis of the interaction between vitronectin and the urokinase receptor. *J Biol Chem*, 2002 Mar 15, 277(11), 9395-9404.

Orlean, P; Menon AK. Thematic review series: lipid posttranslational modifications. GPI anchoring of protein in yeast and mammalian cells, or: how we learned to stop worrying and love glycophospholipids. *J Lipid Res*, 2007 May, 48(5), 993-1011.

Patecki, M; von Schaewen, M; Tkachuk, S; Jerke, U; Dietz, R; Dumler, I; Kusch, A. Tyk2 mediates effects of urokinase on human vascular smooth muscle cell growth. *Biochem Biophys Res Commun*, 2007 Aug 3, 359(3), 679-684.

Paulick, MG; Bertozzi CR. The glycosylphosphatidylinositol anchor: a complex membrane-anchoring structure for proteins. *Biochemistry*, 2008 Jul 8, 47(27), 6991-7000.

Ploug, M; Ellis, V. Structure-function relationships in the receptor for urokinase-type plasminogen activator. Comparison to other members of the Ly-6 family and snake venom alpha-neurotoxins. *FEBS Lett*, 1994 Aug 1, 349(2), 163-168.

Porter, JC; Hogg, N. Integrins take partners: cross-talk between integrins and other membrane receptors. *Trends Cell Biol.*, 1998 Oct, 8(10), 390-396.

Prager, GW; Breuss, JM; Steurer, S; Olcaydu, D; Mihaly, J; Brunner, PM; Stockinger, H; Binder, BR. Vascular endothelial growth factor receptor-2-induced initial endothelial cell migration depends on the presence of the urokinase receptor. *Circ Res*, 2004 Jun 25, 94(12), 1562-1570.

Rabbani, SA; Desjardins, J; Bell, AW; Banville, D; Mazar, A; Henkin, J; Goltzman, D. An amino-terminal fragment of urokinase isolated from a prostate cancer cell line (PC-3) is mitogenic for osteoblast-like cells. *Biochem Biophys Res Commun*, 1990 Dec 31, 173(3), 1058-1064.

Ragno, P. The urokinase receptor: a ligand or a receptor? Story of a sociable molecule. *Cell Mol Life Sci*, 2006 May, 63(9), 1028-1037.

Ragno, P; Montuori, N; Covelli, B; Høyer-Hansen, G; Rossi, G. Differential expression of a truncated form of the urokinase-type plasminogen-activator receptor in normal and tumor thyroid cells. *Cancer Res*, 1998 Mar 15, 58(6), 1315-1319.

Rege, TA; Hagood, JS. Thy-1, a versatile modulator of signalling affecting cellular adhesion, proliferation, survival, and cytokine/growth factor responses. *Biochim Biophys Acta*, 2006 Oct, 1763(10), 991-999.

Rege, TA; Pallero, MA; Gomez, C; Grenett, HE; Murphy-Ullrich, JE; Hagood, JS. Thy-1, via its GPI anchor, modulates Src family kinase and focal adhesion kinase phosphorylation and subcellular localization, and fibroblast migration, in response to thrombospondin-1/hep I. *Exp Cell Res*, 2006 Nov 15, 312(19), 3752-3767.

Resnati, M; Guttinger, M; Valcamonica, S; Sidenius, N; Blasi, F; Fazioli, F. Proteolytic cleavage of the urokinase receptor substitutes for the agonist-induced chemotactic effect. *EMBO J*, 1996 Apr 1, 15(7), 1572-1582.

Resnati, M; Pallavicini, I; Wang, JM; Oppenheim, J; Serhan, CN; Romano, M; Blasi, F. The fibrinolytic receptor for urokinase activates the G protein-coupled chemotactic receptor FPRL1/LXA4R. *Proc Natl Acad Sci*, U S A, 2002 Feb 5, 99(3), 1359-1364.

Reverte, CG; Benware, A; Jones, CW; LaFlamme, SE. Perturbing integrin function inhibits microtubule growth from centrosomes, spindle assembly, and cytokinesis. *J Cell Biol*, 2006 Aug 14, 174(4), 491-497.

Ridley, AJ; Schwartz, MA; Burridge, K; Firtel, RA; Ginsberg, MH; Borisy, G; Parsons, JT; Horwitz, AR. Cell migration: integrating signals from front to back. *Science*, 2003 Dec 5, 302(5651), 1704-1709.

Roldan, AL; Cubellis, MV; Masucci, MT; Behrendt, N; Lund, LR; Danø, K; Appella, E; Blasi, F. Cloning and expression of the receptor for human urokinase plasminogen activator, a central molecule in cell surface, plasmin dependent proteolysis. *EMBO J*, 1990 Feb, 9(2), 467-474.

Royer-Zemmour, B; Ponsole-Lenfant, M; Gara, H; Roll, P; Lévêque, C; Massacrier, A; Ferracci, G; Cillario, J; Robaglia-Schlupp, A; Vincentelli, R; Cau, P; Szepetowski, P. Epileptic and developmental disorders of the speech cortex: ligand/receptor interaction of wild-type and mutant SRPX2 with the plasminogen activator receptor uPAR. *Hum Mol Genet*, 2008 Dec 1, 17(23), 3617-3630.

Sahores, M; Prinetti, A; Chiabrando, G; Blasi F; Sonnino, S. uPA binding increases uPAR localization to lipid rafts and modifies the receptor microdomain composition. *Biochim Biophys Acta*, 2008 Jan, 1778(1), 250-259.

Salicioni AM; Gaultier A; Brownlee C; Cheezum MK; Gonias SL. Low density lipoprotein receptor-related protein-1 promotes beta1 integrin maturation and transport to the cell surface. *J Biol Chem*, 2004 Mar 12, 279(11), 10005-10012.

Schwab, W; Gavlik, JM; Beichler, T; Funk, RH; Albrecht, S; Magdolen, V; Luther, T; Kasper, M; Shakibaei, M. Expression of the urokinase-type plasminogen activator receptor in human articular chondrocytes: association with caveolin and beta 1-integrin. *Histochem Cell Biol*, 2001 Apr, 115(4), 317-323.

Selleri, C; Montuori, N; Ricci, P; Visconte, V; Carriero, MV; Sidenius, N; Serio, B; Blasi, F; Rotoli, B; Rossi, G; Ragno, P. Involvement of the urokinase-type plasminogen activator receptor in hematopoietic stem cell mobilization. *Blood*, 2005 Mar 1, 105(5), 2198-2205.

Sid, B; Dedieu, S; Delorme, N; Sartelet, H; Rath, GM; Bellon, G; Martiny, L. Human thyroid carcinoma cell invasion is controlled by the low density lipoprotein receptor-related protein-mediated clearance of urokinase plasminogen activator. *Int J Biochem Cell Biol*, 2006, 38(10), 1729-1740.

Sidenius, N; Andolfo, A; Fesce, R; Blasi, F. Urokinase regulates vitronectin binding by controlling urokinase receptor oligomerization. *J Biol Chem*, 2002 Aug 2, 277(31), 27982-27990.

Sidenius, N; Blasi, F. Domain 1 of the urokinase receptor (uPAR) is required for uPAR-mediated cell binding to vitronectin. *FEBS Lett*, 2000 Mar 17, 470(1), 40-46.

Sier, CF; Sidenius, N; Mariani, A; Aletti, G; Agape, V; Ferrari, A; Casetta, G; Stephens, RW; Brünner, N; Blasi F.Presence of urokinase-type plasminogen activator receptor in urine of cancer patients and its possible clinical relevance. *Lab Invest.*, 1999 Jun, 79(6), 717-722.

Silver, FH; Siperko, LM. Mechanosensing and mechanochemical transduction: how is mechanical energy sensed and converted into chemical energy in an extracellular matrix? *Crit Rev Biomed Eng*, 2003, 31(4), 255-331.

Simon, C; Juarez, J; Nicolson, GL; Boyd, D. Effect of PD 098059, a specific inhibitor of mitogen-activated protein kinase kinase, on urokinase expression and in vitro invasion. *Cancer Res*, 1996 Dec 1, 56(23), 5369-5374.

Sitrin, RG; Johnson, DR; Pan, PM; Harsh, DM; Huang, J; Petty, HR; Blackwood, RA. Lipid rafts compartmentalization of urokinase receptor signalling in human neutrophils. *Am J Respir Cell Mol Biol*, 2004 Feb, 30(2), 233-241.

Sitrin, RG; Pan, PM; Harper, HA; Todd, RF 3rd; Harsh, DM; Blackwood, RA. Clustering of urokinase receptors (uPAR; CD87) induces proinflammatory signalling in human polymorphonuclear neutrophils. *J Immunol*, 2000 Sep 15, 165(6), 3341-3349.

Smith, HW; Marra, P; Marshall, CJ. uPAR promotes formation of the p130Cas-Crk complex to activate Rac through DOCK180. *J Cell Biol*, 2008 Aug 25, 182(4), 777-790.

Stahl, A; Mueller, BM. Melanoma cell migration on vitronectin: regulation by components of the plasminogen activation system. *Int J Cancer*, 1997 Mar 28, 71(1), 116-122.

Stahl, A; Mueller, BM. The urokinase-type plasminogen activator receptor, a GPI-linked protein, is localized in caveolae. *J Cell Biol*, 1995 Apr, 129(2), 335-344.

Stephens, RW; Nielsen, HJ; Christensen, IJ; Thorlacius-Ussing, O; Sørensen, S; Danø, K; Brünner, N. Plasma urokinase receptor levels in patients with colorectal cancer: relationship to prognosis. *J Natl Cancer Inst*, 1999 May 19, 91(10), 869-874.

Sturge, J; Wienke, D; East, L; Jones, GE; Isacke, CM. GPI-anchored uPAR requires Endo180 for rapid directional sensing during chemotaxis. *J Cell Biol*, 2003 Sep 1, 162(5), 789-794.

Tang, H; Kerins, DM; Hao, Q; Inagami, T; Vaughan, DE. The urokinase-type plasminogen activator receptor mediates tyrosine phosphorylation of focal adhesion proteins and activation of mitogen-activated protein kinase in cultured endothelial cells. *J Biol Chem*, 1998 Jul 17, 273(29), 18268-182672.

Tarui, T; Mazar, AP; Cines, DB; Takada, Y. Urokinase-type plasminogen activator receptor (CD87) is a ligand for integrins and mediates cell-cell interaction. *J Biol Chem*, 2001 Feb 9, 276(6), 3983-3990.

Toyoshima, F; Nishida, E. Spindle orientation in animal cell mitosis: roles of integrin in the control of spindle axis. *J Cell Physiol*, 2007 Nov, 213(2), 407-411.

Varma, R; Mayor, S. GPI-anchored proteins are organized in submicron domains at the cell surface. *Nature*, 1998 Aug 20, 394(6695), 798-801.

Vial, E; Sahai, E; Marshall, CJ. ERK-MAPK signalling coordinately regulates activity of Rac1 and RhoA for tumor cell motility. *Cancer Cell*, 2003 Jul, 4(1), 67-79.

Waltz, DA; Chapman, HA. Reversible cellular adhesion to vitronectin linked to urokinase receptor occupancy. *J Biol Chem*, 1994 May 20, 269(20), 14746-14750.

Wang, GJ; Collinge, M; Blasi, F; Pardi, R; Bender, JR. Posttranscriptional regulation of urokinase plasminogen activator receptor messenger RNA levels by leukocyte integrin engagement. *Proc Natl Acad Sci*, U S A, 1998 May 26, 95(11), 6296-6301.

Wang, N; Planus, E; Pouchelet, M; Fredberg, JJ; Barlovatz-Meimon, G. Urokinase receptor mediates mechanical force transfer across the cell surface. *Am J Physiol*, 1995 Apr, 268(4Pt1), C1062-C1066.

Wang, N; Tytell, JD; Ingber, DE. Mechanotransduction at a distance: mechanically coupling the extracellular matrix with the nucleus. *Nat Rev Mol Cell Biol*, 2009 Jan, 10(1), 75-82.

Washington, R; Dore-Duffy, P. Role of cytoskeletal elements in expression of monocyte urokinase plasminogen activator receptor, activation-associated antigen Mo3. *Clin Diagn Lab Immunol*, 1994 Nov, 1(6), 714-721.

Weaver, AM; Hussaini, IM; Mazar, A; Henkin, J; Gonias, SL. Embryonic fibroblasts that are genetically deficient in low density lipoprotein receptor-related protein demonstrate increased activity of the urokinase receptor system and accelerated migration on vitronectin. *J Biol Chem*, 1997 May 30, 272(22), 14372-14379.

Webb, DJ; Nguyen, DH; Gonias, SL. Extracellular signal-regulated kinase functions in the urokinase receptor-dependent pathway by which neutralization of low density lipoprotein receptor-related protein promotes fibrosarcoma cell migration and matrigel invasion. *J Cell Sci*, 2000 Jan, 113(Pt1), 123-134.

Webb, DJ; Nguyen, DH; Sankovic, M; Gonias, SL. The very low density lipoprotein receptor regulates urokinase receptor catabolism and breast cancer cell motility in vitro. *J Biol Chem*, 1999 Mar 12, 274(11), 7412-7420.

Wei, Y; Tang, CH; Kim, Y; Robillard, L; Zhang, F; Kugler, MC; Chapman, HA. Urokinase receptors are required for alpha 5 beta 1 integrin-mediated signalling in tumor cells. *J Biol Chem*, 2007 Feb 9, 282(6), 3929-3939.

Wei, Y; Waltz, DA; Rao, N; Drummond, RJ; Rosenberg, S; Chapman, HA. Identification of the urokinase receptor as an adhesion receptor for vitronectin. *J Biol Chem*, 1994 Dec 23, 269(51), 32380-32388.

Wei, Y; Yang X; Liu, Q; Wilkins, JA; Chapman, HA. A role for caveolin and the urokinase receptor in integrin-mediated adhesion and signalling. *J Cell Biol*, 1999 Mar 22, 144(6), 1285-1294.

Weinand, RG; Rosenspire, AJ; Petty, HR. Modeling the influence of ectodomain affinities on the spatial distribution of membrane receptors. *J Theor Biol*, 1999 Mar 21, 197(2), 217-225.

Wickström, SA; Veikkola, T; Rehn, M; Pihlajaniemi, T; Alitalo, K; Keski-Oja, J. Endostatin-induced modulation of plasminogen activation with concomitant loss of focal adhesions and actin stress fibers in cultured human endothelial cells. *Cancer Res*, 2001 Sep 1, 61(17), 6511-6516.

Wieduwilt, MJ; Moasser, MM. The epidermal growth factor receptor family: biology driving targeted therapeutics. *Cell Mol Life Sci*, 2008 May, 65(10), 1566-1584.

Wilson, AJ; Gibson, PR. Epithelial migration in the colon: filling in the gaps. *Clin Sci (Lond)*, 1997 Aug, 93(2), 97-108.

Yu, W; Kim, J; Ossowski, L. Reduction in surface urokinase receptor forces malignant cells into a protracted state of dormancy. *J Cell Biol*, 1997 May 5, 137(3), 767-777.

Zaidel-Bar, R; Itzkovitz, S; Ma'ayan, A; Iyengar, R; Geiger, B. Functional atlas of the integrin adhesome. *Nat Cell Biol*, 2007 Aug, 9(8), 858-867.

Zijlstra, A; Lewis, J; Degryse, B; Stuhlmann, H; Quigley, JP. The inhibition of tumor cell intravasation and subsequent metastasis via regulation of in vivo tumor cell motility by the tetraspanin CD151. *Cancer Cell*, 2008 Mar, 13(3), 221-234.

In: Cytoskeleton: Cell Movement...
Editors: S. Lansing et al., pp. 37-68

ISBN: 978-1-60876-559-1
© 2010 Nova Science Publishers, Inc.

Chapter II

LIMK1, The Key Enzyme of Actin Remodeling Bridges Spatial Organization of Nucleus and Neural Transmission: From Heterochromatin Via Non-Coding RNAs to Complex Behavior

*Anna V. Medvedeva, Alexander V. Zhuravlev and Elena V. Savvateeva-Popova**

Pavlov Institute of Physiology Russian Academy of Sciences,
Laboratory of Neurogenetics, 6, Makarova nab.,
199034 St. Petersburg, Russia

Abstract

According to present knowledge, systemic realization of genetic activity in the dynamic spatial organization of the genome in the nucleus provides such a level of plasticity of complex biological systems that allows them to adequately respond to environmental stimuli or signals during the development, modulate and shift the balance of contacting components and dimensions of their interactions, resulting in structural rearrangements. The chromosome positions within the nucleus determine both normal development and progression of genomic diseases, i.e., changes according to the environmental requirements, current needs of the organism, and its individual experience. At the same time, the striking output of the evolution of higher organisms, largely ignored to date, is that only 1.2% of the mammalian genome encodes proteins and the vast majority of the expressed information is in RNA. There are hundreds of thousands of non-coding (nc) RNAs, as well as many other yet-to-be-discovered small regulatory RNAs . A new paradigm envisions the interactions between these two worlds,

---

* Corresponding author: Tel +7 (812) 946 38 13, Email esavvateeva@mail.ru

the one of protein and the other of RNA, as providing a dynamic link between the transcriptome and the environment and, therefore, the progressive maturation and functional plasticity of the nervous system in health and disease. Also, a wide repertoire of ncRNAs plays an important role in chromatin organization, gene expression, and disease etiology via a signal cascade of actin remodeling (LIMK1, cofilin, actin). The activity of the protein kinase LIMK1 that controls spine development, local dendritic translation at postsynaptic sites and ionotropic glutamate receptor trafficking is regulated by a brain-specific miRNA miR-134. This miRNA is localized to the synapto-dendritic compartment of rat hippocampal neurons and negatively regulates the size of dendritic spines--postsynaptic sites of excitatory synaptic transmission. Moreover, LIMK1 hemizygosity is considered to cause cognitive defects in a genome disorder Williams syndrome. Drosophila is a helpful model organism to determine the sequence of events in this system of hierarchical relationships. Drosophila LIMK1 gene (*agnostic*) with a specific chromosome architecture around the gene capable of generating miRNAs, recapitulates many features both of Williams syndrome and of neurodegenerative disorders. Mutants in the gene have increased expression of LIMK1 and cofilin, modified chromosome packaging and homologous and nonhomologous pairing, implemented in different rates of unequal recombination. Also, they display congofilic inclusions both in the adult brain and larval tissues presumably leading to severe defects in learning and memory during courtship conditioning.

Introduction

Recent findings both in neurobiology and genetics promote an outbreak in our traditional notion of neural transmission. Nowadays in our understanding of synaptic plasticity, long term potentiation (LTP) and long term depression (LTD) presumed to comprise a fine cellular basis for learning and memory we have to address the whole spectrum of purely genetic topics of neuron–specific transcription, epigenetic chromatin remodeling, trafficking of mRNAs from soma to the remote sites of their local translation in axons and dendrites. Our pursuit of unraveling the etiology of neural diseases posed a problem of a multilevel organization of the genetic material in the nucleus of a nerve cell (van Driel et al., 2003). The first level is a linear arrangement of the sequence in the chromosome. The second is belonging to a particular structural–functional chromosome block. The third is the spatial association of these blocks in the nucleus and their belonging to a particular nuclear domain. Therefore, the notion of gene activity *per se* is meaningless, since it the result of a network of genetic and biological relationships. Consequently, the view on systemic realization of genetic activity, whose critical aspect is the spatial organization of the genome in the nucleus, became crucial. This dynamic nuclear medium emphasizes the significance of the role of self-organization in the formation of its structure, when the chromatin domains located far apart in the linear DNA, as well as chromosome arms, can have physical contacts or terminate them. This provides such level of plasticity of complex biological systems that allows them to adequately respond to environmental stimuli or signals during the development, modulate and shift the balance of contacting components and dimensions of their interactions, resulting in structural rearrangements. The chromosome positions within the nucleus determine both normal development and progression of genomic diseases (O'Brien et al., 2003), i.e., changes according to the environmental requirements, current needs of the organism, and its individual experience.

The role of the main factor of bridging all of the genomic levels is fulfilled by nuclear actin, which is capable to: (1) regulate transcription by activating all three classes of RNA polymerases; (2) participate in chromatin remodeling, interacting with numerous proteins; and (3) line the nuclear membrane, determining the sites of chromosome attachment and the formation of nuclear pores, regulating export from the nucleus (Olave et al., 2002; Pederson and Aebi, 2005; Sjolinder et al., 2005; Grummt, 2006; Percipalle and Visa, 2006; Chen and Shen, 2007; Percipalle et al., 2003; 2009). Actin is not only a major cytoskeletal component in all eukaryotic cells but also a nuclear protein that accompanies the mRNA through the entire RNA biogenesis pathway, from gene to polysomes. To this point, Percipalle (2009) rises three important questions: 1) if actin is associated with all eukaryotic RNA polymerases, actin is also likely to be located at gene promoter; 2) how does actin mediate polymerase assembly at the promoter and 3) is this function independent from the observation that actin is also in chromatin remodeling complexes? Indeed, chromatin immunoprecipitation experiments confirmed the presence of actin at rDNA promoter, promoters of inducible and constitutively expressed RNA polymerase II genes, as well as its association with the promoter of the RNA polymerase III U6 snRNA gene and also demonstrated that actin is present at the coding region of constitutively active genes, coupled to elongating RNA polymerases I and II (Percipalle, 2009 and ref therein). These findings put forward an intriguing possibility that actin performs a chaperone function in the molecular interplay between RNA polymerase and the machines involved in chromatin reorganization at the gene promoter to facilitate the establishment of transcription- competent RNA polymerases (Louvet and Percipalle, 2009). This is in accord with ideas in a new and rapidly evolving field - an assembly of a neuron-specific chromatin remodeling complexes (Olave et al., 2002; Aigner et al., 2007; Schleicher and Jockusch, 2008; de la Torre-Ubieta and Bonni, 2008) which appeared to be linked to the role of epigenetic promoter remodeling of actin cytoskeleton proteins like Reelin and GABAergic promoter hypermethylation in schizophrenia (Niu et al., 2008; Gregório et al., 2009; Costa et al., 2009).

The next important step in RNA biogenesis is mRNA transport and its localization in a certain cell compartment for a proper function. For this, immediately upon transcription, pre-messenger RNA molecules become associated with hnRNPs to form RNP complexes. hnRNPs influence RNA stability, cytoplasmic localization and mRNA translation. As shown in Diptera *C.tentans*, actin is incorporated in nascent pre-mRNPs, is associated with hnRNP proteins (Percipalle et al., 2001; 2009). The *D. melanogaster* hnRNP A1-like Squid protein (hrp40) governs the specific localization of the grk mRNA to the dorsoanterior corner of the oocyte during mid-oogenesis (Neuman-Silberberg et al., 1993; Matunis et al., 1994). These early findings have paved a road for a newly-emerged field of local translation in axons and dendrites (Lin and Holt, 2007) which, according to present notion, is regulated by ever growing number of noncoding (nc) RNAs (Mattick, 2007; Savvateeva-Popova et al., 2008).

Since both the neuron-specific chromatin remodeling and local translation in neurons shed a new light on the mechanisms of action of actin in modern studies on neural transmission, let's first introduce the main players in actin remodeling and second – follow up the *Drosophila* model which enables a journey along the way from a gene in the cascade of actin remodeling to complex behavior.

The Main Players in the Signal Cascade of Actin Remodeling

The signal cascade of actin remodeling: receptors of neurotransmitters – small Rho GTPases (RhoA, Cdc42 and Rac1) –LIM kinase 1 (LIMK1) -cofilin – actin – is believed to play the main role in dendrite- and synaptogenesis. LIMK1 being the key enzyme of actin remodeling (da Silva and Dotti, 2002; Miller and Kaplan, 2003), phosphorylates cofilin on a conserved serine residue, Ser3. Thereby LIMK1 inactivates ADF/cofilin, whereas phosphatases such as slingshot can activate ADF/ cofilin by dephosphorylating Ser3. LIMK1 contains two LIM domains, a PDZ domain, and a protein kinase domain, as well as a domain for binding to SRP-α_N (Signal Recognition Particle). Inactivation of the second LIM domain by site-specific mutagenesis or deletion of the PDZ domain increase the activity of LIMK1 in vivo (Birkenfeld et al., 2001). Since the role of the PDZ domains is to organize supramolecular complexes of signal transduction, they are crucial for functioning of many receptors, such as NMDA NR2/D, AMPA, GluR2, mGluR5, beta-AR, melatonin and for ion channels Shaker K^+, voltage-gated Na^+, N-type $Ca2^+$ (te Velhuis and Bagowski, 2007). Cofilin, a ligand for both monomeric and polymeric actin, contains a nuclear location sequence, and in its dephosphorylated state can transport actin into the nucleus. When bound to actin polymers, it distorts their conformation such that these filaments do not bind the diagnostic stain for actin, RHODAMIN- phalloidin anymore. Among other nuclear proteins which form complexes with actin and interfere with the formation of conventional actin filaments is profilin which binds to monomeric actin. Nuclear profilin is apparently involved in the regulation of the level of nuclear actin, as profilin –actin complexes are recognized and exported from mammalian nuclei by a specific exportin, while actin free of profilin can apparently be exported by a different exportin, due to its nuclear export sequences Thus, these proteins might be critical in creating forms specific for nuclear actin, as detected by specific antibodies (reviewed in Lee-Hoeflich et al., 2004; Schleicher and Jockusch, 2008). The "actin cascade" is particularly important in dendrites, since LIMK1 null mice display defects in the formation of actin-based dendritic spines in hippocampal neurons and decreased levels of cofilin phosphorylation (Meng et al, 2002). Moreover, the hemizigosity of LIMK1 contributes to Williams syndrome, a genome disorder characterized by a strong cognitive defect in visuospatial cognition (Donnai and Karmiloff-Smith, 2000). Another LIMK1-dependent signaling pathway is involved in synaptogenesis which is crucial for normal learning acquisition and memory formation. The tail region of BMPR-II (bone morphogenetic protein receptor II) was isolated during a search for LIMK1-interacting proteins and this finding highlighted the dual roles of the BMP signaling (Foletta et al., 2003). BMPs are involved in axon pathfinding, morphological differentiation of dendrites and many other cellular processes. Their signals are transduced by the kinase receptors BMPR-I and BMPR-II, leading to Smad transcription factor activation via BMPR-I. A second, parallel pathway, involves a two-step mechanism: binding of LIMK1 to BMPRII relieves an autoinhibitory effect of LIM and PDZ domains on the catalytic domain of

LIMK1, thereafter BMP-dependent activation of Cdc42 results in phosphorylation of the activation loop Thr residue, thereby increasing LIMK1 catalytic activity (Lee-Hoeflich et al., 2004). In *Drosophila*, BMP-like molecules regulate neuromuscular synapse morphology and neuropeptide cell identity via the BMPRII-like receptor, *wishful thinking* (*Wit*), required for synapse stabilization (Marque's et al, 2002; Eaton and Davis, 2005). Moreover, a BMP7 gradient elicits bidirectional turning responses from nerve growth cones by acting through LIM kinase (LIMK) and Slingshot (SSH) phosphatase to regulate actin-depolymerizing factor (ADF)/cofilin-mediated actin dynamics (Wen et al., 2007). Interestigly, manipulation of LIMK1 activity failed to alter dendrite growth in Xenopus retinal ganglion cells, but was critical for axon extension (Hocking et al., 2009). This brings us to a problem of directional steering in axons and dendrites which appears to be closely intermingled with a new topic of local translation in these nerve cell extensions. But first we have to address more traditional problem of transcriptional regulation in soms of the nerve cells.

From Chromatin Remodeling to Neurogenesis

The packaging of genomic DNA into chromatin is crucial step in the regulation of gene expression. Chromatin remodelling complexes which alter local chromatin structure operate as large, multiunit machines in mammals, insects, yeast and plants to reorganize the genetic material by unravelling nucleosomes and converting the genetic material into a form suitable for transcription. Though the details of organization of such machines are far from clear, it is already evident that actin and nuclear actin-related proteins (Arps) are involved in chromatin remodeling. Actin was identified in complex with specific subunits of most ATPases (Gangarajuand Bartholomew, 2007) together with four nuclear Arps (4, 5, 6 and 8) in all organisms, with the exception of yeast (Olave et al. 2002a; Percipalle and Visa 2006; Schleicher and Jockusch, 2008). Another fascinating finding was the identification of a polymorphic, neuron-specific chromatin remodeling complex (Olave et al. 2002b). This was done in assumption that "the expected characteristics of such a chromatin remodeling complex would be that it be expressed in all neuronal cell types, not be expressed outside the nervous system and that it be activated at or near the time of neuronal subtype differentiation" (Olave et al. 2002b). As shown, vertebrate neurons have a specialized chromatin remodeling complex, bBAF, specifically containing the actin-related protein, BAF53b, which is first expressed in postmitotic neurons at. BAF53b is combinatorially assembled into polymorphic complexes with ubiquitous subunits including the two ATPases BRG1 and BRM. Brahma-related gene-1 (BRG1), the central catalytic subunit of the SWI/SNF chromatin-modifying enzymatic complexes, shows neural-enriched expression (Seo et al., 2005), uses the energy derived from ATP-hydrolysis to disrupt the chromatin architecture of target promoters and is believed to be a major coregulator of transcription (Trotter and Archer, 2008). Pretty soon it has been shown, that actin-related proteins at chromatin level not only ubiquitously control of the cell cycle and developmental transitions (Meagher et al., 2007), but neural development itself is based on a switch in subunit composition of a chromatin remodeling complex (Lessard, 2007). For example, global chromatin changes accompany the transition from proliferating mammalian neural stem cells to committed neuronal lineages. While proliferating neural stem and progenitor cells express complexes in which BAF45a, a Krüppel/PHD domain protein and the actin-related protein BAF53a are quantitatively associated with the SWI2/SNF2-like ATPases, Brg and Brm, the neuronal differentiation requires the replacement of these subunits by the homologous BAF45b, BAF45c, and BAF53b. However, combinatorial assembly appears to be unique to vertebrates, because *Drosophila* and *C. elegans* have only one gene encoding each subunit including BAF53 and there is yet no evidence of combinatorial assembly of the *Drosophila* complex (Olave et al., 2002b). Nevertheless, this has brought to awareness, that combinatorial assembly of subunits in SWI/SNF-like complexes in vertebrates is necessary to achieve biological specificity in generation and refinement of dendrites during normal brain development and neural plasticity in response to neuronal activity (Wu et al., 2007; de la Torre-Ubieta and Bonni, 2008). For instance, a novel element which constitutes the SWI/SNF complex, is activity-dependent neuroprotective protein (ADNP), a heterochromatin 1-binding protein, and its complete deficiency leads to dramatic changes in gene expression, neural tube closure defects, and death at gestation day 9 in mice (Mandel and Gozes, 2007). Thus, the statements "From chromatin to dendrites" (de la Torre-Ubieta and Bonni, 2008), "A novel model for an older remodeler" (Aigner et al., 2007) and the question "How many remodelers does it take to make a brain?" (Brown et al., 2007) shed a new light on the old and purely genetic issue of chromatin organization. Moreover, epigenetic mechanisms have been implicated in different aspects of brain development, such as neuronal differentiation and plasticity (Hsieh and Gage, 2005).

Regulation of Gene Activity at Posttranslation Level

Protein synthesis underlying synaptic plasticity mediated by activity or experience and memory is controlled at the level of mRNA translation. About 1-4% of the neuron transcriptome is found in RNA granules and the characterization of bound mRNAs reveal that they encode proteins of the cytoskeleton, the translation machinery, vesicle trafficking, and/or proteins involved in synaptic plasticity. ncRNAs and microRNAs (miRNAs) are also found in dendrites and likely regulate RNA translation (Sánchez-Carbente-Mdel and Desgroseillers, 2008). Also, axons and their growth cones are specialized neuronal sub-compartments that possess translation machinery and have distinct mRNAs (Yoon et al., 2009). Therefore, the axonal pathfinding and activity-dependent synaptic plasticity utilize the similar mechanisms of regulating local translation.

Lin and Holt (2007) raise an interesting question - why regulate protein activity by translation rather than posttranslational modifications? This question is especially important because quite unexpectedly the topics of chromosome structure and of regulation of epigenetic processes by ncRNAs have appeared to be intimately related. Therefore, the authors give a number of very reasonable answers.

(1) From a theoretical standpoint, cells have limited volume, and further crowding with macromolecules might slow diffusion or alter reaction rates unacceptably;

(2) Since an mRNA can be a template for theoretically unlimited translation, it may be more efficient in the face of this biophysical limit to store mRNA rather than inactive proteins;
(3) A constant turnover of proteins that tightly regulates the levels of specific proteins may occur in synaptic plasticity;
(4) Regulation of proteins by mRNA translation rather than protein modification provides more flexibility, because the activity of a protein can be regulated by arbitrary mRNA sequences rather than constituent domains of the protein;
(5) Proteins do not always contain the information necessary for their localization;
(6) Axonal mRNA splicing might provide an additional layer of regulation for axonally translated proteins.

Different axonal guidance cues induce rapid translation of cytoskeletal proteins or regulators based on whether they are attractive or repulsive: proteins induced by attractive cues build up the cytoskeleton, whereas proteins induced by repulsive cues break it down. For example, an attractive gradient of netrin-1 or BDNF induces asymmetrical translation of b-actin in axonal growth cones within 5 min. Contrary to attractive cues, the repellent Slit2 induces a protein synthesis-dependent increase in growth cone cofilin within 5 min. Another repellent, Semaphorin3A (Sema3A), induces axonal synthesis of the small GTPase RhoA, which is required for Sema3A-induced growth cone collapse. RhoA mediates neurite retraction through regulation of the actin cytoskeleton (reviewd in Lin and Holt, 2007). Moreover, evidence from the *Drosophila* midline axon guidance system suggests that the F-actin-microtubule cross-linker Short stop (Shot) might link the translation machinery to the cytoskeleton in the growth cone (Van Horck and Holt, 2008). mRNA transport and translation are coupled and regulated by RNA-binding proteins, which transport mRNAs in "granules", large ribonucleoprotein (RNP) complexes that hold mRNAs repressed at the initiation or elongation stage (Bramham, 2008). Interestingly, RNA-binding protein Fragile X Mental Retardation Protein (FMRP) is reqired both for axonal growth cones (Antar et al, 2006) and for regulation of local translation in dendrites (Zalfa et al, 2006). Moreover, the 3'UTR of RhoA mRNA contains a possible binding site for FMRP (Wu et al, 2005). Therefore, Long-term potentiation and depression (LTP and LTD) might be considered analogous to attractive and repulsive turning (Lin and Holt, 2007).

What proteins ate locally translated? Using proteomics methodologies as a novel means to catalog axonally synthesized proteins from injury-conditioned adult rat dorsal root ganglion (DRG) neurons, it was possible to demonstrate that microtubule, intermediate filament and microfilament proteins, several heat shock proteins (HSPs) and heat shock-like proteins, endoplasmic reticulum (ER)-resident chaperone proteins, proteins linked to neurodegenerative disorders including those with proteolytic functions, and metabolic proteins were locally synthesized in axons (Willis et al., 2005). By RT-PCR was possible to detect peripherin, vimentin, and cofilin mRNAs in DRG axonal preparations. Also, the stress-response proteins B crystallin, HSP27, HSP60, HSP70, HSP90, grp75 and grp78/BiP are synthesized in the DRG axons. Among mRNAs whose translation modulates the ability of the dendrite to receive and integrate presynaptic information are those encoding CamKIIalpha, NMDA receptor subunits, and the postsynaptic density (PSD) scaffolding protein Homer2.

Local translation of these previously dormant mRNAs may be inhibited until neurons are exposed to appropriate extracellular stimuli such as a neurotrophic factor (for example, brain-derived neurotrophic factor (BDNF) or neurotransmitter release at the synapse (Schratt et al, 2004). Three of the BDNF-regulated mRNAs (discs large homologue 2 (DLG2), Neurod2, LIMK1were found to contain conserved 3'UTR sequence elements that were partially complementary to mouse miR-134. Presumably, the association of LIMK1 mRNA with miR-134 keeps the LIMK1 mRNA in a dormant state while it is being transported within dendrites to synaptic sites. In the absence of synaptic activity, miR-134 may recruit a silencing complex that has a key role in repressing LIMK1 mRNA translation. This then limits the synthesis of new LIMK1 protein and restricts the growth of dendritic spines. At the same time miR-134 was proposed to be not the single miRNA capable to regulate LIMK1 expression. (Schratt et al, 2006). According to our bioinformatics analyses, dme-miR-210 is the only miRNA in miRBASE Targets database computationally predicted to bind with LIMK1 gene mRNA transcripts of *Drosophila melanogaster* (Figure 1). However, in agreement with above proposal, a great number of miRNAs was detected using MicroInspector software to bind to *D. melanogaster* LIMK1 mRNA with different specificity and free binding energy (Zhuravlev et al., 2009, to be published elsewhere).

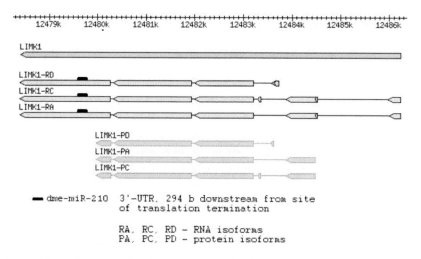

Figure 1. *Drosophila melanogaster* LIMK1 gene transcripts in complex with micro RNA dme-miR-210.

Chromatin Structure: Studies in *Drosophila*

What was long ago learned from studies on the *Drosophila* polytene chromosomes, became evident only after the completion of Genome projects in different species. *Drosophila melanogaster* offers a unique system in which one can study the whole scope of aformentioned phenomena. The design of recombination maps of the *Drosophila* genes in its 4 chromosomes started as early, as 1913 (Surtevant, 1913). Due to the fact that the giant polytene chromosomes can be found in larval tissues, especially in salivary glands, a high proportion of the genes have also been located cytogenetically taking the advantage of numerous chromosome aberrations. In the detailed map of the polytene chromosomes established by Bridges (1935) each of approximately 5000 polytene bands is assigned a unique code, which identifies each band within one of 102 numbered chromosomal divisions, each with up to six lettered subdivisions. This has been one of the decisive starting steps to the *Drosophila* Genome project which finally helped to create detailed and highly correlated genetic, cytogenetic and molecular maps, down to the nucleotide level (Kafatos et al, 1991).

In general, *Drosophila* chromosomes are homologous associated in the early stages of development in addition to their association observed during meiosis. The giant polytene chromosomes exhibit a close synapsis of homologues along their entire lengths and a given locus occupies a discrete subregion within the nucleus (Marshall et al., 1996). Therefore, homologous pairing is believed to be crucial for the establishment of 3-D architecture of the nucleus. This organization stems from a combination of an overall centromere–telomere spatial organization (the classical "**Rabl**" **configuration**), as well as more specific patterning (Fung et al., 1998). What is important, this homologous chromosome pairing proceeds through multiple independent initiations. When the chromosome synapsis is distorted due to either specific chromosome architecture or to the response to any type of stressful conditions, different chromosome aberrations, deletions, duplications and inversions arise in the *Drosophila* polytene chromosomes. When the results of the Human genomic projects have started to be thoroughly analyzed, this phenomenon known for a long time from the *Drosophila* studies, appeared to be quite common to the human genome. It has turned out that chromosome-specific low-copy repeats, or duplicons, occur in multiple regions of the human genome. Homologous recombination between different duplicon copies leads to chromosomal rearrangements, such as deletions, duplications, inversions, and inverted duplications, depending on the orientation of the recombining duplicons (Purandare and Patel, 1997; Ji et al., 2000). When such rearrangements cause dosage imbalance of a developmentally important gene(s), this results in genetic diseases now termed genomic disorders which arise at a frequency exceeding this of single gene mutations (Lupski, 1998; 2009; Stankiewicz and Lupski, 2006). Among such syndromes with multiple manifestations are Prader-Willi syndrome at 15q11–q13, Di- George syndrome at 22q11, Charcot-Marie-Tooth syndrome type 1A(CMT1A) at 7p12, Smith-Magenis syndrome (SMS) at 17p11.2 which is a mental retardation/multiple congenital anomalies syndrome and Williams syndrome due to deletion at 7q11.23. WS, due to a contiguous 1.5 Mb gene deletion at 7q11.23, is associated with a distinctive facial appearance, cardiac abnormalities, infantile hypercalcemia, and growth and developmental retardation. More than 17 genes are uncovered by the deletion and two adjacent, one for elastin and the other for LIMK1 are believed to have a major impact on WS manifestations (Donnai and Karmiloff-Smith, 2000). Thus, elastin hemizygosity is associated with supravalvular aortic stenosis and other vascular stenoses and LIMK1 hemizygosity may contribute to the characteristic cognitive profile – defects in visual-spatial processing. The WBS deletion is flanked by large repeats containing genes and pseudogenes. The deletions arise spontaneously by inter- or intrachromosomal crossover events within misaligned duplicated regions of high sequence identity that flank the typical deletion (Francke, 1999). Also, the WS region can generate duplications: the 7q11.23 duplication could be involved in complex clinical phenotypes, ranging from developmental or language delay to mental retardation and autism (Depienne et al., 2007).

We have designed a model for the Williams syndrome, using spontaneous and mutant variants of the *Drosophila* locus *agnostic* containing the *CG1848*gene for the LIMK1 located on the X chromosome in region 11 AB. Alleles of the *agnostic* locus differently determine (1) the structure of LIMK1 gene; (2) the chromosome architecture in the region of the locus location; (3) chromosome packaging; (4) features of homologous and nonhomologous pairing, implemented in different rates of unequal recombination; (5) activities of the components of cascade LIMK1– cofilin–actin; (6) the appearance of cytoplasmic amyloid-like inclusions; and (7) the capability of learning acquisition and preserving memory (Medvedeva et al., 2008) Locus *agnostic* was found by screening for temperature-sensitive mutations induced by ethyl methane sulphonate (EMS) on the background of strain CantonS (CS), which could impair the activity of enzymes for cAMP synthesis and degradation (Savvateeva et al., 1978). A mutant of this locus, agn^{ts3}, exhibit extremely high activity of Ca^{2+}/CaM phosphodiesterase, elevated ability of females for classical olfactory learning with negative reinforcement at 25°C and inability to learn at 29°C (Savvateeva and Kamyshev, 1981). Immunofluorescent staining of the adult brain sections with antibodies to LIMK1 reveals its predominant localization in the central complex and optic lobes in normal flies. The agn^{ts3} mutants demonstrate a drastic increase of anti-LIMK1 in all brain structures which can be seen in normal flies only after their exposure at 29° C (Figure 2). Similarly to WS, the hemizygosity for the gene leads to a loss of LIMK1 temperature dependency and its predominant localization in the visual system. PCR analysis of the LIMK1 gene detected polymorphism both in strains carrying mutations in the *agnostic* locus, and in the wild-type strains. However, the polymorphic sites are unevenly distributed over the gene, occurring more often at the 3' end of the region examined. As to agn^{ts3}, it shows a putative insertion (Figure 3). Presumably, this insertion might result from a specific chromatin architecture in the region where approximately 6 kb from the end of LIMK1 gene starts a 20kb-long AT-rich repeats stretching to the telomere (Figure 4). Therefore, it is not surprising, that standard genetic mapping procedures reveal 3-fold map expansion around the agn^{ts3} mutation (Savvateeva-Popova et al., 2002).

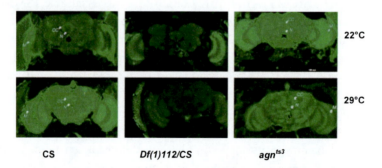

Figure 2. Expression of LIMK1 in the imaginal brain as revealed by immunofluorescence. Paraffin sections of the brain of adult flies of (a, c) the wild-type Canton-S strain and (b, d) the *agnts3* mutant were stained with antibodies against LIMK1 (dilution 1:500) and secondary FITC-conjugated (dilution 1:400) antibodies. (goat LIMK1, donkey-anti-goat IgG-FITC, donkey serum, Santa Cruz)
Flies were kept at a permissive temperature of 22°C or exposed at 29°C for 2 h. Brain structures: CC, central complex; N, noduli; M, medulla.

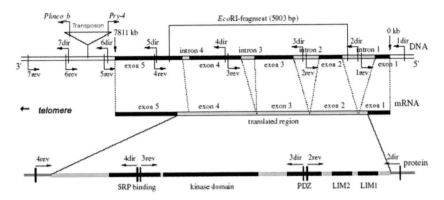

Figure 3. Insertion of genetic material in 3'UTR of LIMK1 gene agn^{ts3} sites of primer binding are indicated relative to DNA, RNA and protein sequences

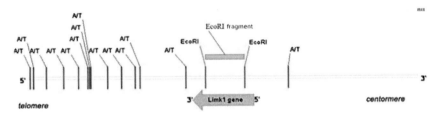

Figure 4. A/T-rich regions in vicinity of the Drosophila LIMK1 gene (The National Centre for Biotechnology Information, NCBI)

The aforementioned similarities with WS are in accord with the recent trend to identify *Drosophila* genes related to human disease genes in assumption that cross-genomic analysis of human disease genes using the power of modern *Drosophila* databases which combine the data of classic and molecular genetics, is very promising (Reiter et al., 2001). Undoubtedly, such an approach refers only to considering the first level of organization of the genetic material, i.e. a linear arrangement of the sequence in the chromosome. However, the demonstration of high frequency of occurrence of genomic disorders exceeding that of single gene mutations requires considering the second level – belonging of a certain gene sequence to a particular structural–functional chromosome block.

Second Level of Genome Organization: Structural Organization of a Chromosome, Euchromatic and Heterochromatic Regions of the *Drosophila* Polytene Chromosomes

The specificity of genome architecture is providing substrates for homologous recombination between nonhomologous regions of chromosomes which harbor different types of repetitive sequences, segmental duplications with a certain level of homology (Prokofyeva-Belgovskaya and Khvosotova, 1939; Shaw and Lupski, 2004). Since in humans this can result in DNA rearrangements that cause disease, the problem of chromosome organization deserves a special attention. The *Drosophila melanogaster* genome consists of four chromosomes that contain 165 Mb of DNA, 120 Mb of which are euchromatic. It is possible to differentiate in the polytene chromosomes their euchromatin from heterochromatin: banding patterns, distribution of satellite DNAs and location of the rDNA. In polytene chromosomes, condensed (bands), decondensed (interbands), genetically active (puffs), and silent (pericentric and intercalary heterochromatin (IH) as well as areas subjected to position effect variegation (PEV) regions were found long ago and their features were described in detail (Bridges, 1935; Prokofyeva-Belgovskaya and Khvosotova, 1939; Prokofyeva-Belgovskaya, 1945, 1986; Khesin and Leibovitch, 1976; reviwed in Zhimulev et al., 2004). Long thought to be inert, heterochromatin is now recognized to give rise to small ncRNAs, which, by means of RNA interference, direct the modification of proteins and DNA in heterochromatic repeats and transposable elements (Lippman and Martienssen, 2004). Heterochromatin has thus emerged as a key factor in epigenetic regulation of gene expression, chromosome behavior and evolution.

IH consists of extended chromosomal domains which are interspersed throughout the euchromatin and contain silent genetic material. These domains comprise either clusters of functionally unrelated genes or tandem gene duplications and possibly stretches of noncoding sequences. Also, IH harbors homeotic genes. Repeats of various kinds have been localized in the IH, such as transposable elements or the tRNA genes; and tandem, such as histone or the ribosomal RNA genes, satellite DNA, and oligonucleotide tracts (Wimber and Steffensen, 1973). Strong repression of genetic activity means that IH displays properties that are normally attributable to classic pericentric heterochromatin: high compaction, late replication and underreplication in polytene chromosomes, and the presence of heterochromatin-specific proteins (Zhimulev, 1998; Grewal et al., 2002; Huisinga et al, 2006; Belyaeva et al., 2008). Moreover, IH regions are often considered to be the so called weak spots (Zhimulev et al., 1982). Low temperature considerably promotes the expression of chromosome "fragility" in the weak spots. Decrease in heterochromatin amount (removal of the Y chromosome) in the nucleus produces a sharp increase in break frequencies. There is circumstantial evidence concerning the action of genetic modifiers of PEV. A comparison of strains contaning En-var(3)2 and Su-var(3)9 releaved higher break frequencies in larvae having an enhancer of PEV. This allows concluding that treatments increasing PEV also increase the heterochromatin fragility. Indeed, peaks of the highest frequencies of spontaneous and induced aberrations were observed mainly in the IH regions. For the X-chromosome these are regions 1F, 3C, 4E, 7B, 9A, 11A, 12D, 12E, 16F, 19E (Kaufmann, 1946; Ilyinskaya et al., 1988). Interestingly, some of these regions coincide with recombinational boundaries found in the X-chromosome: 3C4–6/7, 7A–7E, 11A, and a region proximal of 18C (Hawley, 1980). The most unusual is region 11A involved in Kosikov duplication, which is characterized by homology between 11A and 12D and between 11B and 12E (Kosikov, 1936). Region 11A is a hot spot of chromosome breaks, ectopic contacts, underreplication, and recombination, which take place on exposure to common chemical mutagen ethyl methanesulfonate (EMS) in particular (Xamena et al., 1985). Owing to these properties, the region may be used as a marker of intercalary heterochromatin or as a test system suitable for analyzing various cytological phenomena in *D. melanogaster* (Belyaeva et al., 1998). It is this region that contains the *agnostic* locus harboring a gene for LIMK1. Note again that WS results from chromosome aberrations arising because of the specific chromosome architecture; namely, the relevant region contains numerous complex duplicons, which allow unequal meiotic crossing over. Likewise, many repeats are characteristic of region 11A–11B9 of the *D.*

melanogaster X chromosome on evidence of Southern hybridization analysis of P1 phages containing *D. melanogaster* genome material (Savvateeva-Popova et al., 2002; 2004).

Gene Silencing

Soon after its discovery 75 years ago, heterochromatin was found to silence genes. Zhimulev and Belyaeva (2003) envision IH regions as comprising stable inactivated genes, whose silencing is developmentally programmed. Moreover, post-translational modification of histones and the specific nonhistone protein complexes participate in the establishment and maintenance of silencing for all heterochromatin types (Grewal and Rice, 2004). Studies in the fission yeast have begun to highlight the genetic pathways critical for the assembly and epigenetic maintenance of heterochromatin, including key roles played by the RNAi machinery, H3 lysine 9 methylation and heterochromatin protein 1 (HP1) (Horn and Peterson, 2006). Although it is known that chromatin architecture is altered by methylation of theDNA and by various types of modifications to histones (the so-called 'histone code'), including compound patterns of methylation, acetylation, phosphorylation, ubiquitinylation, sumoylation, ADP-ribosylation, carbonylation, deimination and proline isomerization at various residues, a rapidly emerging notion that "epigenetic memory" is mainly based on the fuction of different types of ncRNAs, such as miRNA, siRNA, piRNA (Moazed et al., 2006; Kutter and Svoboda, 2008; Scott and Li, 2008; Obbard et al., 2009). They are genome-encoded, endogenous negative regulators of translation and mRNA stability originating from long primary transcripts with local hairpin structures. RNAi is triggered by the processing of long double-stranded RNA (dsRNA) into small interfering RNAs (siRNAs), which mediate sequence-specific cleavage of nascent mRNAs. The third common class of repressive small RNAs, PIWI-associated RNAs (piRNAs), is produced in a Dicer-independent manner. Current data suggest that piRNAs protect the germline from mobile genome invaders such as transposons. A small RNA involved in RNA silencing associates with proteins in an effector ribonucleoprotein complex usually referred to as RNA-Induced Silencing Complex (RISC). Key components of RISC complexes are proteins of the Argonaute family, which determine RISC functions. Argonaute-2 (ago-2) is required for proper nuclear migration, pole cell formation, and cellularization during the early stages of embryonic development in *Drosophila* (Deshpande et al., 2005). Why this newly-emerging preference of ncRNAs-regulated silencing pathways is so promising? The most reasonable explanation is as follows (Mattick et al., 2009). There are only a limited number of enzymes (DNA methyltransferases, histone methyltransferases, acetylases, deacetylases etc.) and repressive and permissive (Polycomb-group and Trithorax-group) chromatin-modifying complexes involved, very few of which are known to have affinity for particular DNA sequences. Also, it is known that RNA is an integral component of chromatin and that many of the proteins involved in chromatin modifications, as well as transcription factors have the capacity to bind RNA or complexes containing RNA. These include DNA methyltransferases and methyl DNA binding domain proteins, heterochromatin protein 1 (HP1), the multi-KH domain protein DPP1 which suppresses heterochromatin-mediated silencing in *Drosophila*, and domains commonly found in chromatin remodelling enzymes and effector proteins such as SET domains, tudor domains and chromodomains. Moreover, signal-induced ncRNAs can act as selective ligands to modulate histone acetyltransferase activity at specific genomic positions (for references see Mattick et al., 2009). The nuclear organization of chromatin insulators and chromatin domains is also affected by the RNAi machinery and recent deep sequencing studies have shown that double-stranded RNAs formed by sense-antisense transcript pairs originating from inverted repeats, bidirectional/antisense transcripts from retrotransposons, pseudogenes and mRNAs in mouse oocytes and *Drosophila* somatic cells are processed into large numbers of small RNAs that may have regulatory functions in epigenetic pathway (Watanabe et al., 2008; Tam et al., 2008; Ghildiyal et al., 2008). However, though endogenous *Drosophila* siRNAs have not yet been identified, siRNAs can be derived from long hairpin RNA genes (hpRNAs). The *Drosophila* hpRNA pathway is a hybrid mechanism that combines canonical RNA interference factors (Dicer-2, Hen1 known as CG12367 and Argonaute 2) with a canonical miRNA factor (Loquacious) to generate approximately 21-nucleotide siRNAs. These novel regulatory RNAs reveal unexpected complexity in the sorting of small RNAs, and open a window onto the biological usage of endogenous RNA interference in *Drosophila* (Okamura et al., 2008). This is in accord with our finding of a hairpin structure which simultaneously serves as a site for integrating of transposons in vicinity of the *agnostic* gene (Medvedeva et al., 2008). It is possible that the impairment of the *agn^{ts3}* gene 3'UTR might affect miRNA –dependent post-translational regulation of the *agnostic* gene due to mRNA-miRNA complementation defects. Normally, miRNA binding to mRNA 3'UTR prevents from translational termination leading to a transcript degradation (Mathieu and Bender, 2004). In the *agn^{ts3}* mutants this putative complementation defect might lead to an increase in number of LIMK1 transcripts which, in comparison to the wild type, would much more successfully pass through translation.

How these ncRNA regulatory pathways can control LIMK1 gene expression at the level of chromatin organization? As detected by immunofluorescence techniques in larval salivary glands the extremely high activity of LIMK1 and p-cofilin in *agn^{ts3}*, normally exceeding those of the wild type, decrease only after HS. In wild type HS results in an increase of the LIMK1 and p-cofilin levels (Medvedeva et al., 2008). How does this potent change in the activity of both the LIMK1 gene product and p-cofilin affect homologous and nonhomologous chromosome pairing?

Table 1 presents the data on revealing a sensitive period of forming non-homolog contacts. In the wild type these are the first 4.5 hrs after egg laying. Following fertilization, the *Drosophila* embryo progresses through 13 synchronous mitotic cycles to create a syncitial blastoderm with thousands of nuclei arrayed just below the surface of the outer membrane (Foe et al. 1993). These mitotic divisions are initially just a few minutes long and then slow down during cycles 11–13 before finally pausing for at least 60 min during interphase 14, at which time the syncitial blastoderm cellularizes (Foe et al., 1993).Temperature treatment administered during second half of embryogenesis (Table 1) does not affect frequency of ectopic contacts (FEC). This is in accord with the finding that the last few syncitial divisions are of particular interest, since the homolog pairing is first observed during this time, progressing to appreciable but locus-specific levels of pairing during the long interphase of cycle 14 (Hiraoka et al., 1993; Fung et al., 1998; Gemkowet al., 1998).

Interestingly, the onset of homolog pairing during the late syncitial mitotic cycles coincides with the critical period of embryogenesis when many aspects of the developmental program switch from maternal to zygotic control, known as the maternal-to zygotic transition (MZT, Bateman and Wu, 2008). At the moment of beginning of the zygotic gene transcription occurs the formation of the heterochromatic regions which might be influenced by temperature treatments (Lippman and Martienssen, 2004; 2006). This is in accord with our data.

Table 1. Frequency of ectopic contacts between regions of intercalary heterochromatin in the 2L arm of the polytene chromosome 2 in wild type Canton-S (CS) and agn^{ts3} following low and high temperature treatments.

	CS	agn^{ts3}
intact	0,48±0,033	0,71±0,022
15° C, 24 hr of embryonic development	0,702±0,042*	0,78±0,049
29° C, 24 hr of embryonic development	0,67±0,035*	0,62±0,027*
37° C, first 2,5 hrs of embryonic development	0,72±0,044*	0,74±0,064
37° C, 2,5 hrs beginning from 8th hr of embryonic development	0,55±0,033	0,65±0,08
15° C, 24 hr I instar larva	0,48±0,024	0,65±0,018*
15° C, 24 hr II instar larva	0,66±0,036*	0,58±0,028*

* $P < 0,05$ differences from the intact animals from each strain, **Student's t criterion**

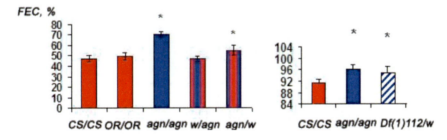

Figure 5. Frequency of ectopic contacts in 2L-arm.

Interestingly, agn^{ts3} mutants show a maternal effect on FEC in 2L (Figure 5). Presumably, mRNAs for LIMK1 are maternally transmitted to the zygote. Therefore, the absence of temperature response results from prolonged survival of the mutant mRNA, since the degradation of maternal mRNAs is directed by miRNAs (Schier, 2007). This might be the aforementioned consequence of altered regulatory interaction between miRNAs and LIMK1 mRNA in agn^{ts3}.

Our results on forming of non-homolog contacts at the blastoderm stage are in accord with findings that temperature treatments during first 3 hrs of embryogenesis enhance PEV-dependent (Vlassova et al., 1991). The coincidence of the onset of these two phenomena point to both their interrelations and to an increase of heterochromatic silencing in response to temperature treatment. Therefore, we can conclude that:

(1) similarly to PEV, the frequency of ectopic contacts can indicate the rate of silencing
(2) the *agnostic* gene is involved into repressive mechanisms leading to gene silencing

The distribution of FECs (Figure 6) shows that certain IH blocks demonstrate the most sharp differences in agn^{ts3} mutants. The insertion in AT-rich region adjacent to LIMK1 gene might be the source of small ncRNAs which can stimulate RNA-directed methylation of heterochromatic regions known to contain sequences complementary to those of anti-viral defense (Mathieu and Bender, 2004). The increase in the repressive properties of these chromatin regions might lead to an increase in FEC.

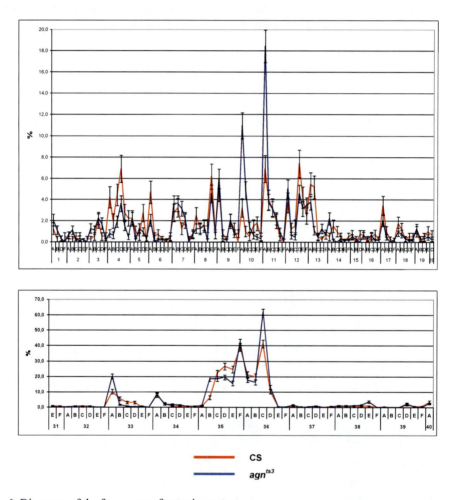

Figure 6. Diagrams of the frequency of ectopic contacts.

Third Level of Genome Organization: Spatial Organization of Chromosomes in the Nucleus

The long-lasting awareness derived from findings on fixed preparations is that chromosomes in the nucleus are motionless, finally begun to expire. First, functional studies of chromosome behavior suggested that many essential processes, such as recombination, require interphase chromosomes to move around within the nucleus (Belmont et al., 1997; Vasquez et al., 2001; Marshall, 2002). Since chromosomes occupy discrete territories within the nucleus, individual loci have to undergo limited movement to reach a suitable environment for gene regulation (Heard and Bickmore 2007). Further studies from diverse organisms have shown that distinct interchromosomal interactions are associated with many developmental events, since stable interchromosomal contacts must be formed between maternal and paternal homologous chromosomes (Bateman and Wu, 2008). Although communication between chromosomes was first postulated long ago in *Drosophila* and other dipteran insects (Stevens, 1908; Lewis, 1954), the importance of the three-dimensional organization of the genome has started to draw attention only recently. Somatic pairing in *Drosophila*, especially in the giant polytene chromosomes, provides an excellent model for understanding interchromosomal interactions and their effect on gene expression . Importantly, somatic pairing or synapsis is initiated by multiple independent associations rather than by "zippering" the chromosomes from a discrete pairing initiation site (Fung et al., 1998). At present, at least two mechanisms that bring homologous sequences together within the nucleus are considered: those that act between dispersed homologous sequences and those that act to align and pair homologous chromosomes (Blumenstil et al., 2008). The most profound study of such mechanisms in so called non-homologous, ectopic pairing comes from the Zhimulev's lab. Ectopic contacts may arise simultaneously in several regions of different chromosomes. Zhimulev *and co-workers* have classified the centers of ectopic pairing of polytene chromosomes in the early 1980s. According to our data, the ectopic contact matrix constructed for the wild-type X chromosome confirmed this early observation and in the case of the mutant X chromosome, a dramatic increase was also established for ECFs of regions 11A and 11B with regions 9A, 10A, 10B, 12A, 12D–F, 13AB, and 14A (Savvateeva-Popova et al., 2004). Interestingly, such X-chromosomal regions contain genes for components of signal transduction and ionic channels (Adams et al., 2000). Like LIMK1, many of these proteins have PDZ domains, which mediate multiple protein–protein interactions in supramolecular complexes involved in signal transduction. It is probably regions of ectopic chromosome pairing that harbor these genes and brings them close together to ensure their efficient and rapid transcription. For instance, region 10B7-8 contains the *Disc large* gene, whose product first allowed a discovery of the PDZ domain. Region 10B4-5 contains the *disheveled* gene, whose product is involved in the Wnt–frizzled signaling cascade. It is noteworthy that deletion causing WS involves several genes, including a homolog of the *D. melanogaster frizzled* gene. Such regions are scattered all over *Drosophila* chromosomes. For instance, Rossi et al., (2007) report that 70% of heterochromatic gene models of chromosome 2 encode putative proteins sharing significant similarity with human proteins, such as specific RNA pol II Specific RNA pol II transcription factors, voltage-gated potassium channel, MAP-kinase and different protein kinases, serine/threonine phosphatase and proteins of RNA biogenesis.

Also, there is strong positive correlation between increased Suppressor of Underreplication (SuUR) gene expression extent, amount of DNA truncation, and formation of ectopic contacts in IH regions (Belyaeva et al., 2006). Only when induced during early stages of chromosome polytenization, SuUR overexpression results in the formation of partial chromosomal aberrations whose breakpoints map exclusively to the regions of intercalary and pericentric heterochromatin. IH underreplication in polytene chromosomes results in free double-stranded ends of DNA molecules; ligation of these free ends is the most likely mechanism for ectopic pairing between intercalary heterochromatic and pericentric heterochromatic regions.

A strong SUUR interactor is HP1, the well-studied heterochromatin protein, and the C-terminal part of HP1, which contains the hinge and chromoshadow domains interact with the central region of SUUR. In addition, recruitment of SUUR to ectopic HP1 sites on chromosomes provides evidence for their association in vivo (Pindyurin et al., 2008). Notably, the SuUR protein, which is bound in regions of ectopic pairing of IH, has the N-terminal region homologous to the N-terminal domain of the SW12/SNF2 family proteins (Ambach et al., 2000). Since actin plays a dual role as a component of complexes of remodeling and premRNA- binding proteins, any change in the actin dynamics, resulting from a mutational lesion of LIMK1 activity, should affect the properties of heterochromatin and the spatial features of the organization of the whole chromosome. This can be characterized by asynapsis of polytene chromosomes of salivary glands. Furthermore, physical interactions between homologous sequences have been either directly observed or implicated in many epigenetic phenomena, including transvection, paramutation in plants and in mice, repeat induced point mutation and methylation induced premeiotically, meiotic silencing of unpaired DNA ,meiotic sex chromosome inactivation and X inactivation (reviewed in Bateman and Wu, 2008).

Moreover, homologous chromosome pairing is essential for creating prerequisites for unequal crossing over. The intercalary heterochromatin itself provides association with the nuclear membrane by filaments of ectopic contacts in sites referred to as terminal asynapsis points (Mathog, et al., 1984). Consequently, a change in the distribution of asynaptic regions along the agn^{ts3} chromosome may show change in nuclear localization of the corresponding chromosome region. As follows from (Figure 7), strong interstrain differences in asynapsis characteristics were found between chromosomes of strains CS and agn^{ts3}. The frequency of asynapsis occurs in agn^{ts3} mutants is nearly threefold lower than that in CS flies. As agn^{ts3} flies are characterized by higher frequency of ectopic contacts, this suggests association between the characters examined, the involvement of IH in homologous pairing, and participation of the *agnostic* gene in these processes. Our data on the distribution of the asynaptic regions along chromosome arms (Figure 8) allow to suppose their localization within the nucleus. Assuming that some nuclear compartments favor homologos pairing while others do not, we can arbitrary consider the frequency of asynapsis occurrence equal to 40%±5 as high asynaptic level and assign «+». Consequently, the low frequency of assynapsis may be assigned as «-». Then, the frequencies of asynapsis in proximal regions of the polytene chromosome is as follows: in the X - CS«+», agn«-»; in 2R - CS«+», agn«-»; in 3L - CS«+», agn«+»; in 3R - CS«+», agn«-»; in 2L- CS«-», agn«-». Therefore, we can suggest that in wild type proximal regions of the X, 2R, 3R and 3L are localized in a compartment disfavoring homologous pairing. As for agn^{ts3} the proximal regions of the X, 2R and 3R occupy the same compartment, as 2L in CS.

The frequencies of asynapsis in distal regions might be the following: in 2R - CS«+», agn«+»; in X - CS«-», agn«-»; in 2L- CS«-», agn«+»; in 3L – CS«-», agn«-»; in 3R - CS«-», agn«-». In this case, only 2L-arm in agn^{ts3} shows another localization than in wild type. The possibility of occurrence of two alternative values of frequencies of asynapsis in neighboring regions of the same chromosome might indicate that a certain region can occupy different nuclear compartments.

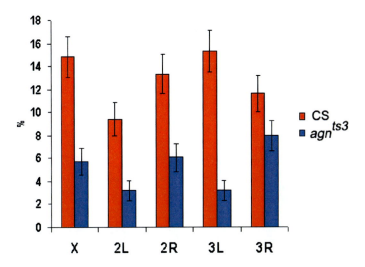

Figure 7. Interstrain differences in asynapsis frequencies in the *Drosophila* chromosomes.

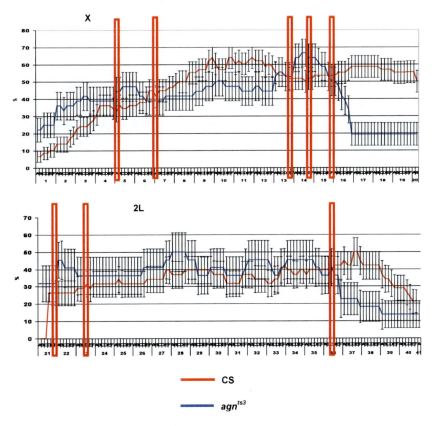

Figure 8. Asynaptic profile of *Drosophila* chromosome
Red bars mark the boundaries of regions demonstrating alternative interstrain asynaptic values.

Several types of distribution of asynaptic regions along the chromosome can be distinguished (Figure 9). We classify these distributions into type 1 and type 2. Type 1 is characterized by prevalence of short asynapses with a gradual decrease in frequency of each subsequent gradation. This type includes the X chromosome, 2L in CS and agn^{ts3}, as well as 2R in agn^{ts3} and 3R in CS. In type 2 distribution, the frequency of long asynapses is enhanced. The examples of this type are 2R in CS, 3L in CS and agn^{ts3}, and especially 3R in agn^{ts3}.

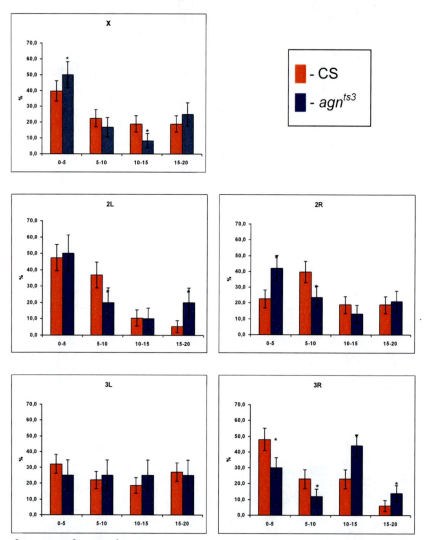

Ordinate – frequency of asynapsis, per cent
Abscissa – number of asynaptic sections

Figure 9. Interstrain differences in asynapsis lengths in *Drosophila* chromosomes.

In view of the above, one can assume that modification of asynaptic state constitutes two mutually dependent actors: (1) if the distributions of long and short asynapses are similar, interstrain differences in asynapsis frequencies would depend on the nuclear compartment, into which falls the interstitial region flanked by terminal asynapsis points; the nucleus may have advantageous and disadvantageous conditions for homologous synapsis; (2) if the distributions of asynapsis lengths are different, the heterochromatin state and the degree of its attachment to the membrane and nuclear matrix are of importance. Our results demonstrate association between ectopic and homologous pairing. In agn^{ts3} with high FEC, far closer homologous synapsis is observed, which confirms the role of mutational LIMK1 impairment in the organization of genetic apparatus.

Epigenetic Mechanisms in Memory Formation

Long-term potentiation (LTP) of synaptic transmission is a primary experimental model of memory formation in neuronal circuits (Lynch, 2004; Raymond, 2008). Although the research on the molecular basis of memory is very intensive, it still focuses mainly on proteins despite of the fact that nc RNAs are predominantly enriched in the brain where they can direct epigenetic modifications (Mercer et al., 2008).

Models of synaptic plasticity comprise at least three sequential but mechanistically distinct components which involve different compartments of a nerve cell and different levels of regulation (Raymond 2007). The first or early phase, which lasts up to 3 hours and is manifested in synapse, is dependent on modifications of existing proteins. This early phase is thought to relate to the formation of short–term memories and is unaffected by protein-synthesis inhibitors (Lynch 2004). The intermediate phase, lasting 2 to 8 hours, is dependent on local translation in dendrites from pre-existing RNA, but independent of gene transcription. The final or late phase that produces a sustained response is dependent on gene transcription in soma of the nerve cell in addition to protein synthesis. These three phases have been identified in both vertebrates and invertebrates and are believed to represent a general feature of synaptic plasticity.

Epigenetic changes including chromatin modifications and DNA methylation play important roles in regulating networks of gene expression underlying memory formation and maintenance (Levenson and Sweatt, 2006). Histones associated with genes involved in synaptic plasticity are dynamically acetylated in response to L-LTP induction and memory formation is also blocked by the inhibition of DNA methyltransferase. These observations show that epigenetic changes are integral to memory formation and indeed the processes of acetylation and methylation seem to function in a combined and coordinated manner. Chromatin modifications are additionally coordinated with the transcriptional cascades induced by changes in synaptic plasticity. For example, the CREB binding protein (CBP) is a transcriptional co-activator that may also act as a histone acetyltransferase, providing a direct link between chromatin modification and CREB-dependent pathways. Non-coding RNAs may provide an additional link between transcriptional networks such as CREB-dependent pathways and epigenetic modifications.

We tested the learning acquisition and memory formation in 5 day-old wild type and agn^{ts3} males in conditioned courtship suppression paradigm (Kamyshev et al., 1999). Earlier, we have developed a design of heat shock treatment of adult flies and during their development to affect them in the period of the formation of brain structures responsible for learning (HS1, the late embryonic–early larval stage, the time of formation of mushroom bodies) and the memory formation (HS2, prepupal stage, the formation of the central complex), as well as in adults (HS) (Nikitina et al., 2003). The results were surprising and paradoxical: intact agn^{ts3} mutants showed 3-h (intermediate) memory and learning ability that were threefold lower than those in Canton S flies. The agn^{ts3} mutants treated with heat shock during the mushroom body formation exhibited even more drastic, six -fold, reduction in these parameters. However, after a heat shock treatment of adult agn^{ts3} or a heat shock at the prepupal stage, during the formation of the brain central complex, the memory and learning indices were not only the same as in CS flies, but showed a trend for increase. As to long-term memory, when it is tested 2 and 8 days after 5 hrs training at day 5, it is also severely suppressed in intact agn^{ts3} compared to wild type. Again, heat shock administration to adult males somehow improves the poor performance of agn^{ts3}, and heat shock at the stage of formation of the central complex of the brain (HS2) brings the long-term memory practically to the wild type level (Nikitina et al., 2009, unpublished). The studies aimed to correlate these findings with CREB level are underway but as we have already shown (Medvedeva et al., 2008), the altered intermediate memory depends on the rate of formation of amyloid-like inclusions in the brain. In case of agn^{ts3} mutational change of each of the analyzed levels disrupts systemic regulation of genetic and cytogenetic processes, which results in the formation of amyloid-like inclusions.

In the wild-type strain, heat shock decreases the spontaneous level of amyloid-like inclusions in larvae and does not lead to the formation of inclusions in the adult brain, which is diagnostic for many neurodegenerative diseases. By contrast, in the agn^{ts3} mutant, the amount of inclusions in all larvae examined at normal temperature significantly decreases after heat shock. In adult flies, amyloid-like inclusions were recorded at both temperatures (Medvedeva et al., 2008).

Such factors as actin and cofilin have been shown to be involved in the formation of inclusions (mostly cytoplasmic, less frequently, nuclear) in manyneurodegenerative diseases, including all varieties of prionic conditions (Minamide et al., 2000; Maselli et al., 2003). Granules of the actin–cofilin complex are preferentially found in postmortem sections of patients with the Alzheimer disease; in them, all amyloid-like inclusions are surrounded by actin-cofilin comple, but not all inclusions of these complexes contain amyloid aggregates. In the case of the Alzheimer disease, the earliest events occur on the cell membrane, where multiprotein complexes are formed with participation of integrins and LIMK1. Its activation by neurotoxic fragments of the amyloid protein and the subsequent cofilin phosphorylation result in rearrangement of the actin cytoskeleton and the formation of actin filaments (Heredia et al., 2006). It is believed (Lee at al., 2004) that the cytoplasmic aggregates block axonal transport, contributing to neurophysiological dysfunction presumably due to synaptic pathology which is also common to human AD brain (Masliah et al., 1989). In terms of genetics, upon analysis of mutant and spontaneous variants of the *agnostic* locus, this series of events is as follows: the LIMK gene structure—disruption of LIMK1 and cofilin expression—the formation of Congophilic (amyloid-like) inclusions surrounded by the actin–cofilin complex—the resultant cognitive level.

Conclusion

Recent combined efforts of neurobiology and genetics has brought to a new notion that epigenetic changes leading to chromatin remodeling play important roles in regulating networks of gene expression during development of the nervous system, when they determine the switch from nerve stem cells to dendrite development and axon path finding, and in the adult brain where they underlie memory formation and maintenance (Lin and Holt, 2007). Though the detailed mechanisms are still far from clear, it is already possible to conceive that directional steering in axons and dendrites based on attractive and repulsive turning is analogous to long-term potentiation and depression (LTP and LTD). Chromatin modifications in soma of the nerve cell are coordinated with the transcriptional cascades induced by changes in synaptic plasticity which can also promote local translation in dendrites and axons of dormant mRNAs for neurotransmitter receptors and components of actin cytoskeleton. At the protein level actin and actin related proteins appear to be the main players in the game, at the level of RNA its flexibility and a vast number of non-coding RNAs predominantly enriched in the brain enable the RNA machinery to set the rules of this game. Both non-coding RNAs and actin-dependent processes orchestrate the responses of an organism to environmental requirements, current needs of the organism, and its individual experience. The critical aspect of this response is the spatial organization of the genome in the nucleus when the chromatin domains located far apart in the linear DNA, as well as chromosome arms, can have physical contacts thereby predisposing to unequal recombination which results in structural rearrangements. The chromosome positions within the nucleus determine both normal development and progression of genomic diseases. For example, hemizygosity for LIMK1, the key enzyme of actin remodeling (small GTPases of Rho family – LIMK1 – cofilin – actin) leads to cognitive pathology of the Williams syndrome and the mostly studied details of the crosstalk of non-coding RNAs and signaling cascades refer to LIMK1 (Schratt et al, 2006). The signaling cascade of actin remodeling acts downstream of different receptors including those for neurotransmitters and is tightly involved in the feedback regulation of different receptors and ion channels. Notably, many human and *Drosophila* genes coding for neurotransmitter receptors, ion channels and components of different signaling cascades map to heterochromatic region. Our findings on structural impairments of the *agnostic* locus harboring the *Drosophila* gene for LIMK1, its belonging to intercalary heterochromatic regions, its role in heterochromatin formation, spatial organization of the chromosomes in the nucleus, and cognitive process allow the extrapolation of these peculiarities on aforementioned genes mapping to heterochromatin. Probably, the genes from signaling cascades which are localized in heterochromatin like LIMK1 gene can regulate gene expression during memory formation not only via activation of effector molecules, but also via chromatin remodeling due to specificity of their localization. The heterochromatic genes containing repeats in 3'UTRs similarly to LIMK1 gene might serve as a source of non-coding RNAs. This could lead both to silencing and to ectopic contacts of the heterochromatic regions complementary to sequences of these non-coding RNAs. It seems plausible that LIMK1 itself can act as a regulatory factor in bridging three hierarchic levels of genome organization, the first being the linear organization of transcriptionally active and regulatory DNA sequences; the second being the chromatin level mediating switching between different functional states of transcriptional activity or repression of gene clusters and the third being the nuclear level, a dynamic, three-dimensional spatial organization of the chromosomes, epigenetically regulating gene clusters of different chromosomes.

References

Adams, M. D., Celniker, S. E., Holt, R. A., et al. (2000). The Genome Sequence of *Drosophila melanogaster*, *Science*, *287*, 2185-2195.

Aigner, S., Denli, A. M. & Gage, F. H. (2007). A Novel Model for an Older Remodeler: The BAF Swap in Neurogenesis. *Neuron*, *55*, 171-173

Ambach, A., Saunus, J., Konstandin, M., et al. (2000). The Serine Phosphatases PP1 and PP2A Associate with and Activate the Actin-Binding Protein Cofilin in Human T Lymphocytes. *Eur. J. Immunol.*, *30*, 3422-3431.

Antar, L. N., Li, C., Zhang, H., Carroll, R. C. & Bassell, G. J. (2006). Local functions for FMRP in axon growth cone motility and activity-dependent regulation of filopodia and spine synapses. *Mol Cell Neurosci*, *32*, 37-48.

Aravin, A. A., Lagos-Quintant, M., Yalcin, A., Zavolan, M., Marks, D., et al. (2003). The small RNA profile during *Drosophila melanogaster* development. *Dev Cell*, *5*, 337-350.

Bateman, J. R. & Wu, C. t. (2008). A Genomewide Survey Argues That Every Zygotic Gene Product Is Dispensable for the Initiation of Somatic Homolog Pairing in *Drosophila*. *Genetics*, *180*, 1329-1342.

Bateman, J. R. & Wu, C. t. (2008). A Genomewide Survey Argues That Every Zygotic Gene Product Is Dispensable for the Initiation of Somatic Homolog Pairing in *Drosophila*. *Genetics*, *180*, 1329-1342,

Belyaeva, E. S., Andreyeva, E. N., Belyakin, S. N., Volkova, E. I. & Zhimulev, I. F. (2008). Intercalary heterochromatin in polytene chromosomes of *Drosophila melanogaster*. *Chromosoma.*, *117*, 411-8.

Belyaeva, E. S., Demakov, S. A., Pokholkova, G. V., Alekseyenko, A. A., Kolesnikova, T. D. & Zhimulev, I. F. (2006). DNA underreplication in intercalary heterochromatin regions in polytene chromosomes of *Drosophila melanogaster* correlates with the formation of partial chromosomal aberrations and ectopic pairing. *Chromosoma*, *115*, 355-66.

Belyaeva, E. S., Zhimulev, I. F., Volkova, E. I., et al. (1998). Su(UR)ES: A Gene Suppressing DNA Underreplication in Intercalary and Pericentric Heterochromatin of *Drosophila melanogaster* Polytene Chromosomes. *Proc. Natl. Acad. Sci.*, USA, *95*, 7532-7537.

Birkenfeld, J., Betz, H. & Roth, D. (2001). Inhibition of Neurite Extension by Overexpression of Individual Domains of LIM Kinase1. *J. Neurochem.*, *78*, 924-927.

Blumenstiel, J. P., Fu, R., Theurkauf, W. E. & Hawley, R. S. (2008). Components of the RNAi Machinery That Mediate Long-Distance Chromosomal Associations Are Dispensable for Meiotic and Early Somatic Homolog Pairing in *Drosophila melanogaster*. *Genetics*, *180*, 1355-1365.

Blumenstiel, J. P., Fu, R ., Theurkauf, W. E., Hawley, R. S., Hiraoka, Y., Dernburg, A. F., Parmelee, S. J., Rykowski, M. C., Agard, D. A., et al. (1993). The onset of homologous chromosome pairing during *Drosophila melanogaster* embryogenesis. *J. Cell Biol., 120,* 591-600.

Blumenstiel, J. P., Fu, R., Theurkauf, W. E. & Hawley, R. S. (2008). Components of the RNAi Machinery That Mediate Long-Distance Chromosomal Associations Are Dispensable for Meiotic and Early Somatic Homolog Pairing in *Drosophila melanogaster*. *Genetics, 180,* 1355-1365.

Bramham, C. R. (2008). Local protein synthesis, actin dynamics, and LTP consolidation. *Curr Opin Neurobiol., 18,* 524-31.

Bridges, C. B. (1935). Salivary chromosome maps with a key to the banding of the chromosomes of *Drosophila melanogaster*. *J. Hered., 26,* 60-64.

Brown, E., Malakar, S. & Krebs, J. E. (2007). How many remodelers does it take to make a brain? Diverse and cooperative roles of ATP-dependent chromatin-remodeling complexes in development. *Biochem Cell Biol., 85,* 444-62.

Chen, M. & Shen, X. (2007). Nuclear actin and actin-related proteins in chromatin dynamics. *Curr Opin Cell Biol., 19,* 326-30.

Costa, E., Chen, Y., Dong, E., Grayson, D. R., Kundakovic, M., Maloku, E., Ruzicka, W., Satta, R., Veldic, M., Zhubi, A. & Guidotti, A. (2009). GABAergic promoter hypermethylation as a model to study the neurochemistry of schizophrenia vulnerability. *Expert Rev Neurother., 9,* 87-98.

da Silva, J. S. & Dotti, C. G. (2002). Breaking the neuronal sphere: regulation of the actin cytoskeleton in neuritogenesis. *Nat Rev Neurosci, 3,* 694-704.

de la Torre-Ubieta, L. & Bonni, A. (2008). Combinatorial assembly of neurons: from chromatin to Dendrites. *Trends in Cell Biology, 18,* 48-51.

Depienne, C., Heron, D., Betancur, C., Benyahia, B., Trouillard, O., Bouteiller, D., Verloes, A., LeGuern, E., Leboyer, M. & Brice, A. (2007). Autism, language delay and mental retardation in a patient with 7q11 duplication. *Journal of Medical Genetics, 44,* 452-458.

Deshpande, G., Calhoun, G. & Schedl, P. (2005). *Drosophila* argonaute-2 is required early in embryogenesis for the assembly of centric/centromeric heterochromatin, nuclear division, nuclear migration, and germ-cell formation. *Genes Dev., 19,* 1680-5.

Donnai, D. & Karmiloff-Smith, A. (2000). Williams syndrome: from genotype through to the cognitive phenotype. *Am. J. Med. Genet., 97,* 64-71.

Eaton, B. A. & Davis, G. W. (2005). LIM Kinase1 controls synaptic stability downstream of the type II BMP receptor. *Neuron, 47,* 695-708.

Foe, V. E., Odell, G. M. & Edgar, B. A. (1993) *Mitosis and morphogenesis in the Drosophila embryo: point and counterpoint pp. 149-300 in The Development of Drosophila melanogaster*. Cold Spring Harbor, Cold Spring Harbor Laboratory Press, NY

Foletta, V. C., Lim, M. A., Soosairajah, J., Kelly, A. P., Stanley, E. G., Shannon, M., He, W., Das, S., Massague, J. & Bernard, O. (2003). Direct signaling by the BMP type II receptor via the cytoskeletal regulator LIMK1. *J Cell Biol., 162,* 1089-98.

Francke, U. (1999). Williams-Beuren syndrome: genes and mechanisms. *Hum. Mol. Genet., 8,* 1947-1954.

Fung, J. C., Marshall, W. F., Dernburg, A., Agard, D. A. & Sedat, J. W. (1998). Homologous chromosome pairing in *Drosophila melanogaster* proceeds through multiple independent initiations. *J Cell Biol. 141,* 5-20.

Gangaraju, V. K. & Bartholomew, B. (2007). Mechanisms of ATP Dependent Chromatin Remodeling. *Mutat Res.*, *618*, 3-17.

Gemkow, M. J., Verveer, P. J. & Arndt-Jovin, D. J. (1998). Homologous association of the Bithorax-Complex during embryogenesis: consequences for transvection in *Drosophila melanogaster*. *Development*, *125*, 4541-4552.

Ghildiyal, M., Seitz, H., Horwich, M. D., Li, C., Du, T., et al. (2008). Endogenous siRNAs derived from transposons and mRNAs in *Drosophila* somatic cells. *Science*, *320*, 1077-1081.

Gregório, S. P., Sallet, P. C., Do, K. A., Lin, E., Gattaz, W. F. & Dias-Neto, E. (2009). Polymorphisms in genes involved in neurodevelopment may be associated with altered brain morphology in schizophrenia: preliminary evidence. *Psychiatry Res.*, *165*, 1-9.

Grewal, S. I. & Rice, J. C. (2004) Regulation of heterochromatin by histone methylation and small RNAs. *Curr Opin Cell Biol*, *16*, 230-238.

Grewal, S. I. S. & Elgin, S. C. R. (2002). Heterochromatin: new posibitis for the inheritance of structure. *Curr. Opin. Cell. Genet. Devel.*, *12*, 17-187.

Grummt, I. (2006). Actin and myosin as transcription factors. *Curr Opin Genet Dev.*, *16*, 191-6.

Hawley, R. S. (1980). Chromosomal Sites Necessary for Normal Levels of Meiotic Recombination in *Drosophila melanogaster*: I. Evidence for and Mapping of the Sites. *Genetics*, *94*, 625-646.

Heard, E. & Bickmore, W. (2007). The ins and outs of gene regulation and chromosome territory organisation. *Curr. Opin. Cell Biol.*, *19*, 311-316.

Heredia, L., Helguera, P., de Olmos, S., et al. (2006). Phosphorylation of Actin-Depolymerizing Factor/Cofilin by LIM-Kinase Mediates Amyloid Beta-Induced Degeneration: A Potential Mechanism of Neuronal Dystrophy in Alzheimer's Disease. *J. Neurosci.*, *26*, 6533-6542.

Hocking, J. C., Hehr, C. L., Bertolesi, G., Funakoshi, H., Nakamura, T. & McFarlane, S. (2009). LIMK1 acts downstream of BMP signaling in developing retinal ganglion cell axons but not dendrites. *Dev Biol.*, [Epub ahead of print]

Horn, P. J. & Peterson, C. L. (2006). Heterochromatin assembly: a new twist on an old model. *Chromosome Res.*, *14*, 83-94.

Hsieh, J. & Gage, F.H. (2005). Chromatin remodeling in neural development and plasticity. *Curr. Opin. Cell Biol.*, *17*, 664-671.

Huisinga, K. L., Brower-Toland, B. & Elgin, S. (2006). The contradictory definitions of heterochromatin: transcription and silencing. *Chromosoma*, *115*, 110-122.

Ilyinskaya, N. B., Petrova, N. A. & Demin, S. Yu., (1988). Seasonal dynamics of chromosomal polymorphism in Chironomus plumosus L. (Diptera. Chironomidae). *Genetika*, *24*, 1393-1401. [In Russian].

Ji, Y., Eichler, E. E., Schwartz, S. & Nicholls, R. D. (2000). Structure of chromosomal duplicons and their role in mediating human genomic disorders. *Genome Res.*, *10*, 597-610.

Ji, Y., Eichler, E. E., Schwartz, S. & Nicholls, R. D. (2000). Structure of chromosomal duplicons and their role in mediating human genomic disorders. *Genome Res.*, *10*, 597-610.

Kafatos, F. C., Louis, C., Savakis, C., Glover, D. M., Ashburner, M., Link, A. J., Sidén-Kiamos, I. & Saunders, R. D. (1991). Integrated maps of the *Drosophila* genome: progress and prospects. *Trends Genet.*, *7*, 155-61.

Kamyshev, N. G., Iliadi, K. G. & Bragina, J. V. (1999). *Drosophila* Conditioned Courtship: Two Ways of Testing Memory. *Learn. Mem.*, *6*, 1-20.

Kaufmann, B. P. (1946). Organization of chromosome. 1. Break distribution and chromosome recombination in *Drosophila melanogaster*. *J. Exp. Zool.*, *102*, 293-320.

Khesin, R. B. & Leibovitch, B. A. (1976) Structure of chromosomes, histones and gene activity in *Drosophila*. *Molecular.biol.*, *10*, 3-34. [In Russian].

Kosikov, K. V. (1936). A New Duplication in the *Drosophila melanogaster* X Chromosome and Its Evolutionary Significance. *Dokl. Akad. Nauk SSSR*, *3*, 297-300.

Kutter, C. & Svoboda, P. (2008). miRNA, siRNA, piRNA: Knowns of the unknown. *RNA Biol.*, *5*, 181-8.

Lee, W., Yoshihara, M. & Littleton, J. T. (2004). Cytoplasmic aggregates trap polyglutamine-containing proteins and block axonal transport in a *Drosophila* model of Huntington's disease. *Proc. Nat. Acad. Sci., USA.*, *101*, 3224-3229.

Lee-Hoeflich, S. T., Causing, C. G., Podkowa, M., Zhao, X., Wrana, J. L. & Attisano, L. (2004). Activation of LIMK1 by binding to the BMP receptor, BMPRII, regulates BMP-dependent dendritogenesis. *The EMBO Journal*, *23*, 4792-4801

Lessard, J., Wu, J. I., Ranish, J. A., Wan, M., Winslow, M. M., Staahl, B. T., Wu, H., Aebersold, R., Graef, I. A. & Crabtree, G. R. (2007). An essential switch in subunit composition of a chromatin remodeling complex during neural development. *Neuron*, *55*, 201-15.

Levenson, J. M. & Sweatt, J. D. (2006). Epigenetic mechanisms: a common theme in vertebrate and invertebrate memory formation. *Cell Mol Life Sci.*, *63*, 1009-16.

Levenson, J. M., Qiu, S. & Weeber, E. J. (2008). The role of reelin in adult synaptic function and the genetic and epigenetic regulation of the reelin gene. *Biochim Biophys Acta.*, *1779*, 422-31.

Lin, A. C. & Holt, C. E.(2007). Local translation and directional steering in axons. *EMBO J.*, *26*, 3729-3736.

Lippman, Z. & Martienssen, R. (2004). The role of RNA interference in heterochromatic silencing. *CNature*, *431*, 364-70.

Louvet, E. & Percipalle, P. (2009). Transcriptional control of gene expression by actin and myosin. *Int Rev Cell Mol Biol.;272*, 107-47.

Lupski, J. R. (1998). Genomic disorders: structural features of the genome can lead to DNA rearrangements and human disease traits. *Trends Genet.*, *14*, 417-22.

Lupski, J. R. (2009). Genomic disorders ten years on. *Genome Med.*, *1*, 42.

Lynch, M. A. (2004). Long-term potentiation and memory. *Physiol. Rev.*, *84*, 87-136.

Mande, S. & Gozes, I. (2007). Activity-dependent Neuroprotective Protein Constitutes a Novel Element in the SWI/SNF Chromatin Remodeling Complex. *J. Biol. Chem.*, *282*, 34448-34456.

Marqués, G., Bao, H., Haerry, T. E., Shimell, M. J., Duchek, P., Zhang, B. & O'Connor, M. B. (2002). The *Drosophila* BMP type II receptor Wishful Thinking regulates neuromuscular synapse morphology and function. *Neuron.*, *33*, 529-43.

Marshall, W. F. (2002). Order and Disorder in the Nucleus. *Review Current Biology, 12,* 724-8.

Marshall, W. F., A. Straight, J. F., Marko, J. R., Swedlow, A. F., Dernburg, B. A., Belmont, A. W., Murray, D. A. & Sedat, J. W. (1997). Interphase chromosomes undergo constrained diffusional motion in living cells. *Curr. Biol., 7,* 930-939.

Marshall, W. F., Straight, A., Marko, J. F., Swedlow, J., Dernburg, A., Belmont, A., Murray, A. W., Agard, D. A. & Sedat, J. W. (1997). Interphase chromosomes undergo constrained diffusional motion in living cells. *Current Biology, 7,* 930-9.

Maselli, A., Furukawa, R., Thomson, S. A., et al. (2003). Formation of Hirano Bodies Induced by Expression of an Actin Cross-Linking Protein with a Gain-of-Function Mutation. *Eukaryot Cell, 2,* 778-787.

Masliah, E., Terry, R. D., DeTeresa, R. M. & Hansen, L. A. (1989). Immunohistochemical quantification of the synapse-related protein synaptophysin in Alzheimer disease. *Neurosci. Lett., 103,* 234-239.

Mathieu, O. & Bender, J. (2004). RNA-directed DNA methylation. *J. Cell Sci., 117,* 4881-4888.

Mathog, D., Hochstrasser, M., Gruenbaum, Y., et al. (1984). Characteristic Folding Pattern of Polytene Chromosomes in *Drosophila* Salivary *Gland Nuclei. Nature, 308,* 414-421.

Matsumoto, M., Setou, M. & Inokuchi, K. (2007). Transcriptome analysis reveals the population of dendritic RNAs and their redistribution by neural activity. *Neurosci Res., 57,* 411-23.

Mattick, J. S. (2007). A new paradigm for developmental biology. *Exp. Biol., 210,* 1526-1547.

Mattick, J. S., Amaral, P. P., Dinger, M. E., Mercer, T. R. & Mehler, M. F. (2009). RNA regulation of epigenetic processes. *Bioessays., 31,* 51-9.

Matunis, E. L., Kelley, R. L. & Dreyfuss, G. (1994) Essential role for a heterogeneous ribonucleoprotein (hnRNP) in oogenesis: hrp40 is absent form the germ line in the dorso-ventral mutant squid. *Proc Natl Acad Sci.,* USA, *91,* 2781-2784.

Meagher, R. B., Kandasamy, M. K., Deal, R. B. & McKinney, E. C. (2007). Actin-related proteins in chromatin-level control of the cell cycle and developmental transitions. *Trends Cell Biol., 17,* 325-32.

Medvedeva, A. V., Molotkov, D. A., Nikitina, E. A., Popov, A. V., Karagodin, D. A., Baricheva, E. M. & Savvateeva-Popova, E. V. (2008). Systemic regulation of genetic and cytogenetic processes by a signal cascade of actin remodeling: Locus agnostic in *Drosophila. Russian Journal of Genetics, 44,* 669-681

Meng, Y., Zhang, Y., Tregoubov, V., Janus, C., Cruz, L., Jackson, M., Lu, W. Y., MacDonald, J. F., Wang, J. Y., Falls, D. L. & Jia, Z. (2002). Abnormal spine morphology and enhanced LTP in LIMK-1 knockout mice. *Neuron, 35,* 121-133.

Mercer, T. R., Dinger, M. E., Mariani, J., Kosik, K. S., Mehler, M. F. & Mattick, J. S. (2008). Noncoding RNAs in Long-Term Memory Formation. *Neuroscientist, 14,* 434-45.

Miller, F. D. & Kaplan, D. R. (2003) Signaling mechanisms underlying dendrite formation. *Curr Opin Neurobiol, 13,* 391-398.

Minamide, L. S., Striegl, A. M., Boyle, J. A., et al. (2000). Neurodegenerative Stimuli Induce Persistent ADF/Cofilin-Actin Rods That Disrupt Distal Neurite Function, *Nature Cell Biol.*, *2*, 628 - 636.

Moazed, D., Bühler M., Buker, S. M., Colmenares, S. U., Gerace, E. L., Gerber, S. A., Hong, E. J., Motamedi, M. R., Verdel, A., Villén, J. & Gygi, S. P. (2006) Studies on the mechanism of RNAi-dependent heterochromatin assembly. *Cold Spring Harb Symp Quant Biol.*, *71*, 461-71.

Muotri, A. R. & Gage, F. H. (2006). Generation of neuronal variability and and complexity. *Nature*, *441*, 1087-93.

Nagata, K., Ohashi, K., Yang, N. & Mizuno, K. (1999). The N-terminal LIM domain negatively regulates the kinase activity of LIM-kinase 1. *Biochem J.*, *343*, 99-105.

Neuman-Silberberg, F. S. & Schupbach, T. (1993) The *Drosophila* dorsoventral patterning gene gurken produces a dorsally localized RNA and encodes a TGFa-like protein. *Cell*, *75*, 165

Nikitina, E. A., Tokmacheva, E. V. & Savvateeva-Popova, E. V. (2003). Heat Shock during the Develorment of Central Structures of the *Drosophila* Brain: Memory Formation in the *l(1)ts403* Mutant of Drosophila melanogaster. *Russ. J. Genet.*, *39*, 25-31.

Niu, S., Yabut, O. & D'Arcangelo, G. (2008). The Reelin signaling pathway promotes dendritic spine development in hippocampal neurons. *J Neurosci.*, *28*, 10339-48.

O'Brien, T. P., Bult, C. J., Cremer, C., et al. (2003). Genome Function and Nuclear Architecture: From Gene Expression to Nanoscience. *Genome Res.*, *13*, 1029-1041.

Obbard1, D. J., Gordon, K. H. J., Buck, A. H. & Jiggins, F. M. (2009). The evolution of RNAi as a defence against viruses and transposable elements. *Phil. Trans. R. Soc.*, *364*, 99-115.

Okamura, K., Chung, W. J., Ruby, J. G., Guo, H., Bartel, D. P. & Lai, E. C. (2008). The *Drosophila* hairpin RNA pathway generates endogenous short interfering RNAs. *Nature*, *453*, 803-6.

Olave, I., Wang, W., Xue, Y., Kuo, A. & Crabtree, G. R. (2002). Identification of a polymorphic, neuron-specific chromatin remodeling complex. *Genes Dev*, *16*, 2509-2517.

Olave, I. A., Reck-Peterson, S. & Crabtree, G. R. (2002). Nuclear Actin and Actin-Related Proteins in Chromatin Remodeling. *Annu. Rev. Biochem.*, *71*, 755-781.

Pederson, T. & Aebi, U. (2005). Nuclear Actin Extends, with no Contraction in Sight. *Mol. Biol. Cell*, *16*, 5055-5060.

Percipalle, P. & Visa, N. (2006). Molecular functions of nuclear actin in transcription. *J Cell Biol.*, *172*, 967-71.

Percipalle, P. (2009). The long journey of actin and actin-associated proteins from genes to polysomes. *Cell Mol Life Sci.*, *Mar 20*. [Epub ahead of print]

Percipalle, P., Jonsson, A. & Nashchekin, U. (2003,). Actin in the Nucleus: What Form and What for? *J. Struct. Biol.*, *140*, 3-9.

Percipalle, P., Raju, C. S. & Fukuda N. (2009). Actin-associated hnRNP proteins as transacting factors in the control of mRNA transport and localization. *RNA Biol.*, *6*, [Epub ahead of print]

Percipalle, P., Zhao, J., Pope, B., Weeds, A., Lindberg, U. & Daneholt, B. (2001) Actin bound to the heterogeneous nuclear ribonucleoprotein hrp36 is associated with Balbiani ring mRNA from the gene to polysomes. *J Cell Biol, 153,* 229-236.

Pindyurin, A. V., Boldyreva, L. V., Shloma, V. V., Kolesnikova. T. D., Pokholkova, G. V., Andreyeva, E. N., Kozhevnikova, E. N., Ivanoschuk, I. G., Zarutskaya, E. A., Demakov, S. A., Gorchakov, A. A., Belyaeva, E. S. & Zhimulev, I. F. (2008). Interaction between the *Drosophila* heterochromatin proteins SUUR and HP1. *J Cell Sci., 121,* 1693-703.

Prokofyeva-Belgovskaya, A. A. (1945). Heterochromatinization as a change in chromosome cycle. *Zhurnal Obshch. Biologii, 6,* 93-124. [In Russian].

Prokofyeva-Belgovskaya, A. A. & Khvosotova, V. V. (1939). Distribution of chromosome rearrangement breaks in *Drosophila melanogaster* X chromosome. *Doklady Acad. Nauk SSSR, 23,* 269-271, [In Russian].

Prokofyeva-Belgovskaya, A. A. (1986) *Heterochromatic regions of chromosomes.* Moscow., Nauka, [In Russian].

Purandare, S. M. & Patel, P. I. (1997). Recombination hot spots and human disease. *Genome Res., 7,* 773-786.

Rando, O. J., Zhao, K., Janmey, P. & Crabtree, G. R. (2002). Phosphatidylinositol-dependent actin filament binding by the SWI/SNF-like BAF chromatin remodeling complex. *Proc. Natl. Acad. Sci.,* USA, *99,* 2824-2829.

Raymond, C. R. (2007). LTP forms 1, 2 and 3: different mechanisms for the "long" in long term potentiation. *Trends Neurosci., 30,* 167-75.

Raymond, C. R. (2008). Different requirements for action potentials in the induction of different forms of long-term potentiation., *The Journal of Physiology, 586,* 1859-65.

Reiter, L. T., Potocki, L., Chien, S., Gribskov, M. & Bier, E. (2001). A systematic analysis of human disease-associated gene sequences in *Drosophila melanogaster. Genome Res., 11,* 1114-25.

Rusinov, V., Baev, V., Minkov, I. N. & Tabler, M. (2005). MicroInspector: a web tool for detection of miRNA binding sites in an RNA sequence. *Nucleic Acids Res., 33,* (Web Server issue):W696-700.

Sánchez-Carbente, M. R. & Desgroseillers, L. (2008). Understanding the importance of mRNA transport in memory. *Prog Brain Res., 16,* 41-58.

Savvateeva, E. V. & Kamyshev, N. G. (1981). Behavioral Effects of Temperature Sensitive Mutations Affecting Metabolism of cAMP in D. melanogaster. *Pharm. Biochem. Behav., 14,* 603-611.

Savvateeva, E. V., Kamyshev, N. G. & Rosenblyum, S. R. (1978). Isolation of Temperature-Sensitive Mutations that Impair Metabolism of Cyclic-3.5.-Adenosine Monophosphate in D. melanogaster, *Dokl. Akad. Nauk SSSR, 240,* 1443-1445.

Savvateeva-Popova, E. V., Peresleni, A. I., Sharagina, L. M., et al., (2002). Complex Study of *Drosophila* Mutants in the agnostic Locus: A Model for Connecting Chromosomal Architecture and Cognitive Functions. *Zh. Evolyuts. Biokhim. Fiziol., 38,* 557-577.

Savvateeva-Popova, E., Medvedeva, A., Popov, A. & Evgen'ev, M. (2008). Role of non-coding RNAs in neurodegeneration and stress response in *Drosophila. Biotechnol. J., 3,* 1010-1021.

Schier, A. F. (2007). The maternal-zygotic transition: death and birth of RNAs. *Science, 316*, 406-7.

Schleicher, M. & Jockusch, B. M. (2008). Actin: its cumbersome pilgrimage through cellular compartments. *Histochem Cell Bio, 129*, 695-704.

Schratt, G. M., Nigh, E. A., Chen. W. G., Hu, L. & Greenberg, M. E. (2004). BDNF regulates the translation of a select group of mRNAs by a mammalian target of rapamycin-phosphatidylinositol 3-kinase-dependent pathway during neuronal development. *J Neurosci., 24*, 7366-77.

Schratt, G. M., Tuebing, F., Nigh, E. A., Kane, C. G., Sabatini, M. E., Kiebler, M. & Greenberg, M. E. (2006). A brain-specific microRNA regulates dendritic spine development. *Nature, 439*, 283-289.

Scott, M. J. & Li, F. (2008). How do ncRNAs guide chromatin-modifying complexes to specific locations within the nucleus? *RNA Biol., 5*, 13-6.

Seo, S., Richardson, G. A. & Kroll, K. L. (2005). The SWI/SNF chromatin remodeling protein Brg1 is required for vertebrate neurogenesis and mediates transactivation of Ngn and NeuroD. *Development., 132*, 105-15.

Shaw, C. J. & Lupski, J. R. (2004). Implications of genome architecture for rearrangement-based disorders: the genomic basis of disease. *Human Mol. Gen., 13*, 57-64.

Sjolinder, M., Bjork, P., Soderberg, E., et al. (2005). The Growing Pre-mRNA Recruits Actin and Chromatin-Modifying Factors to Transcriptionally Active Genes. *Genes Dev., 19*, 1871-1884.

Stankiewicz, P. & Lupski, J. R. (2006). The genomic basis of disease, mechanisms and assays for genomic disorders. *Genome Dyn., 1*, 1-16.

Stevens, N. M. (1908). A study of the germ cells of certain Diptera with reference to the heterochromosomes and the phenomena of synapsis. *J. Exp. Zool., 5*, 359-374.

Surtevant, A. H. (1913). The linear arrangement of six sex-linked factors in Drosophila, as shown by their mode of association. *Jour. Exp. Zool., 14*, 43-59.

Tam, O. H., Aravin, A. A., Stein, P., Girard, A., Murchison, E. P., et al. (2008). Pseudogene-derived small interfering RNAs regulate gene expression in mouse oocytes. *Nature, 453*, 534-538.

te Velthuis, A. J. & Bagowski, C. P. (2007). PDZ and LIM domain-encoding genes: molecular interactions and their role in development. *Scientific World Journal, 7*, 1470-92.

Trotter, K. W. & Archer, T. K. (2008). The BRG1 transcriptional coregulator. *Nucl Recept Signal., 6*, e004.

Van Driel, R., Fransz, P. F. & Verschure, P. J. (2003). The Eukaryotic Genome: A System Regulated at Different Hierarchical Levels. *J. Cell Sci., 116*, 4067-4075.

Van Horck, F. P. & Holt, C. E. (2008). A cytoskeletal platform for local translation in axons. *Sci Signal., 1*, 11.

Vazquez, J., Belmont, A. S. & Sedat, J. W. (2001). Multiple regimes of constrained chromosome motion are regulated in the interphase *Drosophila* nucleus. *Current Biology, 11*, 1227-1239.

Vlassova, I .E., Graphodatsky, A. S., Belyaeva, E. S. & Zhimulev, I. F. (1991). Constitutive heterochromatin in early embryogenesis of *Drosophila melanogaster*. *Mol. Gen. Genet., 229*, 316-318.

Watanabe, T., Totoki, Y., Toyoda, A., Kaneda, M., Kuramochi-Miyagawa, S., et al. (2008.). Endogenous siRNAs from naturally formed dsRNAs regulate transcripts in mouse oocytes. *Nature, 453*, 539-543.

Wen, Z., Han, L., Bamburg, J. R., Shim, S., Ming, G. L. & Zheng, J. Q. (2007). BMP gradients steer nerve growth cones by a balancing act of LIM kinase and Slingshot phosphatase on ADF/cofilin. *J Cell Biol., 178*, 107-19.

Willis, D., Li, K. W., Zheng, J. Q., Chang, J. H., Smit, A., Kelly, T., Merianda, T. T., Sylvester, J., van Minnen, J. & Twiss, J. L. (2005). Differential Transport and Local Translation of Cytoskeletal, Injury-Response, and Neurodegeneration Protein mRNAs in Axons. *The Journal of Neuroscience, 25*, 778-791.

Wimber, D. E. & Steffensen, D. M.(1973). Localization of gene function. *Annu. Rev. Genet., 7*, 205-223.

Wu, J. I., Lessard, J., Olave, I. A., Qiu, Z., Ghosh, A., Graef, I. A. & Crabtree, G. R. (2007). Regulation of dendritic development by neuron-specific chromatin remodeling complexes. *Neuron., 56*, 94-108.

Wu, K. Y., Hengst, U., Cox, L. J., Macosko, E. Z., Jeromin, A., Urquhart, E. R. & Jaffrey, S. R. (2005). Local translation of RhoA regulates growth cone collapse. *Nature, 436*, 1020-1024.

Xamena, N., Creus, A. & Macros, R., (1985). Effect of Intercalating Mutagens on Crossing Over in *Drosophila melanogaster* Females. *Experientia, 41*, 1078-1081.

Yoon, B. C., Zivraj, K. H. & Holt, C. E. (2009). Local Translation and mRNA Trafficking in Axon Pathfinding. *Results Probl Cell Differ.*, [Epub ahead of print]

Zalfa, F., Achsel, T. & Bagni, C. (2006). mRNPs, polysomes or granules: FMRP in neuronal protein synthesis. *Curr Opin Neurobiol, 16*, 265-269.

Zhimulev, I. F. & Belyaeva, E. S. (2003). Intercalary heterochromatin and genetic silencing. *Bioessays, 25*, 1040-51.

Zhimulev, I. F. (1998). Polytene chromosomes, heterochromatin, and position effect variegation. *Advances in Genetics., 37*, 566.

Zhimulev, I. F., Belyaeva, E. S., Semeshin, V. F., Koryakov, D. E., Demakov, S. A., Demakova, O.V., Pokholkova, G. V. & Andreyeva, E. N. (2004). Polytene chromosomes: 70 years of genetic research. *Int Rev Cytol., 241*, 203-75.

Zhimulev, I. F., Semeshin, V. F., Kulichkov, V. A. & Belyaeva, E. S. (1982). Intercalary Heterochromatin in *Drosophila*: Localization and General Characteristics, *Chromosoma, 87*, 197-228.

In: Cytoskeleton: Cell Movement...
Editors: S. Lansing et al., pp. 69-100

ISBN: 978-1-60876-559-1
© 2010 Nova Science Publishers, Inc.

Chapter III

Common Tasks of Cytoskeleton and Dystrophin in Muscular and Neurological Functions: Perpectives in Gene Therapy

Joel Cerna Cortés[*,1]*, Dominique Mornet*[2]*, Doris Cerecedo*[3]*,
Francisco García-Sierra*[4]*, Janet Hummel*[6]*,
Eliud Alfredo García Montalvo*[8]*, Olga Lidia Valenzuela Limón*[8]*,
Valery Melnikov*[1]*, Sergio Adrián Montero Cruz*[1]*,
Juan Alberto Osuna Castro*[7]*, Alejandra Mancilla*[7]*,
Rafael Rodríguez-Muñoz*[4] *and Bulmaro Cisneros*[5]

[1] Facultad de Medicina. Universidad de Colima, Avenida Universidad 333 Col. Las Viboras, C.P. 28040, Colima, Col., México.
[2] ERI 25 "Muscle et Pathologies" EA 4202, Université Montpellier 1, Hopital Arnaud de Villeneuve, 395 Avenue du Doyen G. Giraud, 34295, Montpellier, France.
[2] Departamento de Genética y Biología Molecular.
[3] Laboratorio de Hematología, Escuela Superior de Medicina y Homeopatía, I.P.N., Wilfrido Massieu Helguera 239, Frac. La Escalera Ticomán. México, D.F. 07320, México
[4] Departamento de Biología.
[5] Departamento de Genética y Biología Molecular. Centro de Investigación y Estudios Avanzados del IPN. Av. I.P.N. 2508, Col. San Pedro Zacatenco, México D.F., C.P 07360.

---

[*] correspondence to: Dr. Joel Cerna Cortés, Facultad de Medicina de la Universidad de Colima. Avenida Universidad 333 Col. Las Viboras, C.P. 28040, Colima, Col., México. Tel: (52) 312 3161000 ext 47552, Fax: (52) 312 3161129, E-mail: joelcerna@ucol.mx

[6] Facultad de Medicina Veterinaria y Zootecnia. [7] Facultad de Ciencia Biológicas y Agropecuarias de la Universidad de Colima, Km 40 autopista Colima-Manzanillo, C.P. 28100.
[8] Facultad de Ciencias Químicas, Universidad Veracruzana, Avenida Oriente 6 1009, Apartado Postal 215, C.P. 94340, Orizaba, Veracruz, México.

Abstract

Duchenne Muscular Dystrophy (DMD) is an inherited disorder characterized by progressive muscular degeneration and cognitive impairment due to mutations in the DMD gene. This disease seriously affects the quality of life of DMD patients causing death due to cardiac and respiratory complications before 30 years of age. Elucidation of the molecular basis for this illness has determined that cytoskeleton and the product of the DMD gene called dystrophin works in a coordinated way to maintain fibre muscle integrity. It is known that cytoskeleton via its association with the integrin complexes modulates migration of stem cells during embryogenesis to give rise to diverse tissues and organs. This association is also important in performing basic neurological processes such as synaptogenesis. Recent findings have shown that the DMD gene is also manifested in the central nervous system where it has different functions from that seen in muscle. Among the most clearly defined tasks of DMD gene in neurons is its involvement in modulating the formation of beta 1-integrin complexes. This chapter describes the scientific path that allowed elucidation of the molecular basis for Duchenne Muscular Dystrophy. The up dated knowledge to explain the role of the DMD gene in neurological functions is also described together with the advances in the design of therapeutic strategies focused on restoration of the DMD gene function in patients.

Historical Background

Duchenne Muscular Dystrophy (DMD) is a neuromuscular genetic disease in which the muscle of a patient (young male) suffers progressive damage, due to lack of dystrophin protein. DMD patient muscles become gradually weaker which subsequently effects essential physiological mechanisms such as: respiratory system, nervous system, cardiovascular system, etc. By nine years old, DMD boys have need of a wheelchair for at least part of the time as mobility becomes more difficult and his weakened muscles will cause him to tire easily. In most cases, adolescent years are when the most significant loss of skeletal muscle strength takes place. It is at this point that activities involving the arms, legs, or trunk of the body will require assistance or mechanical support. Heart complications become the main threat to both health and life due to damage and loss of respiratory muscle. The muscle layer of the heart (called 'myocardium') begins to deteriorate, similar to the skeletal muscles which puts them at risk of a heart attack. Major symptoms of myocardium impairment include: shortness of breath, fluid in the lungs, or swelling in the feet and lower legs (caused by fluid retention). Finally the death is caused by heart failure before thirty years old.

Duchenne de Boulogne (Figure 1), a French doctor (Born at Boulogne-sur-Mer, 1806-1875) was the first to identify clinically a muscular pathology and his discovery in 1868 gives a clinical identification to this particular muscle disorder, that will be named the DMD (Duchenne Muscular Dystrophy[1,2] More recently but about 100 years later, the German doctor, Peter Emil Becker reported in 1955 a less strict but related pathology that will be identify as the Muscular Dystrophy of Becker BMD[3]. During the seventies of 20th century, scientific efforts focused on describing muscle tissue abnormalities displayed by DMD patients by using electron microscopy and histochemical studies[4-10]. During the same time period, investigations also focused on identifying biochemical markers in blood to diagnose the disease. Some of them included: serum aldolase activity, creatine kinase, the electrophoretic pattern of the enzyme lactic dehydrogenase (LDH), ATP:creatine phosphotransferase levels[11-15].

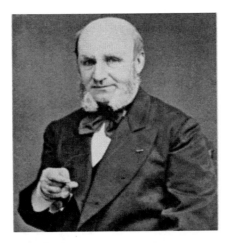

Figure 1. Duchenne de Boulogne identified clinically for the first time the DMD.

In 1963, a study attempting to establish a link between the genes for Duchenne Muscular Dystrophy and the Xg blood group was reported[16]. However, the observation about the way by which the illness appears along the generations allowed to define the DMD as a X-linked recessive inheritance disease[17]. Further studies showed the possibility that an aberrant protein synthesis could be responsible for triggering the disease[18]. In parallel, several drugs such as prednisone were evaluated with the purpose to improve the patient conditions[19]. DMD patient's satellite cells were also analyzed with electron microscopy[20] and through electrophysiological methods the muscle motor-units[21]. Some other works took the erythrocyte as a model to study alterations on cell membrane with the aim to establish an extrapolable celular mechanism for the muscular units of contraction called sarcomers[22,23]. In 1976 the first study that showed the association of DMD with learning difficulties was published[24]

Later, a study performed by Rowland LP[25], helped to focus the investigations on the molecular mechanisms causing DMD. This author established that DMD appears due to a biochemical abnormality that alters the skeletal muscle membrane. His study showed that an aberrant permeability of muscular fibers causes an abnormal seeping out of soluble enzymes and other proteins from muscle tissue. An altered property, of certain enzymes that binds the muscle membrane was also observed. This author proposed that the development of DMD is caused by a genetic alteration that results in an abnormal regulation of the intracellular calcium content of muscular fibers.

In 1981, the identification of a gene translocation allowed the locating of the DMD locus in the short arm of the X chromosome[26]. Other data showed that the DMD gene locus is on the X chromosome short arm, between Xp11 y and Xp22[27]. When analysis of a genetic linkage using two DNA polymorphisms was performed on women carrying X chromosome gene translocations. Several studies employing RFLP (Restriction Fragment Length Polymorphism) analysis support the theory that mutations in a gene on the X chromosome were responsible for the development of the disease[5,6,28]. At that time, the epidemiology of DMD was assessed establishing that 1 out of 3,300 newborn males has DMD[29].

The DMD GENE and Dystrophy

The year 1987 was a trascendental time in the path to establish the molecular bases of the DMD. During this year, Kunkel and collaborators determined the DMD gene sequence, which resulted to be the largest human gene until now described. These authors established that the mRNA encoded by this gene in mice and humans has a 14 kb in length. They also predicted that the aminoacid sequence of the protein produced by the gen is 90 % conserved in both mammals[30] and shows structural characteristics similar to other muscle proteins[31]. Another study, published in the same year defined the preliminary genomic organization of the DMD gene in healthy people and DMD patients. This report described that the DMD transcript comprises 60 exons (currently, it is known that the gene is made up of 79 exons). This work was of great importance since the cDNA sequence of the DMD gene was tested with the DNA isolated from 104 DMD boys for detection of deletions. By means of this experiments it was determined that more than 60% of DMD patients carry gene deletions[32]. Furthermore, the first polyclonal antibody against the protein produced by the DMD gene was generated which permited for the first time its visualization. This protein of 427 kDa that represents 0.002% of the total striated muscle was called dystrophin[33]. The analysis of dystrophin expresion using an anti-dystrophin antibody showed that muscle tissue of both DMD children and mdx mouse do not contain this protein. This result suggested that both genetic disorders were similar. Since this report, the mdx mouse was taken as an animal model to study DMD. Later, studies performed by Koening in 1988[34] proposed that the 3685 aminoacids of Dp427 can be separated into four domains; a N-terminal of 240 aminoacids that presents homology with the actin-binding of α–actinin; a large second domain denominated rod, formed by a succession of 25 triple-helical segments similar to the repeat domains of spectrin; a rich cysteine that has similarity to the carboxyl-terminus of Dictyostelium α-actinin and finally, a carboxi-terminal, formed by the last 420 amino acids of dystrophin which, does not show any similarity with previously reported proteins. Between 1988 and 1990, several works were focused on identifying mutations all through the DMD gene in patients[35-37]. In this respect, the polymerase chain reaction (PCR) represented a powerful diagnostic tool for the identification of new mutations[38,39].

Identification of the Dystrophin Associated Glycoprotein Complex and Molecular Basis for the DMD

The identification of protein partners to which dystrophin binds was an essential step in establishing its function in the muscular cells and to having a better understanding of the pathological processes leading from the absence of dystrophin to the muscular degeneration. The Campbell's research group established in 1990[40] that dystrophin forms an oligomeric complex with four glycoproteins and that one of these proteins was poorly expressed in DMD patients. This suggested that the absence of dystrophin could lead to a complex instability due to dystrophin-dependent negative modulation of a dystrophin associated protein. A further work showed that the Dystrophin Associated Glycoprotein Complex (DAPC) is highly enriched in muscle skeletal membranes and is located specifically in the plasmatic membrane of sarcomers[41]. Based on this evidence, a model was proposed on the organization of the DAPC[42,43], which established that the glycoproteins alpha sarcoglycan (50 kDa), beta dystroglycan (43 kDa) and gamma sarcoglycan (35 kDa) as well as the 25 kDa dystrophin-associated protein (later called sarcospan) are integral membrane proteins, whereas dystrophin, alpha dystroglycan (156 kDa) and alpha syntrophin (59 kDa) are peripheral proteins. Dystrophin and alpha syntrophin are cytoskeletal elements that bind alpha dystroglycan via the transmembrane proteins of the DAPC. The mdx mouse model of human Duchenne Muscular Dystrophy showed that the DAPC proteins were poorly expressed in muscular tissue, suggesting that an absence of dystrophin and not the indirect effect due to the degradation of the muscular fiber, affected the stability of these proteins[44]. Later (1992) the analysis of alpha dystroglycan and beta dystroglycan expression revealed that both proteins come from a common RNA messenger and that the alpha dystroglycan binds to the extracellular matrix protein laminin. This finding supported the notion that DAPC forms a bridge between the sarcolema (via the interaction of the carboxy-terminal domain of dystrophin with actin) and the extracellular matrix (via the interaction of alpha dystroglycan with the extracellular matrix protein laminin), acting as a spring or like a shock absorber during the process of muscular contraction and relaxation. Therefore, dystrophin transmits the mechanical energy produced by the actin-myosin "contraction apparatus" to the muscle cell membranes and the outside structures of the muscle, the connective tissue and the sinews, in an well-balanced way that does not overstresses them (Figure 2A). In this way, the loss or dysfunction of dystrophin and the subsequent instability of one or several DAPC would cause the loss of the bridge that binds the sarcolem with the extracellular matrix (Figure 2B), which would finally cause the necrosis of muscular fibers in patients with DMD[45].

The importance of the DAPC in the functioning of muscular tissue was reinforced with the finding that mutations in the genes that codify for alpha and gamma sarcoglycans cause the severe childhood autosomal recessive muscular dystrophy (SCARMD)[46,47,48]. These authors demonstrated that the DAPC disintegrates, which indicates that DAPC formation is affected by the absence of only one member.

In the last decade, several new DAPC members have been identified and the DAPC model shows new modifications. Currently, it is known that the carboxyl-terminal portion of dystrophin binds to beta dystroglycan, alpha syntrophin and alpha distrobrevin[49]. On the other hand, alpha syntrophin recruits the enzyme neuronal nitric oxide synthase (nNOS)[50]. This finding displays the potential implication of DAPC in signaling events. In this sense, it has also been demonstrated that the carboxyl-terminal portion of dystrophin is responsible for the binding of calmodulin[51]. The current sarcoglycan subcomplex includes: alpha, beta, gamma, delta, epsilon and zeta sarcoglycans and sarcospan[52,53]. Caveolin 3, (which performs functions such as clathrin mediated endocytosis, the potocytosis and signal transduction)[54], and syncoilin, (an intermediate filament protein) which interacts with alpha dystrobrevin[55] are also DAPC members (Figure 2A). A Type-VI intermediate filament which plays an important cytoskeletal role within the muscle cell cytoskeleton has also been identified. It forms heteropolymeric intermediate filaments with desmin and/or vimentin, and via its interaction with cytoskeletal proteins alpha-dystrobrevin, dystrophin, talin-1, utrophin and vinculin, is able to link these heteropolymeric intermediate filaments to adherens-type junctions, such as to the costameres, neuromuscular junctions, and myotendinous junctions within striated muscle cells. Mutations leading to defects in intermediate filament assembly, network formation compromise in vivo functions of intermediate filaments as protectors against environmental stress[56,57].

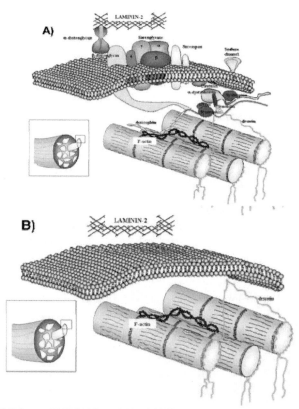

Adapted from J of Cell Science 2002 [110 pp 2501-2503].

Figure 2. A) The dystrophin associated protein complex in a healthy person allows the interaction of the extracellular matrix with the sarcomeric cytoskeleton. B) Loss of the DAPC complex in a patient with Duchenne Muscular Dystrophy.

Current Definition of Duchenne Muscular Dystrophy

Duchenne Muscular Dystrophy is an X-link recessive disorder due to mutations in the DMD gene or in DAPC components. Duchenne boys have none or very little dystrophin in their muscular fibers. When their protective and organizing effects are absent, muscle contraction causes the rupture of the muscle membranes, and thus allows that larger amounts of calcium circulate through the fibers. Excessive calcium influx in cells activates enzymes like calpain and other proteases that break down muscular proteins and initiate cell-death programs. The destroyed muscular cells are replaced by connective and fatty tissue; with the consequent loss of muscular function. The space produced by destruction of muscular tissue become sections with fibrosis that restrict the contraction process, causing contractures and muscular rigidity with subsequent loss of muscle function and ability of movement. Among the substances that escape from the interior of the muscular cell towards the sanguineous torrent, the one with the greatest relevance is the enzyme denominated: creatine kinase CK, also named creatine phosphokinase (CPK), which participates in the process for energy production, the energy that is essential for proper muscle function. When the amount of CPK diminishes, the muscle looses its functional capacity causing muscular weakness. This results in a double damage; on the one hand: the amount of muscular cells diminishes while on the other hand, the surviving cells progressively lose their functional capacity, thus causing the muscles to become debilitated in a progressive and continuous way. Liberation of muscle CPK into the circulatory system increases its blood levels to greater than 10-100 times the normal blood values. The excessive amount of CPK in the blood does not cause any additional damage and can be used as a parameter to diagnose muscle problems. As the Muscular Dystrophy Duchenne progresses, many physical symptoms are developed. This complex disorder can affect a multitude of muscle groups and body's systems, including the back (spine), hips, legs, joints, sinews, heart, lungs and brain.

Transcriptional Regulation of DMD Gene Expression: Identification of New Isoforms

The genomic analysis of the DMD gene, the largest and complex of the human genes until now described [32, 58], showed a functional complexity. From different internal promoters, the DMD gene produces a group of transcripts that codify for different size isoforms of dystrophin (Figure 3). The first identified DMD gene transcripts were those corresponding to three full-length dystrophin isoforms, denominated Dp427 (M), Dp427 (B), Dp427 (P). Subsequently, four short transcripts were found; in chronological order of their finding these are: Dp71, Dp116, Dp140 and Dp260. The characteristics of each one of these isoforms as well as the location of its respective promoters are described in the following paragraphs (Figure 3).

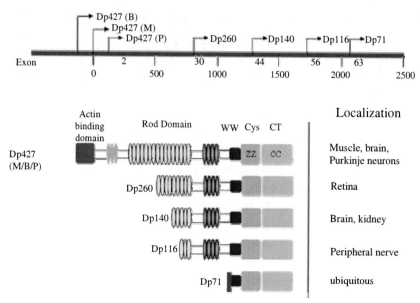

Adapted from J Child Neurol 2005 BC Decker, INC.

Figure 3. The scheme shows the seven promoters of the DMD gene, the domains of each one of the generated isoforms as well as their differential expression.

Dp427 (M) This isoform is expressed in cardiac muscular tissue and skeletal muscle and its expression increases during the differentiation of the myogenic cells into multinucleate myotubes[59]. It is also present in glial cells and some types of cerebral cells[60].

The promoter of the Dp427 (M) is located 37 base pairs upstream of 5 ' end of the published cDNA sequence for this isoform. This promoter is constituted by 850 base pairs upstream of the initial site of transcription. Nevertheless, the minimum promoter includes the first 149 base pairs located upstream of the inicial site of transcription. This region contains transcription factor binding sites for CArG and the nuclear factor 1, which binds the specific enhancer of myocytes (MSEBNF-1). Both transcription factors regulate the promoter activity[59]. The mRNA generated from this promoter presents a length of 14 kb and differs from the other two full length size transcrips Dp427 (B) and Dp427 (P), in the first bases of its 5 ' end. These three dystrophin isoforms display different initial exons and derive from different promoters [58,60].

Dp427 (B) This isoform is specific of brain. The Dp427 (B) is expressed neither in the muscle nor in the glial cells[60]. Its promoter is located 90 Kb upstream of 5' end of the muscular promoter and to 400 kb of exon 2, from which its transcript is processed by splicing[61]. This promoter is neuron-specific and is regulated in a positive way during brain development [61]. Although the function of this isoform is not known, its low expression in human neurons correlates with a deficient expression of the signaling protein nNOS[61].

Dp427 (P) This isoform was identified in the Purkinje cells, which are large neurons of the cerebellum. It is expressed from the denominated P promoter, which generates two transcripts that are processed by splicing: one codifies for the full lenght size dystrophin and the other displays a stop codon located 27 nucleotides after the ATG triplet that represents the translation initiation site. The biological importance of the truncated isoform is unknown.

Nevertheless, its promoter is regulated positively during the development of the cerebral cortex and heart. The transcript that codifies to the complete size isoform is highly expressed in the cerebral cortex of fetus and represents 20% of the transcription generated from DMD gene that is expressed in the skeletal muscle in a healthy adult[58].

Dp260 This isoform is present in the outer plexiform layer of eye retina, which consists of a layer of neuronal synapses. The synapses in the outer plexiform layer are between the rod cell endings or cone cell branched foot plates and horizontal cells. Unlike in most systems, rod and cone cells release neurotransmitters when not receiving a light signal. The 5' end of Dp260 mRNA contains a unique exon that is processed by splicing to generate an open reading frame with exon 30 of the DMD gene. Dp260 contains a unique N-terminal end of 13 amino acids, large part of the rod domain and the rich-cistein and carboxyl-terminus domains. The mouse tissue analysis shows that Dp260 is not only expressed in retina but also in brain and heart. The electrophysiological comparison between the mdx and mdxCv3 mice suggests that Dp260 is required for the normal function of the retina[62]. Mouse retina expresses different dystrophin isoforms. Nevertheless, Dp260 is unique in that it shows a significant increase during the development of this tissue, which correlates with the establishment of the synaptic functions of retina[63]. The Dp260 knockout mice show a delocalisation of the beta dystroglycan in the outer plexiform layer of retina, which suggests that Dp260 is important for the formation of the dystrophin associated protein complex coupled to this tissue. These mice also show an increase in the time of the b wave of Electroretinogram[64]. In the mdx mouse, the ectopic expression of the Dp260 restores the association between costameric actin and sarcolem as well as the assembly of the DAPC complex, which reduces significantly the development of muscular dystrophy[65].

Dp140 This isoform displays the rod and carboxyl-terminus domains of dystrophin and is present in the central nervous system and kidney embryonic tubules, and is located in the basal surface of the epithelial cells [66]. It is believe that Dp140 is important during the process of kidney tubulogenesis [67]. The promoter that transcribes this isoform is located upstream of exon 45 of the DMD gene. DP140 transcript has a 7.5 kb in length and contains a unique exon located in intron 44 of the DMD gene, which is in common between the rat and the human [68,69]. The transcript presents a 5' nontranslated region of 1 kb and first methionine codon locates in exon 51 [68]. Several studies show that an increase in the incidence of cognitive abnormalities exists in patients with Muscular Dystrophy with deletions that affect the codifying region of Dp140 (exons 45-52), which suggests that this isoform is important for the function of the central nervous system [68]: In fact, a statistically significant association exists between the loss of the Dp140 transcript and mental retardation of patients with Duchenne or Becker muscular Dystrophy [70,71]. Dp140 displays an alternative splicing of exons 71-74 and 78 and the isoforms generated by this process are diferencially expressed in the brain and kidney [69]. Exons subjected to alternative splicing codify for domains that binds proteins, which suggests that this process could regulate the association of the Dp140 with integral membrane proteins [69].

Dp116 This isoform has a molecular weight of 116 kDa and is located all through the cellular membrane of the Schwann cells which form the peripheral nerve [72]. Recently, the presence of Dp116 has been detected in skin fibroblasts [73]. This isoform that initially was denominated apo-dystrophin-2 [74], lacks the actin binding domain and large part of the rod domain. The promoter that regulates its expression generates a transcript of 5.2 Kb, which initiates with a unique exon located 850 base pairs upstream of exon 56 of DMD gene [72].

The Schwann cells express dystroglycan complex[75], the sarcoglycans (without sarcospan)[73, 76-79], syntrophins and alpha dystrobrevin[80]. With these proteins, the Dp116 forms the DAPC complex of the Schwann cells, which is associated with the cholesterol transporter[80]. Through this complex, Dp116 establishes a bridge between the cytoskeleton and the extracellular matrix[75,78,81]. The interaction between the Dp116 and the beta dystroglycan is mediated by the last 15 amino acids present in the carboxyl-terminus domain of this last protein[75]. On the other hand, beta dystroglycan interacts with the extracellular protein alpha dystroglycan which contacts the extracellular matrix protein laminin-2. [76]. The presence of mutations or deletions in portions of DMD gene that codify for Dp116, Dp140 and Dp71 have been correlated with the mental retardation of patients with DMD or Becker muscular dystrophy [76]. The overexpression of Dp116 in mice with null expression of Dp427 denominated mdx (4cv) does not improve the phenotype of dystrophy [77].

Dp71 The Dp71 protein has a molecular weight of 70.8 kDa and represents the smallest and most abundant product of the DMD gene in the majority of non-muscular tissues, especially in the brain[82]. This isoform displays a unique actin binding domain that allows its interaction with the cellular cytoskeleton[83] and contains the carboxyl-terminus and rich-cysteine domains present in the rest of dystrophins. However, lacks of the rod and the actin binding domains both present in the Dp427 [82]. Dp71 is codified by a mRNA of 6.5 Kb and is the first transcript of the DMD gene that is detected in the stage of pluripotent embryonic stem cells during development [84]. In myogenic cells, the expression of Dp71 diminishes [85], whereas in the brain its expression increases during the embryonic development. In this organ It is glycosylated and locates in the synaptic plasmatic membranes, in microsomes, mitocondries and in an smaller proportion in synaptic vesicles [86]. This isoform is also expressed in the dentate gyrus as well as in the olfactory bulb [87], the inner membrane of the retina (where it interacts with the beta dystroglycan), the blood vessels [88,89] and the hippocampus [90]. In the spermatozoa, its expression helps to maintain the flagellar morphology as well as the distribution of ionic channels and nNOS protein [91]. The promoter that regulates the expression of Dp71, does not contain TATA box and displays a high proportion of GC base pairs as well as several potential transcription factor-binding sites for Sp1. This promoter is located more than 2000 Kb downstream of 3' end to the muscle and brain type dystrophin promoters and only 150 kb from the 3' end of the gene [92]. In mice, the absence of Dp71 induces a reduction in the expression of the dystrophin associated proteins [93]. On the other hand, its over-expression in the muscle of mdx mice restores the expression of all the members of DAPC complex as well as its assembly. Nevertheless, it does not improve the muscular function [94,95]. The over-expression of Dp71 in wild type mice damages the skeletal muscle in a similar manner to that produced by the absence of Dp427 (M) which suggests that Dp71 competes with the Dp427 for the binding to the DAPC complex [96].

Distinctive DAPC complexes that contain Dp71 have been determined in different tissues. These complexes differ from each other since the expression of dystrophin associated glycoproteins varies from one cell type to another [97-103]. Because of their heterogeneity, it is thought that the Dp71 complexes have differential functions. For example, in the rat retina DAPC complex, Dp71 works as a scaffold protein to anchor the potassium channel kir 4.1 [104].

The Dp71 mRNA experiences alternative splicing of exons 71 and 78, which are expressed in a variable manner in different tissues such as heart, kidney, lung, testicles and liver [105]. Alternative splicing of exon 78 regulates the subcellular distribution of this protein. In this sense, the isoform which contains it, displays a predominant nuclear localization, whereas the one that lacks it, presents a predominant cytoplasmic localization [106,107]. In the brain, the DMD transcripts show an alternative splicing of exons 71-74. This region is important since exons 73 and 74 represents the binding domain for syntrophin [108]. This region is present in the majority of the Dp71 and Dp140 transcripts expressed in the brain [106].

The isoform of Dp71 that lacks of the binding site for syntrophin are expressed during the early stages of the neuronal development [109] and can shows alternative splicing of exon 78 [110].

Gene Therapy to Cure the Duchenne Muscular Dystrophy

The gene therapy is defined as the restitution of a gene by inducing its expression in somatic tissue with the aim of curing a disease [111]. The experimental approach of these studies with the DMD gene has been performed by using the murine mdx model (which does not express Dp427 M). The muscular injection of these animal with cDNA of the dystrophin gene, using recombinant plasmid vector as well as attenuated replication-competent retroviruses resulted in a deficient delivery of the muscle fibers since less than 10% of fibers of the injected muscle expressed dystrophin [112]. Although the adenovirus is more efficient in its capacity to infect mamalian cells [113], a small proportion of infected cells is still obtained when using this vector, showing that adenovirus is not a good candidate to be used as a gene therapy vector for DMD patients [113].

Other contemplated strategies for DMD gene therapy is the restitution of Dp427 (M) with the expression of its well-known analogous protein called utrophin or with the expression of Dp71. The idea to over-express utrophin in DMD patients, arose after it was observed that a considerable reversion of the dystrophic phenotype occurred in transgenic mdx mice over-expressing utrophin [114]. On the other hand, in the mdx mouse, the transgenic expression of Dp71 was able to restitute and locate all the DAPC components at the membrane of sarcolema [94].

Other efforts in the path to develop gene therapy for DMD patients have exploited the antisense RNA technology to correct specific mutations leading to stop codons or mutations leading to exon skipping [115]. In this respect, it is important to remember that a wide range of mutations can give rise to the development of Duchenne Muscular Dystrophy. Due to the heterogeneity of the genetic alterations that cause the DMD, in economic terms, it is desirable that the restoration of the DMD gene function be by using the complete cDNA sequence of Dp427 (M).

In the development of the gene therapy for DMD patients, the design of viral vectors or of plasmidic DNA with a specific transcripcional activity to express Dp427 (M) that can be injected intravenously and caught specifically by the muscle (specific tissue-tropism) are still required.

Molecular Bases for the Mental Retardation Manifested in DMD Patients

One third of Duchenne patients suffer a moderate to severe, non-progressive form of mental retardation. [116]. This observation has raised the interest of several research groups to establish the molecular mechanisms through which mutations in the DMD gene induce mental delay. Scientific evidence indicate the role of dystrophin Dp71 as an important molecule for the functions that the DMD carries out in brain. In this regard, it has been ascertained that Dp71 is the DMD gene isoform with the most abundant expression in the brain [117]. In addition, its expression increases in this organ during the embryonic development [86]. Perhaps, the background research about Dp71 in the development of cerebral functions bases its implications on a correlation between mental impairment and DMD gene mutations located in regions that codify for the rich-cysteine and carboxyl-terminus domains of this isoform [76, 116, 118].

In order to approach the neuronal function of the Dp71, the PC12 cells have been used as a cellular model [119-121] since these cells differentiate into sympathetic-like neurons by exposure to the nerve growth factor (NGF) [122]. In PC12 cells, the expression of Dp71 increases during the process of cellular differentiation induced by NGF [120]. These cells express two Dp71 isoforms, one of which contains exon 78 and shows a predominant nuclear subcellular localization (Dp71d); the other lacks exon 78 (Dp71f) and localizes predominantly in the cellular cytoplasm [121]. To approach the role of Dp71 during the neuronal differentiation, the inhibition of its expression was performed by using antisense RNA in NGF-stimulated PC12 cells. Through these studies, it was observed that Dp71 deficiency inhibits the neuronal differentiation of PC12 cells when stimulated by nerve growth factor [119]. The inhibition of the neuronal differentiation induced by the absence of Dp71 could be explained if it is considered that the Dp71f associates with the β1-integrin mediated adhesion complex [123,124] stabilizing it [123].

The integrin complex-mediated cellular adhesion modulates neuronal migration, as well as the synaptogenesis during the development of central nervous system. This evidence was obtained from experiments in which the genic deleción of the β1-integrin subunit resulted in an aberrant migration of the neuronal precursor cells of the brain's crust [125]. The participation of the Dp71f as a key protein for the formation of the integrin complex, represents an important advance toward understanding the potential function of Dp71 during the neuronal development [126]. In this sense, it has been determined that Dp71f associates with several components of the integrin complex in neurites and that these associations are stronger in growth cones. For this reason, it is thought that this isoform modulates the functions that the integrin complexes have during navigation, elongation and the maintenance of neurites. Dp71f also modulates the recruitment of the signaling protein GSK3-β to the β1-

integrin adhesion complex probably to be inactivated by ILK. GSK3-β is a negative regulator of the Wnt signaling route [127]. The inhibition of GSK3-β by ILK induces the activation of transcription factors such as AP-1 and β-catenin/LEF-1 [127-129]. This signaling performs important functions during the embryonic development, including: the determination of the cellular types, development of the extremities, nervous system, skeleton, lungs, hair, teeth and gonads. On the other hand, it is probable that mental retardation is also tied to the recently discovered function of Dp71d in the nucleus. Nuclear import of this isoform is modulated by CaMKII phosphorylation [130]. In the nucleus, Dp71d associates with the nuclear matrix, which is a structure that serves as a scaffold for nuclear processes, including: genic transcription, chromatin modeling and splicing. Therefore, Dp71 might modulate nuclear-matrix-associated processes [90].

Integrins and Types of Integrins Expressed by PC12 Cells

Integrins include a large family of glycoproteins located on the cellular surface that mediates cell-cell interactions as well as interactions between the extracellular matrix (ECM) and the cytoskeleton working as a transmembranal bridge and performing signaling through the cellular membrane [131]. Integrins regulate many aspects of the cellular behavior, such as death, proliferation, migration and differentiation. They are expressed as a surface heterodimers, which consist of an α subunit and a β subunit that are non-covalently bound (Figure 4). In mammals, at least 16 α and 8 β different subunits have been identified, which associate to form 22 αβ heterodimers. These heterodimers have been classified into three groups and each heterodimer recognizes specific ligands in the ECM molecules (for example: laminin and fibronectin) or other immunoglobulin superfamily receptors as the intercellular adhesion molecule 1 (ICAM-1). Some integrins bind only one specific ligand while others are more promiscuous, binding several different ligands and conversely, some ECM ligands bind to multiple integrins. This confers a great specificity since one ECM ligand can elicit a variety of cellular signaling pathways via the different bound integrins. In the CNS, integrins of the β1 and αV classes are expressed on a variety of different cell types, including neurons, glial cells, meningeal cells and endothelial cells [132,133]. β2 integrins are expressed specifically by leukocytes, and within the CNS are found on microglia and on infiltrating leukocytes [134].

The cellular line PC12 expresses two classes of heterodimers: β1α1 and β1α3 [134]. Both heterodimers recognize the ECM proteins collagen and laminin. Since the adhesion to these extracellular matrices is affected by the absence of the Dp71, it was logical to think that Dp71f (the cytoplasmic isoform) modulated the β1-integrin adhesion complex in this cellular line. These antecedents together with the previous finding about the interaction of α-actinin-2 with the carboxyl-terminus of dystrophin [135] moved us to look for the possible association of Dp71f with the β1-integrin adhesion complex in the neuronal cell line PC12.

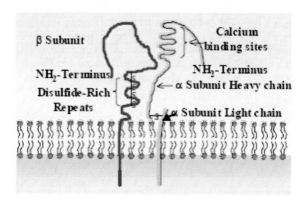

Figure 4. Integrins are expressed as a surface heterodimers, which consist of an α-subunit and a β-subunit that are non-covalently bound.

Molecular Structure of the Focal Adhesions and Point Contacts

The transmembrane connection between the actin cytoskeleton and the extracellular matrix through the integrin family occurs at sites called focal adhesions localized on the plasma membrane. These sites are the specialized structures at the ends of stress fibers, up to 10 μm in length and 0.5 μm in width[136-138]. Originally, focal adhesions or focal contacts were described in living or fixed fibroblasts cultured on glass or plastic. Molecularly, focal adhesions consist of integrin mediated complexes. The interaction of integrins with proteins of the ECM leads to integrin clustering (Figure 5A) and recruitment of actin filaments and signaling proteins to the cytoplasmic domain of integrins. Clustering of integrins, leads to tyrosine phosphorylation of several cellular proteins, including members of the Src-family kinases, FAK, MAPK (Erk1/2, c-Jun kinase, and p38) as well as the Rho GTPase family members: RhoA, Rac1 and CDC42. These important molecules regulate cellular survival and morphologic changes of diverse cell types [139] (Figure 5B).

It is possible to discriminate between small focal points through which the movable cells adhere transitorily to their matrices (podosomas) and the extensive focal adhesions which often last for hours or days, as observed in cultures of epithelial, endothelial, or fibroblastic cells. Typical focal contacts are mainly developed in cultured cells and are rarely found in the organism. However, since cultured cells are amenable to microscopic and biochemical analyses and can be experimentally manipulated, the focal contacts in cultured cells have been extensively studied as a model system for cell-matrix interactions. Another important cellular model to study the focal adhesions is the activated blood plateles. [140].

In the neuronal PC12 cell model the integrins α1, α3 y β1 are expressed and distributed with a punctuate pattern on the cell surface in contact with the ECM protein collagen. These sites are called point contacts which are functional sites of adhesion, structurally different from the typical focal adhesions observed in nonneuronal cells [141].

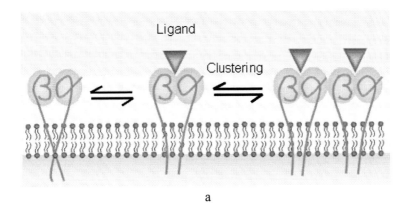

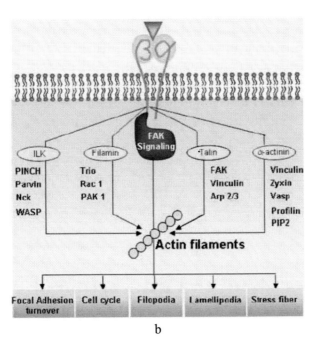

Figure 5. A) Interaction of integrins with proteins of the ECM leads to integrin clustering B) After integrin clustering, the recruitment of actin filaments and signaling proteins to the cytoplasmic domain of integrin occurs, modulating diverse physiological cell mechanisms.

Integrin Functions During the Neural Development

Historically, integrins have been shown to be critical determinants of basic morphogenesis in many developmental events including implantation, gastrulation, and formation of the cardiovascular system [142]. One aspect of CNS development that has been extensively studied is the migration of neurons during establishment of the cerebral cortex [143]. In this process, neurons are born in the ventricular zone and after exiting the cell cycle they attach to radial glial fibers to migrate radially into more superficial positions. At the cortical plate they detach from the glial fibers and form into separate layers. Later-born neurons migrate to more superficial positions in the cerebral cortex, which results in an "inside-out" laminar organization. Several studies support the notion that the β1 integrins may be important in mediating the adhesion and migration of neuronal cell populations within the developing CNS. In one of these studies the β1 integrins were deleted specifically from neurons and glia [125]. This was achieved by creating one strain of transgenic mice expressing the Cre recombinase under the control of the nestin promoter, and crossing these animals with another transgenic strain in which the β1 integrin subunit had been flanked by two LoxP sites. This study showed that the development of the cerebral cortex is perturbed. The developing neurons still form adhesive interactions with the glial fibers, are able to migrate along the fibers, and then detach to take up their positions in the appropriate layer. However, the most superficial layer of the cortex, the marginal zone, appears to be grossly disorganized. In the normal CNS the radial glial fibers terminate on the basement membrane produced by meningeal cells and a specific cell population called the Cajal-Retzius cells form a chain immediately below the basement membrane, and secrete the ECM molecule reelin [144]. In β1-deficient mice, the glial fibers fail to form contacts with the meningeal basement membrane, and terminate at random positions throughout the different cortical layers. In addition, the linear chain of Cajal-Retzius cells is disrupted and the cells are arranged in clusters, and expression of both the basement membrane and Reelin show an abnormal discontinuous distribution. As a result, the migrating neurons invade the marginal zone at breaks in the Cajal-Retzius cell layer, to produce aberrant cellular organization in this zone.

The Recent finding about the role of Dp71f as a key component of the β1 integrin adhesion complex in the neuronal cell line PC12 shows the potential function of this dystrophin isoform during the neural development.

Details About the Interaction of DP71F with the Integrin Complex

In order to study the neural role of Dp71, our research group adopted the PC12 neuronal cell line. By means of a treatment on PC12 cells with plasmids that carry the sequence of Dp71 cDNA in antisense orientation, we generated transfected clones that displayed a reduced expression of Dp71f in 80-90% (antisense-Dp71 clones). The antisense-Dp71 clones present an altered phenotype of cellular adhesion when they are grown on different ECM proteins such as laminin, collagen and fibronectin[123].

Through this study we observed the following experimental evidence showing that Dp71f is a new component of the β1-integrin adhesion complex of PC12 cells, and that its presence is necessary for the formation and/or stability of this protein complex [123]

1) By using double staining immunofluorescence assays and confocal microscopy we demonstrated that in non differentiated PC12 cells, Dp71f colocalized in filopodias and periphery of the cellular bodies with the adhesion proteins β1-integrin, α- actinin, talin and vinculin. Colocation was more evident at the basal part of the cell that contacts with the extracellular matrix[123]. In NGF-differentiated PC12 cells, Dp71f colocalizes with the

components of the adhesion complex β-integrin, talin, vinculin and α-actinin in growth cones, which suggests that such interactions are important for neuritogenesis.

2) A reduced fluorescent signal of β1-integrin, α- actinin, talin and vinculin was observed in Dp71-antisense cells, specifically at the basal portion of cells that makes contacts with the ECM[123].

3) By immunoprecipitation experiments it was established that Dp71f associates with the adhesión proteins β1-integrin, α- actinin, talin, actin, FAK and GSK3- β (figure 4A). Paxillin and the vinculin were not detected in Dp71f inmunoprecipitates. Nevertheless, in the β1-immunoprecipitates paxillin was observed but not vinculin[123]. It is probable that the ionic strength used during the immunoprecipitation tests could have affected the interaction between the vinculin and the adhesion complex.

4) The deficiency of Dp71f in the antisense cells provokes a significant reduction in the levels of talin, FAK, actin, α-actinin and GSK3-β that are recruited by the β1-integrin complexes. Consequently, the levels of β1-integrin associated with FAK also diminish remarkably in the Dp71-antisense cells, suggesting that Dp71f modulates the recruitment of structural and signaling proteins. Interestingly, only full-length talin inmunoprecipitated with the β1-integrin subunit. A much greater amount of this full-size protein was obtained from wild type lysates in comparison with the amount obtained from the Dp71-antisense cells, which suggests that a larger amount of stable β1-integrin complexes were present in wild type PC12 cells. On the other hand, in our results a similar amount of paxillin was detected in the β1 immunoprecipitates obtained from the wild type strain as well as from the Dp71-antisense clone[123]. It is probable that the paxillin is recruited to the focal adhesions through their LIM domains, possibly through a direct association with the β1-integrin cytoplasmic domain. However, experimental evidences show the role of some kinases in regulating paxillin recruitment to focal adhesions throughout LIM domains [145]. Given the adhesion deficiency of antisense cells, it was expected that a smaller amount of paxillin could be associated to the β1-integrin subunit. We do not know why the integrin-paxillin interaction is not altered by the deficiency of the levels of Dp71f, or why when the cells detach from the substrate this interaction is not disrupted.

An alternative hypothesis to explain the deficient adhesion of the Dp71-antisense cells would be that the deficient formation of the adhesion complex was caused by a negative regulation in the expression of adhesion proteins in these cells. Nevertheless, by performing western blot analysis it was determined that these cells express similar protein levels of the adhesión complex members: β1-integrin, talin, vinculin, α-actinin, FAK y paxillin. In fact, an overexpression of integrin, paxillin and vinculin was observed in the deficient Dp71f clones maybe as a compensatory cell response to overcome the adhesion failure.

Because our results indicate a clear interaction of Dp71f with the β1-integrin adhesion complex, an interesting question arises: How does Dp71f interact with this group of proteins? Dp71f consists of a N-terminal actin binding domain and a carboxyl-terminal domain that can be subdivided into two termed WW and ZZ; these domains along with the EF-hand region form the rich cysteine region. The WW domain is a protein-protein interacting module that binds to proline-rich sequences [146], whereas the ZZ region is a Zinc finger domain also involved in mediating protein-protein interactions [147]. Taking into account that FAK contains a proline-rich domain near its carboxyl-terminal region that recruits proteins containing SH3 domains [139], it is probable that through this region this protein interacts directly with Dp71f WW domain. Although the results of in vitro pull down assays [123] and immunofluorescence experiments (Figure 6) reinforce this hypothesis, it is important to consider that the Dp71f WW domain is truncated. However this domain appears to be functional since the association between Dp71f and β-dystroglycan was demonstrated. This interaccion occurs through the binding of the Dp71f WW domain with the β-dystroglycan proline-rich domain. Thus a competition between FAK and β-dystroglycan for binding Dp71f WW domain apparently takes place since both proteins do not interact with Dp71f at the same time.

With regards to the possible binding between Dp71f and talin, it is known that talin contains a 47 kDa N-terminal domain and a carboxyl 190-kDa rod domain[148]. Nevertheless, there are not reports that show that these domains could interact with those present in Dp71f. It is possible that in the PC12 cell point contacts, an indirect interaction between talin and Dp71f occurs through FAK and actin since talin and Dp71f contain actin binding domains and talin interacts directly with FAK. On the other hand, it has been demonstrated that FAK can interact with paxillin. In this way Dp71f could be associated with this protein in the complex also in an indirect manner.

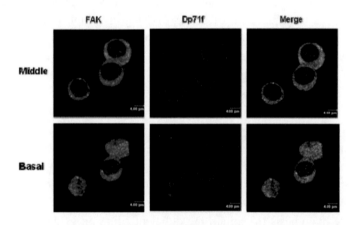

Figure 6. Subcellular distribution of Dp71f and FAK in the wild type and antisense-Dp71 PC12 cells. Cells, plated for 15 h on laminin-coated glass coverslips, were double stained with the anti-distrophin antibody 5F3 (red channel) and with anti-FAK antibody (green channel). Images were analyzed by confocal laser microscopy. Focus was adjusted to the middle or basal portion of cells, as indicated. Merge staining of Dp71f with FAK is shown in yellow (right-hand panels).

Integrin cytoplasmic domains are required for the formation of focal adhesions and cytoskeleton structures. Several studies have mapped functionally important sequences of β1-integrin cytoplasmic domains, which bind specific cytoskeleton molecules, such as α-actinin, paxillin, talin and FAK [139]. A priori, it is difficult to predict if some of the β1-integrin cytoplasmic domains could interact with Dp71f isoform. The immunofluorescence and in vitro interaction results suggest a direct interaction between both proteins. However, since α-actinin can interact with β1-integrin and dystrophin [135,139], it is possible that this protein can serve as a bridge for the interaction between both proteins.

Something that resulted in an interesting finding was the presence of GSK3-β in the Dp71f immunoprecipitates. Co-purification of both proteins was specific since in the Dp71-antisense cells, the amount of GSK3-β that precipitates with the anti-Dp71f antibody was minor compared to that obtained from wild type cells. On the other hand, the amount of GSK3-β recruited by β1-integrin was smaller in the Dp71-antisense cells compared to wild-type cells showing the importance of Dp71f as a β1-integrin adhesion complex scaffolding protein for the recruitment of GSK3-β. It has been determined that the carboxyl-terminal domain of dystrophin Dp427, which is present in Dp71f is a phosphorylated GSK3-β substrate [149] and for its part GSK3-β is an ILK substrate (a component of the β1-integrin complex) [139]. ILK is a 59 kDa serine/threonine kinase, which interacts with the cytoplasmic domains of β1 and β3 integrin subunits [150]. ILK has been shown to be an important effector of both integrin and growth factor receptor signaling, in a PI3K activity dependent manner [127,129]. When ILK is overexpressed in cultured epithelial cells, induces the phosporylation and inhibition of GSK3-β, a negative regulator of the Wnt signaling pathway [127]. The inhibition of GSK3-β by ILK results in the activation of the AP-1 and β-catenin/LEF-1 transcription factors, and the subsequent expression of mesenchymally related genes [127-129]. This signaling performs important functions during the embryonic development: in the determination of the cellular types, the development of the nervous system, the skeleton, lungs, hair, teeth, gonads and extremities. Our research showed for the first time the recruitment of GSK3-β to the β1-integrin adhesion complex and the importance of Dp71f in mediating this interaction [151]. The C-terminal region of dystrophin is a substrate for phosphorylation by casein kinase-2. Phosphorylation of the C-terminal domain of Dp427 (which is present in Dp71f) by casein kinase-2 creates the consensus site required for phosphorylation by GSK3-β. This kind of cooperation between protein kinases has been described as hierarchal phosphorylation, the classic example of which occurs in muscle glycogen synthase [152]. Changes in the phosphorylation status of Dp71f in serine and threonine residues are not observed when PC12 cells are seeded onto ECM laminin which agree with hypothesis that GSK3-β is recruited to the β1-integrin complex to be inactivated by ILK.

The interaction between GSK3-β and Dp71f was also demonstrated by in vitro pulldown assays [151]. These experiments were performed using a GST-Dp71f fusion protein produced in bacteria where phosphorylation of heterologous proteins does not take place. It could be inferred that Dp71f does not need the concensus phosphorylation created by casein kinase-2 required to interact with GSK3-β as described for Dp427 [152]. However, pulldown assays are performed by using total cell lysates with protease inhibitors but with conditions that could allow that enzymes of another class could function [153]. To define the role of Dp71f as a scaffolding protein for GSK3-β recruitment an in vitro translation system assay will be required to establish if a direct interaction between Dp71f and GSK3-β takes place without consensus phosphorylation requirements. In general these results suggest that Dp71f has an important structural role in the recruitment of GSK3-β to the integrin adhesion complex probably to allow the phosphorylation of GSK3-β by ILK and in this way modulate the β1-integrin receptor signaling.

Proteólisis of vinculin and talin disrupt the connection of stress fibers to the plasmatic membrane [154]. This idea is supported from data obtained from platelet activation and thrombin-induced platelet aggregation where a Ca^{2+}-dependent proteolysis of talin and filamin leads to an actin cytoskeleton reorganization [155]. Calpain-mediated proteolysis is a rate-limiting step in the disassembly of focal adhesions. The disassembly of several components of the focal adhesion including paxillin, vinculin and zyxin also depends on calpain-mediated talin cleavage [156]. Vinculin is also a calpain substrate which can be hydrolyzed in fragments of 98, 85 and 26 kDa [157]. Immunohistochemistry studies show that the calpain locates in the plates of focal adhesions [154] suggesting that vinculin fragmentation promotes stress fibers and focal adhesions disassemble. Some results with vinculin-deficient cells indicate that the intact molecule is important for a normal adhesion [158]. Other evidence reveals the importance of vinculin in the formation of lamelipodias, for the efficient promotion of cellular expansion, stress fiber assembly as well as for stabilization of focal adhesions through transferring mechanical stresses that drive cytoskeletal remodeling [159]. According to Arregui CO *et al* 1994 [141], PC12 cells display point contacts and not the typical fibroblast focal adhesion which last days and that are more characteristic of static cells in comparison with the point contacts found in cells presenting a greater migration capacity. If PC12 cells are migranting cells that attach to ECM by forming point contacts, moving across a surface, laying down focal adhesions at the front of the cell and disassembling adhesions at the back, then we hoped that wild type PC12 cells showed a greater fragmention of talin and vinculin with respect to DP71-antisense cells since a large proportion of Dp71f-deficient cells was floating. Protein profile of talin did not show significant changes on proteolysis while vinculin did not display a consistent fragmentation pattern. However most of the experiments showed that there was a significant increase in proteolysis of vinculin in Dp71f-antisense cells compared to wild type PC12 cells [123]. It is possible that Dp71-antisense cells establish anomalous point contacts whose instability leads to a greater activity of calpain on vinculin.

With regards to the possible formation of a macrocomplex formed by the integrins and DAPC complexes in which Dp71f acts as a bridge in the neuronal line PC12, we observed that β-dystroglycan (a DAPC component) interacts with Dp71f but not with β-integrin and FAK (components of the β1-integrin complex)[123]. These results suggest that al least two subpopulations of Dp71f exist, one interacting with the adhesion complex and the other with β-dystroglycan (Figure 7).

Finally, Since there is considerable sequence homology between dystrophin and utrophin, both at the protein and DNA level and both are co-expressed in PC12 cells [119,121]. It is important to determine if utrophin associates with the adhesion complex and if this protein compensates Dp71f deficiency.

β1-integrin-mediated cell adhesion modulates the neuronal migration and the synaptogenesis during the development of the central nervous system [142]. Therefore, the participation of the Dp71f in the modulation of cell adhesión by the β1-integrin receptor constitutes an important advance toward identifying its function in neuronal cells, which could help to establish the molecular bases of mental retardation associated to 30% of the DMD patients.

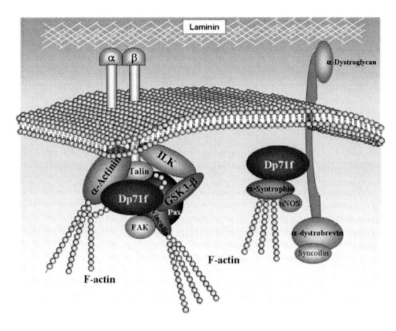

Figure 7. The Dp71f cellular fraction associated with the adhesion complex appears to be different from that interacting with β-dystroglycan or with the whole DAPC

References

[1] Duchenne G. Recherche sur la paralysie musculaire pseudo-hypertrophique ou paralysie myo-sclérosique. *Arch Gen Med.* 1868;142:1461-1471

[2] Pearce J. Some contributions of Duchenne de Boulogne (1806-75). *J Neurol Neurosurg Psychiatry.* 1999;67(3):322.

[3] Becker P, Kiener F. A new x-chromosomal muscular dystrophy. *Arch Psychiatr Nervenkr Z Gesamte Neurol Psychiatr.* 1955;193(4):427-448.

[4] Papadimitriou JM, Mastaglia FL, Kakulas BA. The natural history of Duchenne muscular dystrophy--an ultrastructural study. *Proc Aust Assoc Neurol.* 1969;6:87-92.

[5] Mastaglia FL, Papadimitriou JM, Kakulas BA. Regeneration in Duchenne muscular dystrophy. A histological electron-microscopic and histochemical study. *Proc Aust Assoc Neurol.* 1969;6:93-106.

[6] Davies KE, Speer A, Herrmann F, Spiegler AW, McGlade S, Hofker MH, Briand P, Hanke R, Schwartz M, Steinbicker V, et al. Human X chromosome markers and Duchenne muscular dystrophy. *Nucleic Acids Res.* May 24 1985;13(10):3419-3426.

[7] Bell CD, Conen PE. Change in fiber size in Duchenne muscular dystrophy. *Neurology.* Sep 1967;17(9):902-913.

[8] Bell CD, Conen PE. Histochemical fibre "types" in Duchenne muscular dystrophy. *J Neurol Sci.* Feb 1970;10(2):163-171.

[9] Bell CD, Conen PE. Histopathological changes in Duchenne muscular dystrophy. *J Neurol Sci.* Nov-Dec 1968;7(3):529-544.

[10] Emery AE. Muscle Histology in Carriers of Duchenne Muscular Dystrophy. *J Med Genet.* Mar 1965;42:1-7.

[11] Shepard TH, Gordon LH, Wollenweber JE. Lactic dehydrogenase isoenzymes in muscle from patients with Duchenne muscular dystrophy. *Nature.* Dec 11 1965;208(5015):1107-1108.

[12] Emery AE. Electrophoretic Pattern of Lactic Dehydrogenase in Carriers and Patients with Duchenne Muscular Dystrophy. *Nature.* Mar 7 1964;201:1044-1045.

[13] Thompson MW, Murphy EG, McAlpine PJ. An assessment of the creatine kinase test in the detection of carriers of Duchenne muscular dystrophy. *J Pediatr.* Jul 1967;71(1):82-93.

[14] Soltan HC, Blanchaer MC. Activity of serum aldolase and lactic dehydrogenase in patients affected with Duchenne muscular dystrophy and in their immediate relatives. *J Pediatr.* Jan 1959;54(1):27-33.

[15] Griffiths PD. Serum ATP: creatine phosphotransferase in skeleto-muscular disorders with special reference to duchenne muscular dystrophy. *Guys Hosp Rep.* 1965;114(4):401-420.

[16] Clark JI, Putte RH, Marczynski R, Mann JD. Evidence for the absence of detectable linkage between the genes for Duchenne muscular dystrophy and the Xg blood group. *Am J Hum Genet.* Sep 1963;15:292-297.

[17] Thomson WH. The biochemical identification of the carrier state in X-linked recessive (Duchenne) muscular dystrophy. *Clin Chim Acta.* Nov 1969;26(2):207-221.

[18] Ionasescu V, Zellweger H, Conway TW. Ribosomal protein synthesis in Duchenne muscular dystrophy. *Arch Biochem Biophys.* May 1971;144(1):51-58.

[19] Letter: Prednisone in Duchenne muscular dystrophy. *Lancet.* Feb 15 1975;1(7903):397-398.

[20] Wakayama Y. Electron microscopic study on the satellite cell in the muscle of Duchenne muscular dystrophy. *J Neuropathol Exp Neurol.* Sep-Oct 1976;35(5):532-540.

[21] Panayiotopoulos CP, Scarpalezos S, Papapetropoulos T. Electrophysiological estimation of motor units in Duchenne muscular dystrophy. *J Neurol Sci.* Sep 1974;23(1):89-98.

[22] Howells KF. Structural changes of erythrocyte membranes in muscllar dystrophy. *Res Exp Med (Berl).* Oct 29 1976;168(3):213-217.

[23] Vickers JD, McComas AJ, Rathbone MP. Alterations of membrane phosphorylation in erythrocyte membranes from patients with Duchenne muscular dystrophy. *The Canadian journal of neurological sciences.* Nov 1978;5(4):437-442.

[24] Robinow M. Mental retardation in Duchenne muscular dystrophy: its relation to the maternal carrier state. *J Pediatr.* May 1976;88(5):896-897.

[25] Rowland LP. Biochemistry of muscle membranes in Duchenne muscular dystrophy. *Muscle Nerve.* Jan-Feb 1980;3(1):3-20.

[26] Lindenbaum RH, Clarke G, Patel C, Moncrieff M, Hughes JT. Muscular dystrophy in an X; 1 translocation female suggests that Duchenne locus is on X chromosome short arm. *J Med Genet.* Oct 1979;16(5):389-392.

[27] Moser H. Duchenne muscular dystrophy: pathogenetic aspects and genetic prevention. *Hum Genet.* 1984;66(1):17-40.

[28] Pembrey ME, Davies KE, Winter RM, Elles RG, Williamson R, Fazzone TA, Walker C. Clinical use of DNA markers linked to the gene for Duchenne muscular dystrophy. *Arch Dis Child.* Mar 1984;59(3):208-216.

[29] Ray PN, Belfall B, Duff C, Logan C, Kean V, Thompson MW, Sylvester JE, Gorski JL, Schmickel RD, Worton RG. Cloning of the breakpoint of an X;21 translocation associated with Duchenne muscular dystrophy. *Nature.* Dec 19-1986 Jan 1 1985;318(6047):672-675.

[30] Hoffman EP, Monaco AP, Feener CC, Kunkel LM. Conservation of the Duchenne muscular dystrophy gene in mice and humans. *Science.* Oct 16 1987;238(4825):347-350.

[31] Kunkel LM, Monaco AP, Hoffman E, Koenig M, Feener C, Bertelson C. Molecular studies of progressive muscular dystrophy (Duchenne). *Enzyme.* 1987;38(1-4):72-75.

[32] Koenig M, Hoffman EP, Bertelson CJ, Monaco AP, Feener C, Kunkel LM. Complete cloning of the Duchenne muscular dystrophy (DMD) cDNA and preliminary genomic organization of the DMD gene in normal and affected individuals. *Cell.* Jul 31 1987;50(3):509-517.

[33] Hoffman EP, Brown RH, Jr., Kunkel LM. Dystrophin: the protein product of the Duchenne muscular dystrophy locus. *Cell.* Dec 24 1987;51(6):919-928.

[34] Koenig M, Monaco AP, Kunkel LM. The complete sequence of dystrophin predicts a rod-shaped cytoskeletal protein. *Cell.* Apr 22 1988;53(2):219-228.

[35] Malhotra SB, Hart KA, Klamut HJ, Thomas NS, Bodrug SE, Burghes AH, Bobrow M, Harper PS, Thompson MW, Ray PN, et al. Frame-shift deletions in patients with Duchenne and Becker muscular dystrophy. *Science.* Nov 4 1988;242(4879):755-759.

[36] Kenwrick SJ, Smith TJ, England S, Collins F, Davies KE. Localisation of the endpoints of deletions in the 5' region of the Duchenne gene using a sequence isolated by chromosome jumping. *Nucleic Acids Res.* Feb 25 1988;16(4):1305-1317.

[37] Forrest SM, Cross GS, Flint T, Speer A, Robson KJ, Davies KE. Further studies of gene deletions that cause Duchenne and Becker muscular dystrophies. *Genomics.* Feb 1988;2(2):109-114.

[38] Chamberlain JS, Gibbs RA, Ranier JE, Nguyen PN, Caskey CT. Deletion screening of the Duchenne muscular dystrophy locus via multiplex DNA amplification. *Nucleic Acids Res.* Dec 9 1988;16(23):11141-11156.

[39] Chamberlain JS, Farwell NJ, Chamberlain JR, Cox GA, Caskey CT. PCR analysis of dystrophin gene mutation and expression. *J Cell Biochem.* Jul 1991;46(3):255-259.

[40] Ervasti JM, Ohlendieck K, Kahl SD, Gaver MG, Campbell KP. Deficiency of a glycoprotein component of the dystrophin complex in dystrophic muscle. *Nature.* May 24 1990;345(6273):315-319.

[41] Ohlendieck K, Ervasti JM, Snook JB, Campbell KP. Dystrophin-glycoprotein complex is highly enriched in isolated skeletal muscle sarcolemma. *J Cell Biol.* Jan 1991;112(1):135-148.

[42] Crosbie RH, Heighway J, Venzke DP, Lee JC, Campbell KP. Sarcospan, the 25-kDa transmembrane component of the dystrophin-glycoprotein complex. *J Biol Chem*. Dec 12 1997;272(50):31221-31224.

[43] Ervasti JM, Campbell KP. Membrane organization of the dystrophin-glycoprotein complex. *Cell*. Sep 20 1991;66(6):1121-1131.

[44] Ohlendieck K, Campbell KP. Dystrophin-associated proteins are greatly reduced in skeletal muscle from mdx mice. *J Cell Biol*. Dec 1991;115(6):1685-1694.

[45] Ibraghimov-Beskrovnaya O, Ervasti JM, Leveille CJ, Slaughter CA, Sernett SW, Campbell KP. Primary structure of dystrophin-associated glycoproteins linking dystrophin to the extracellular matrix. *Nature*. Feb 20 1992;355(6362):696-702.

[46] Matsumura K, Tome FM, Collin H, Azibi K, Chaouch M, Kaplan JC, Fardeau M, Campbell KP. Deficiency of the 50K dystrophin-associated glycoprotein in severe childhood autosomal recessive muscular dystrophy. *Nature*. Sep 24 1992;359(6393):320-322.

[47] Fardeau M, Matsumura K, Tome FM, Collin H, Leturcq F, Kaplan JC, Campbell KP. Deficiency of the 50 kDa dystrophin associated glycoprotein (adhalin) in severe autosomal recessive muscular dystrophies in children native from European countries. *C R Acad Sci III*. Aug 1993;316(8):799-804.

[48] Noguchi S, McNally EM, Ben Othmane K, Hagiwara Y, Mizuno Y, Yoshida M, Yamamoto H, Bonnemann CG, Gussoni E, Denton PH, Kyriakides T, Middleton L, Hentati F, Ben Hamida M, Nonaka I, Vance JM, Kunkel LM, Ozawa E. Mutations in the dystrophin-associated protein gamma-sarcoglycan in chromosome 13 muscular dystrophy. *Science*. Nov 3 1995;270(5237):819-822.

[49] Suzuki A, Yoshida M, Hayashi K, Mizuno Y, Hagiwara Y, Ozawa E. Molecular organization at the glycoprotein-complex-binding site of dystrophin. Three dystrophin-associated proteins bind directly to the carboxy-terminal portion of dystrophin. *Eur J Biochem*. Mar 1 1994;220(2):283-292.

[50] Brenman JE, Chao DS, Gee SH, McGee AW, Craven SE, Santillano DR, Wu Z, Huang F, Xia H, Peters MF, Froehner SC, Bredt DS. Interaction of nitric oxide synthase with the postsynaptic density protein PSD-95 and alpha1-syntrophin mediated by PDZ domains. *Cell*. Mar 8 1996;84(5):757-767.

[51] Iwata Y, Pan Y, Yoshida T, Hanada H, Shigekawa M. Alpha1-syntrophin has distinct binding sites for actin and calmodulin. *FEBS Lett*. Feb 20 1998;423(2):173-177.

[52] Yoshida M, Noguchi S, Wakabayashi E, Piluso G, Belsito A, Nigro V, Ozawa E. The fourth component of the sarcoglycan complex. *FEBS Lett*. Feb 17 1997;403(2):143-148.

[53] Estrada FJ, Mornet D, Rosas-Vargas H, Angulo A, Hernandez M, Becker V, Rendon A, Ramos-Kuri M, Coral-Vazquez RM. A novel isoform of delta-sarcoglycan is localized at the sarcoplasmic reticulum of mouse skeletal muscle. *Biochemical and biophysical research communications*. Feb 17 2006;340(3):865-871.

[54] McNally EM, de Sa Moreira E, Duggan DJ, Bonnemann CG, Lisanti MP, Lidov HG, Vainzof M, Passos-Bueno MR, Hoffman EP, Zatz M, Kunkel LM. Caveolin-3 in muscular dystrophy. *Hum Mol Genet*. May 1998;7(5):871-877.

[55] Poon E, Howman EV, Newey SE, Davies KE. Association of syncoilin and desmin: linking intermediate filament proteins to the dystrophin-associated protein complex. *J Biol Chem.* Feb 1 2002;277(5):3433-3439.

[56] Bhosle RC, Michele DE, Campbell KP, Li Z, Robson RM. Interactions of intermediate filament protein synemin with dystrophin and utrophin. *Biochemical and biophysical research communications.* Aug 4 2006;346(3):768-777.

[57] Godsel LM, Hobbs RP, Green KJ. Intermediate filament assembly: dynamics to disease. *Trends in cell biology.* Jan 2008;18(1):28-37.

[58] Holder E, Maeda M, Bies RD. Expression and regulation of the dystrophin Purkinje promoter in human skeletal muscle, heart, and brain. *Human genetics.* Feb 1996;97(2):232-239.

[59] Klamut HJ, Gangopadhyay SB, Worton RG, Ray PN. Molecular and functional analysis of the muscle-specific promoter region of the Duchenne muscular dystrophy gene. *Mol Cell Biol.* Jan 1990;10(1):193-205.

[60] Barnea E, Zuk D, Simantov R, Nudel U, Yaffe D. Specificity of expression of the muscle and brain dystrophin gene promoters in muscle and brain cells. *Neuron.* Dec 1990;5(6):881-888.

[61] Boyce FM, Beggs AH, Feener C, Kunkel LM. Dystrophin is transcribed in brain from a distant upstream promoter. *Proc Natl Acad Sci U S A.* Feb 15 1991;88(4):1276-1280.

[62] D'Souza VN, Nguyen TM, Morris GE, Karges W, Pillers DA, Ray PN. A novel dystrophin isoform is required for normal retinal electrophysiology. *Hum Mol Genet.* May 1995;4(5):837-842.

[63] Rodius F, Claudepierre T, Rosas-Vargas H, Cisneros B, Montanez C, Dreyfus H, Mornet D, Rendon A. Dystrophins in developing retina: Dp260 expression correlates with synaptic maturation. *Neuroreport.* Jul 7 1997;8(9-10):2383-2387.

[64] Kameya S, Araki E, Katsuki M, Mizota A, Adachi E, Nakahara K, Nonaka I, Sakuragi S, Takeda S, Nabeshima Y. Dp260 disrupted mice revealed prolonged implicit time of the b-wave in ERG and loss of accumulation of beta-dystroglycan in the outer plexiform layer of the retina. *Hum Mol Genet.* Dec 1997;6(13):2195-2203.

[65] Warner LE, DelloRusso C, Crawford RW, Rybakova IN, Patel JR, Ervasti JM, Chamberlain JS. Expression of Dp260 in muscle tethers the actin cytoskeleton to the dystrophin-glycoprotein complex and partially prevents dystrophy. *Hum Mol Genet.* May 1 2002;11(9):1095-1105.

[66] Lidov HG, Kunkel LM. Dystrophin and Dp140 in the adult rodent kidney. *Lab Invest.* Dec 1998;78(12):1543-1551.

[67] Durbeej M, Jung D, Hjalt T, Campbell KP, Ekblom P. Transient expression of Dp140, a product of the Duchenne muscular dystrophy locus, during kidney tubulogenesis. *Dev Biol.* Jan 15 1997;181(2):156-167.

[68] Lidov HG, Selig S, Kunkel LM. Dp140: a novel 140 kDa CNS transcript from the dystrophin locus. *Hum Mol Genet.* Mar 1995;4(3):329-335.

[69] Lidov HG, Kunkel LM. Dp140: alternatively spliced isoforms in brain and kidney. *Genomics.* Oct 1 1997;45(1):132-139.

[70] Bardoni A, Felisari G, Sironi M, Comi G, Lai M, Robotti M, Bresolin N. Loss of Dp140 regulatory sequences is associated with cognitive impairment in dystrophinopathies. *Neuromuscul Disord.* Mar 2000;10(3):194-199.

[71] Felisari G, Martinelli Boneschi F, Bardoni A, Sironi M, Comi GP, Robotti M, Turconi AC, Lai M, Corrao G, Bresolin N. Loss of Dp140 dystrophin isoform and intellectual impairment in Duchenne dystrophy. *Neurology.* Aug 22 2000;55(4):559-564.

[72] Byers TJ, Lidov HG, Kunkel LM. An alternative dystrophin transcript specific to peripheral nerve. *Nat Genet.* May 1993;4(1):77-81.

[73] Labarque V, Freson K, Thys C, Wittevrongel C, Hoylaerts MF, De Vos R, Goemans N, Van Geet C. Increased Gs signalling in platelets and impaired collagen activation, due to a defect in the dystrophin gene, result in increased blood loss during spinal surgery. *Hum Mol Genet.* Feb 1 2008;17(3):357-366.

[74] Schofield JN, Blake DJ, Simmons C, Morris GE, Tinsley JM, Davies KE, Edwards YH. Apo-dystrophin-1 and apo-dystrophin-2, products of the Duchenne muscular dystrophy locus: expression during mouse embryogenesis and in cultured cell lines. *Hum Mol Genet.* Aug 1994;3(8):1309-1316.

[75] Saito F, Masaki T, Kamakura K, Anderson LV, Fujita S, Fukuta-Ohi H, Sunada Y, Shimizu T, Matsumura K. Characterization of the transmembrane molecular architecture of the dystroglycan complex in schwann cells. *J Biol Chem.* Mar 19 1999;274(12):8240-8246.

[76] Kumagai T, Miura K, Ohki T, Matsumoto A, Miyazaki S, Nakamura M, Ochi N, Takahashi O. [Central nervous system involvements in Duchenne/Becker muscular dystrophy]. *No to hattatsu.* Nov 2001;33(6):480-486.

[77] Judge LM, Haraguchiln M, Chamberlain JS. Dissecting the signaling and mechanical functions of the dystrophin-glycoprotein complex. *J Cell Sci.* Apr 15 2006;119(Pt 8):1537-1546.

[78] Imamura M, Araishi K, Noguchi S, Ozawa E. A sarcoglycan-dystroglycan complex anchors Dp116 and utrophin in the peripheral nervous system. *Hum Mol Genet.* Dec 12 2000;9(20):3091-3100.

[79] Cai H, Erdman RA, Zweier L, Chen J, Shaw JHt, Baylor KA, Stecker MM, Carey DJ, Chan YM. The sarcoglycan complex in Schwann cells and its role in myelin stability. *Exp Neurol.* May 2007;205(1):257-269.

[80] Albrecht DE, Sherman DL, Brophy PJ, Froehner SC. The ABCA1 cholesterol transporter associates with one of two distinct dystrophin-based scaffolds in Schwann cells. *Glia.* Apr 15 2008;56(6):611-618.

[81] Yamada H, Chiba A, Endo T, Kobata A, Anderson LV, Hori H, Fukuta-Ohi H, Kanazawa I, Campbell KP, Shimizu T, Matsumura K. Characterization of dp6troglycan-laminin interaction in peripheral nerve. *J Neurochem.* Apr 1996;66(4):1518-1524.

[82] Rapaport D, Greenberg DS, Tal M, Yaffe D, Nudel U. Dp71, the nonmuscle product of the Duchenne muscular dystrophy gene is associated with the cell membrane. *FEBS Lett.* Aug 9 1993;328(1-2):197-202.

[83] Howard PL, Klamut HJ, Ray PN. Identification of a novel actin binding site within the Dp71 dystrophin isoform. *FEBS Lett.* Dec 18 1998;441(2):337-341.

[84] Rapaport D, Fuchs O, Nudel U, Yaffe D. Expression of the Duchenne muscular dystrophy gene products in embryonic stem cells and their differentiated derivatives. *J Biol Chem.* Oct 25 1992;267(30):21289-21292.

[85] de Leon MB, Montanez C, Gomez P, Morales-Lazaro SL, Tapia-Ramirez V, Valadez-Graham V, Recillas-Targa F, Yaffe D, Nudel U, Cisneros B. Dystrophin Dp71 expression is down-regulated during myogenesis: role of Sp1 and Sp3 on the Dp71 promoter activity. *J Biol Chem.* Feb 18 2005;280(7):5290-5299.

[86] Jung D, Filliol D, Metz-Boutigue MH, Rendon A. Characterization and subcellular localization of the dystrophin-protein 71 (Dp71) from brain. *Neuromuscul Disord.* Sep-Nov 1993;3(5-6):515-518.

[87] Gorecki DC, Barnard EA. Specific expression of G-dystrophin (Dp71) in the brain. *Neuroreport.* Apr 19 1995;6(6):893-896.

[88] Claudepierre T, Mornet D, Pannicke T, Forster V, Dalloz C, Bolanos F, Sahel J, Reichenbach A, Rendon A. Expression of Dp71 in Muller glial cells: a comparison with utrophin- and dystrophin-associated proteins. *Invest Ophthalmol Vis Sci.* Jan 2000;41(1):294-304.

[89] Howard PL, Dally GY, Wong MH, Ho A, Weleber RG, Pillers DA, Ray PN. Localization of dystrophin isoform Dp71 to the inner limiting membrane of the retina suggests a unique functional contribution of Dp71 in the retina. *Hum Mol Genet.* Sep 1998;7(9):1385-1391.

[90] Fuentes-Mera L, Rodriguez-Munoz R, Gonzalez-Ramirez R, Garcia-Sierra F, Gonzalez E, Mornet D, Cisneros B. Characterization of a novel Dp71 dystrophin-associated protein complex (DAPC) present in the nucleus of HeLa cells: members of the nuclear DAPC associate with the nuclear matrix. *Exp Cell Res.* Oct 1 2006;312(16):3023-3035.

[91] Hernandez-Gonzalez EO, Mornet D, Rendon A, Martinez-Rojas D. Absence of Dp71 in mdx3cv mouse spermatozoa alters flagellar morphology and the distribution of ion channels and nNOS. *J Cell Sci.* Jan 1 2005;118(Pt 1):137-145.

[92] Lederfein D, Yaffe D, Nudel U. A housekeeping type promoter, located in the 3' region of the Duchenne muscular dystrophy gene, controls the expression of Dp71, a major product of the gene. *Hum Mol Genet.* Nov 1993;2(11):1883-1888.

[93] Greenberg DS, Schatz Y, Levy Z, Pizzo P, Yaffe D, Nudel U. Reduced levels of dystrophin associated proteins in the brains of mice deficient for Dp71. *Hum Mol Genet.* Sep 1996;5(9):1299-1303.

[94] Cox GA, Sunada Y, Campbell KP, Chamberlain JS. Dp71 can restore the dystrophin-associated glycoprotein complex in muscle but fails to prevent dystrophy. *Nature genetics.* Dec 1994;8(4):333-339.

[95] Greenberg DS, Sunada Y, Campbell KP, Yaffe D, Nudel U. Exogenous Dp71 restores the levels of dystrophin associated proteins but does not alleviate muscle damage in mdx mice. *Nat Genet.* Dec 1994;8(4):340-344.

[96] Leibovitz S, Meshorer A, Fridman Y, Wieneke S, Jockusch H, Yaffe D, Nudel U. Exogenous Dp71 is a dominant negative competitor of dystrophin in skeletal muscle. *Neuromuscul Disord.* Nov 2002;12(9):836-844.

[97] Blake DJ, Nawrotzki R, Loh NY, Gorecki DC, Davies KE. beta-dystrobrevin, a member of the dystrophin-related protein family. *Proc Natl Acad Sci U S A.* Jan 6 1998;95(1):241-246.

[98] Claudepierre T, Dalloz C, Mornet D, Matsumura K, Sahel J, Rendon A. Characterization of the intermolecular associations of the dystrophin-associated glycoprotein complex in retinal Muller glial cells. *J Cell Sci.* Oct 2000;113 Pt 19:3409-3417.

[99] Haenggi T, Schaub MC, Fritschy JM. Molecular heterogeneity of the dystrophin-associated protein complex in the mouse kidney nephron: differential alterations in the absence of utrophin and dystrophin. *Cell Tissue Res.* Feb 2005;319(2):299-313.

[100] Haenggi T, Soontornmalai A, Schaub MC, Fritschy JM. The role of utrophin and Dp71 for assembly of different dystrophin-associated protein complexes (DPCs) in the choroid plexus and microvasculature of the brain. *Neuroscience.* 2004;129(2):403-413.

[101] Ilarraza-Lomeli R, Cisneros-Vega B, Cervantes-Gomez Mde L, Mornet D, Montanez C. Dp71, utrophin and beta-dystroglycan expression and distribution in PC12/L6 cell cocultures. *Neuroreport.* Oct 29 2007;18(16):1657-1661.

[102] Romo-Yanez J, Ceja V, Ilarraza-Lomeli R, Coral-Vazquez R, Velazquez F, Mornet D, Rendon A, Montanez C. Dp71ab/DAPs complex composition changes during the differentiation process in PC12 cells. *J Cell Biochem.* Sep 1 2007;102(1):82-97.

[103] Royuela M, Chazalette D, Hugon G, Paniagua R, Guerlavais V, Fehrentz JA, Martinez J, Labbe JP, Rivier F, Mornet D. Formation of multiple complexes between beta-dystroglycan and dystrophin family products. *J Muscle Res Cell Motil.* 2003;24(7):387-397.

[104] Fort PE, Sene A, Pannicke T, Roux MJ, Forster V, Mornet D, Nudel U, Yaffe D, Reichenbach A, Sahel JA, Rendon A. Kir4.1 and AQP4 associate with Dp71- and utrophin-DAPs complexes in specific and defined microdomains of Muller retinal glial cell membrane. *Glia.* Apr 15 2008;56(6):597-610.

[105] Austin RC, Howard PL, D'Souza VN, Klamut HJ, Ray PN. Cloning and characterization of alternatively spliced isoforms of Dp71. *Hum Mol Genet.* Sep 1995;4(9):1475-1483.

[106] Garcia-Tovar CG, Perez A, Luna J, Mena R, Osorio B, Aleman V, Mondragon R, Mornet D, Rendon A, Hernandez JM. Biochemical and histochemical analysis of 71 kDa dystrophin isoform (Dp71f) in rat brain. *Acta Histochem.* Apr 2001;103(2):209-224.

[107] Gonzalez E, Montanez C, Ray PN, Howard PL, Garcia-Sierra F, Mornet D, Cisneros B. Alternative splicing regulates the nuclear or cytoplasmic localization of dystrophin Dp71. *FEBS Lett.* Oct 6 2000;482(3):209-214.

[108] Morris GE, Simmons C, Nguyen TM. Apo-dystrophins (Dp140 and Dp71) and dystrophin splicing isoforms in developing brain. *Biochemical and biophysical research communications.* Oct 4 1995;215(1):361-367.

[109] Ceccarini M, Rizzo G, Rosa G, Chelucci C, Macioce P, Petrucci TC. A splice variant of Dp71 lacking the syntrophin binding site is expressed in early stages of human neural development. *Brain Res Dev Brain Res.* Oct 20 1997;103(1):77-82.

[110] Austin RC, Morris GE, Howard PL, Klamut HJ, Ray PN. Expression and synthesis of alternatively spliced variants of Dp71 in adult human brain. *Neuromuscul Disord.* Mar 2000;10(3):187-193.

[111] Mitani K, Clemens PR, Moseley AB, Caskey CT. Gene transfer therapy for heritable disease: cell and expression targeting. *Philos Trans R Soc Lond B Biol Sci.* Feb 27 1993;339(1288):217-224.

[112] Inui K, Okada S, Dickson G. Gene therapy in Duchenne muscular dystrophy. *Brain Dev.* Sep-Oct 1996;18(5):357-361.

[113] Reay DP, Bilbao R, Koppanati BM, Cai L, O'Day TL, Jiang Z, Zheng H, Watchko JF, Clemens PR. Full-length dystrophin gene transfer to the mdx mouse in utero. *Gene Ther.* Apr 2008;15(7):531-536.

[114] Karpati G, Gilbert R, Petrof BJ, Nalbantoglu J. Gene therapy research for Duchenne and Becker muscular dystrophies. *Curr Opin Neurol.* Oct 1997;10(5):430-435.

[115] Muntoni F, Wells D. Genetic treatments in muscular dystrophies. *Curr Opin Neurol.* Oct 2007;20(5):590-594.

[116] Moizard MP, Toutain A, Fournier D, Berret F, Raynaud M, Billard C, Andres C, Moraine C. Severe cognitive impairment in DMD: obvious clinical indication for Dp71 isoform point mutation screening. *Eur J Hum Genet.* Jul 2000;8(7):552-556.

[117] Bar S, Barnea E, Levy Z, Neuman S, Yaffe D, Nudel U. A novel product of the Duchenne muscular dystrophy gene which greatly differs from the known isoforms in its structure and tissue distribution. *Biochem J.* Dec 1 1990;272(2):557-560.

[118] Moizard MP, Billard C, Toutain A, Berret F, Marmin N, Moraine C. Are Dp71 and Dp140 brain dystrophin isoforms related to cognitive impairment in Duchenne muscular dystrophy? *Am J Med Genet.* Oct 30 1998;80(1):32-41.

[119] Acosta R, Montanez C, Fuentes-Mera L, Gonzalez E, Gomez P, Quintero-Mora L, Mornet D, Alvarez-Salas LM, Cisneros B. Dystrophin Dp71 is required for neurite outgrowth in PC12 cells. *Exp Cell Res.* Jun 10 2004;296(2):265-275.

[120] Cisneros B, Rendon A, Genty V, Aranda G, Marquez F, Mornet D, Montanez C. Expression of dystrophin Dp71 during PC12 cell differentiation. *Neurosci Lett.* Aug 2 1996;213(2):107-110.

[121] Marquez FG, Cisneros B, Garcia F, Ceja V, Velazquez F, Depardon F, Cervantes L, Rendon A, Mornet D, Rosas-vargas H, Mustre M, Montanez C. Differential expression and subcellular distribution of dystrophin Dp71 isoforms during differentiation process. *Neuroscience.* 2003;118(4):957-966.

[122] Greene LA, Tischler AS. Establishment of a noradrenergic clonal line of rat adrenal pheochromocytoma cells which respond to nerve growth factor. *Proc Natl Acad Sci U S A.* Jul 1976;73(7):2424-2428.

[123] Cerna J, Cerecedo D, Ortega A, Garcia-Sierra F, Centeno F, Garrido E, Mornet D, Cisneros B. Dystrophin Dp71f associates with the beta1-integrin adhesion complex to modulate PC12 cell adhesion. *J Mol Biol.* Oct 6 2006;362(5):954-965.

[124] Enriquez-Aragon JA, Cerna-Cortes J, Bermudez de Leon M, Garcia-Sierra F, Gonzalez E, Mornet D, Cisneros B. Dystrophin Dp71 in PC12 cell adhesion. *Neuroreport.* Feb 28 2005;16(3):235-238.

[125] Graus-Porta D, Blaess S, Senften M, Littlewood-Evans A, Damsky C, Huang Z, Orban P, Klein R, Schittny JC, Muller U. Beta1-class integrins regulate the development of laminae and folia in the cerebral and cerebellar cortex. *Neuron*. Aug 16 2001;31(3):367-379.

[126] Carri NG, Rubin K, Gullberg D, Ebendal T. Neuritogenesis on collagen substrates. Involvement of integrin-like matrix receptors in retinal fibre outgrowth on collagen. *Int J Dev Neurosci*. Oct 1992;10(5):393-405.

[127] Delcommenne M, Tan C, Gray V, Rue L, Woodgett J, Dedhar S. Phosphoinositide-3-OH kinase-dependent regulation of glycogen synthase kinase 3 and protein kinase B/AKT by the integrin-linked kinase. *Proc Natl Acad Sci U S A*. Sep 15 1998;95(19):11211-11216.

[128] Novak A, Hsu SC, Leung-Hagesteijn C, Radeva G, Papkoff J, Montesano R, Roskelley C, Grosschedl R, Dedhar S. Cell adhesion and the integrin-linked kinase regulate the LEF-1 and beta-catenin signaling pathways. *Proc Natl Acad Sci U S A*. Apr 14 1998;95(8):4374-4379.

[129] Troussard AA, Tan C, Yoganathan TN, Dedhar S. Cell-extracellular matrix interactions stimulate the AP-1 transcription factor in an integrin-linked kinase- and glycogen synthase kinase 3-dependent manner. *Mol Cell Biol*. Nov 1999;19(11):7420-7427.

[130] Calderilla-Barbosa L, Ortega A, Cisneros B. Phosphorylation of dystrophin Dp71d by Ca2+/calmodulin-dependent protein kinase II modulates the Dp71d nuclear localization in PC12 cells. *Journal of neurochemistry*. Aug 2006;98(3):713-722.

[131] Hynes RO. Integrins: versatility, modulation, and signaling in cell adhesion. *Cell*. Apr 3 1992;69(1):11-25.

[132] Jones LS. Integrins: possible functions in the adult CNS. *Trends Neurosci*. Feb 1996;19(2):68-72.

[133] Pinkstaff JK, Detterich J, Lynch G, Gall C. Integrin subunit gene expression is regionally differentiated in adult brain. *J Neurosci*. Mar 1 1999;19(5):1541-1556.

[134] Tomaselli KJ, Hall DE, Flier LA, Gehlsen KR, Turner DC, Carbonetto S, Reichardt LF. A neuronal cell line (PC12) expresses two beta 1-class integrins-alpha 1 beta 1 and alpha 3 beta 1-that recognize different neurite outgrowth-promoting domains in laminin. *Neuron*. Nov 1990;5(5):651-662.

[135] Hance JE, Fu SY, Watkins SC, Beggs AH, Michalak M. alpha-actinin-2 is a new component of the dystrophin-glycoprotein complex. *Arch Biochem Biophys*. May 15 1999;365(2):216-222.

[136] Abercrombie M, Dunn GA. Adhesions of fibroblasts to substratum during contact inhibition observed by interference reflection microscopy. *Exp Cell Res*. Apr 1975;92(1):57-62.

[137] Izzard CS, Lochner LR. Cell-to-substrate contacts in living fibroblasts: an interference reflexion study with an evaluation of the technique. *J Cell Sci*. Jun 1976;21(1):129-159.

[138] Heath JP, Dunn GA. Cell to substratum contacts of chick fibroblasts and their relation to the microfilament system. A correlated interference-reflexion and high-voltage electron-microscope study. *J Cell Sci*. Feb 1978;29:197-212.

[139] Lee JW, Juliano R. Mitogenic signal transduction by integrin- and growth factor receptor-mediated pathways. *Mol Cells*. Apr 30 2004;17(2):188-202.

[140] Jockusch BM, Bubeck P, Giehl K, Kroemker M, Moschner J, Rothkegel M, Rudiger M, Schluter K, Stanke G, Winkler J. The molecular architecture of focal adhesions. *Annu Rev Cell Dev Biol.* 1995;11:379-416.

[141] Arregui CO, Carbonetto S, McKerracher L. Characterization of neural cell adhesion sites: point contacts are the sites of interaction between integrins and the cytoskeleton in PC12 cells. *J Neurosci.* Nov 1994;14(11 Pt 2):6967-6977.

[142] Hynes RO. Targeted mutations in cell adhesion genes: what have we learned from them? *Dev Biol.* Dec 15 1996;180(2):402-412.

[143] Hatten ME. Central nervous system neuronal migration. *Annu Rev Neurosci.* 1999;22:511-539.

[144] Rice DS, Curran T. Role of the reelin signaling pathway in central nervous system development. *Annu Rev Neurosci.* 2001;24:1005-1039.

[145] Turner CE. Paxillin interactions. *J Cell Sci.* Dec 2000;113 Pt 23:4139-4140.

[146] Ilsley JL, Sudol M, Winder SJ. The WW domain: linking cell signalling to the membrane cytoskeleton. *Cell Signal.* Mar 2002;14(3):183-189.

[147] Ponting CP, Blake DJ, Davies KE, Kendrick-Jones J, Winder SJ. ZZ and TAZ: new putative zinc fingers in dystrophin and other proteins. *Trends Biochem Sci.* Jan 1996;21(1):11-13.

[148] Rees DJ, Ades SE, Singer SJ, Hynes RO. Sequence and domain structure of talin. *Nature.* Oct 18 1990;347(6294):685-689.

[149] Michalak M, Fu SY, Milner RE, Busaan JL, Hance JE. Phosphorylation of the carboxyl-terminal region of dystrophin. *Biochem Cell Biol.* 1996;74(4):431-437.

[150] Hannigan GE, Leung-Hagesteijn C, Fitz-Gibbon L, Coppolino MG, Radeva G, Filmus J, Bell JC, Dedhar S. Regulation of cell adhesion and anchorage-dependent growth by a new beta 1-integrin-linked protein kinase. *Nature.* Jan 4 1996;379(6560):91-96.

[151] Cortes JC, Montalvo EA, Muniz J, Mornet D, Garrido E, Centeno F, Cisneros B. Dp71f modulates GSK3-beta recruitment to the beta1-integrin adhesion complex. *Neurochem Res.* Mar 2009;34(3):438-444.

[152] Roach PJ. Control of glycogen synthase by hierarchal protein phosphorylation. *Faseb J.* Sep 1990;4(12):2961-2968.

[153] Tavares F, Sellstedt A. A simple, rapid and non-destructive procedure to extract cell wall-associated proteins from Frankia. *J Microbiol Methods.* Jan 2000;39(2):171-178.

[154] Beckerle MC, Burridge K, DeMartino GN, Croall DE. Colocalization of calcium-dependent protease II and one of its substrates at sites of cell adhesion. *Cell.* Nov 20 1987;51(4):569-577.

[155] Fox JE, Goll DE, Reynolds CC, Phillips DR. Identification of two proteins (actin-binding protein and P235) that are hydrolyzed by endogenous Ca2+-dependent protease during platelet aggregation. *J Biol Chem.* Jan 25 1985;260(2):1060-1066.

[156] Franco SJ, Rodgers MA, Perrin BJ, Han J, Bennin DA, Critchley DR, Huttenlocher A. Calpain-mediated proteolysis of talin regulates adhesion dynamics. *Nat Cell Biol.* Oct 2004;6(10):977-983.

[157] Evans RR, Robson RM, Stromer MH. Properties of smooth muscle vinculin. *J Biol Chem.* Mar 25 1984;259(6):3916-3924.

[158] Goldmann WH, Ingber DE. Intact vinculin protein is required for control of cell shape, cell mechanics, and rac-dependent lamellipodia formation. *Biochemical and biophysical research communications.* Jan 18 2002;290(2):749-755.

[159] Ezzell RM, Goldmann WH, Wang N, Parashurama N, Ingber DE. Vinculin promotes cell spreading by mechanically coupling integrins to the cytoskeleton. *Exp Cell Res.* Feb 25 1997;231(1):14-26.

In: Cytoskeleton: Cell Movement...
Editors: S. Lansing et al., pp. 101-126

ISBN: 978-1-60876-559-1
© 2010 Nova Science Publishers, Inc.

Chapter IV

Measuring Reciprocal Regulation of Mesenchymal Stem Cell and Tumor Cell Motility in Two and Three Dimensions *In Vitro*

Vilma Sardão[1], Teresa Rose-Hellekant[2], Ed Perkins[3], Amy Greene[3] and Jon Holy[4]*

[1]Department of Zoology, Center for Neurosciences and Cellular Biology,
University of Coimbra, Coimbra, Portugal.
[2]Department of Physiology and Pharmacology,
University of Minnesota School of Medicine-Duluth, Duluth, MN USA.
[3]Department of Biomedical Sciences,
Mercer University School of Medicine-Savannah Campus, Savannah, GA USA.
[4]Department of Anatomy, Microbiology, and Pathology,
University of Minnesota School of Medicine-Duluth,
Duluth, MN USA.

Abstract

Cell motility is central to many aspects of cell, tissue, and organ function in both health and disease. Examples include the morphogenetic events of embryogenesis, the functioning of the immune system, wound healing, angiogenesis, and the metastatic spread of cancer. Consequently, numerous methods have been developed to study cell motility. One rapidly growing area of interest in the cell motility field involves the interactions between tumor cells, surrounding stromal cells, and mesenchymal stem cells (MesSCs), which can be recruited to tumor sites. Important motility-related questions include how MesSCs are able to home to tumor sites, and, once present at a tumor site, how they affect the metastatic potential of the tumor cells. This chapter discusses and

---

* Corresponding author: E-mail: jholy@d.umn.edu

compares some of the more popular published experimental approaches to study cell motility, with an emphasis on assays that are suitable for studies of MesSC-tumor cell interactions *in vitro*. Both two-dimensional and three-dimensional cell motility assays are described, along with the specific strengths and weaknesses of each assay for interrogating specific subcomponents of the motility process. We also describe a novel murine breast cancer-MesSC model system that is well suited for *in vitro*, as well as *in vivo* studies of the motility events associated with tumor cell-MesSC interactions.

Introduction

Motility is a fundamental feature of cellular life. The machinery that powers cell motility is responsible for sculpting the shape of cells, tissues, and organs, and alterations in the functioning of this system are responsible for, or contribute to, a wide variety of diseases. Our laboratories have a joint interest in developing cytotherapeutic approaches toward the treatment of cancer, with an emphasis on engineering mesenchymal stem cells (MesSCs) to deliver cytostatic and cytotoxic compounds to primary and metastatic breast tumors. Cell motility events play pivotal roles in this avenue of research, including being required for the homing of MesSCs to tumors, as well as potentially involving effects of engineered MesSCs on the metastatic abilities of the target tumor cells. A number of elegant studies have demonstrated that significant cross-talk occurs between MesSCs and tumor cells, which includes reciprocal effects on motility. Cell motility itself is a complex field, encompassing numerous facets which can each be investigated relatively independently of each other, or in combinations related to specific biological processes. With regards to overall cell movement, a number of different categories are usually defined, including random movements (chemokinesis), directional movements (chemotaxis), and movements stimulated by contact with a surface (haptotaxis). Specific motility assays can be used to measure one or more of these events. For example, one of the most popular types of motility assays, the transwell assay, has been used for diverse purposes, including studies of chemotaxis, separating cells of different motilities from mixed populations, investigating the invasive properties of malignant cells, and testing the roles of specific signaling pathways in cell motility. Because different aspects of cell motility can be studied by distinct assays, and one assay can be adapted to study different aspects of cell motility, researchers new to the field may be somewhat confused when initially faced with the range of methods that have been developed over the years to study motility. The purpose of this review is to introduce and describe a variety of methods that have been used to study a number of processes involved in cell motility. We approach this review from the perspective of using motility assays to investigate MesSC-breast tumor cell interactions, and therefore briefly describe the salient features of metastasis and MesSC migration to tumor sites, prior to discussing the motility assays themselves. Some of the basic features of breast cancer metastasis and MesSC homing to breast tumors are applicable to other types of solid tumor-MesSC interactions, as well.

Cell Motility and Metastasis

The primary cause of mortality in breast cancer patients is metastatic disease. Metastatic tumor cells of epithelial cancers migrate into the stromal compartment after losing their polarity and extracting themselves from their epithelial neighbors [1]. Migration can extend through the lymphatics or vasculature, thereby seeding distant sites; clinical disease occurs when single tumor cells in secondary sites establish growing colonies that impair local tissue function. The favored metastatic sites for primary breast cancers include bone, liver, lung, and brain. Important ongoing clinical goals include the identification of cellular and molecular attributes that distinguish breast cancers with a high probability of metastasis from those with low probability, as well as to determine how local environmental factors influence which metastatic tumor cells establish new tumors.

The value of evaluating tumor morphology and architecture was recognized in the late 1800s and eventually resulted in a system of cancer classification, grading, and staging, based on tumor cell morphology as well as tumor size, inflammatory response, and local invasion into stroma, lymphatics or the vasculature. The latest consensus employs the AJCC system (Breast. In: American Joint Committee on Cancer; AJCC Cancer Staging Manual. 6th ed., New York, NY, Springer, 2002, pp. 171-180). This system has significant prognostic value, with treatment recommendations significantly influenced by whether or not tumor cells are found in local and/or regional lymph nodes.

More recently, breast cancers have been classified by their molecular phenotype, of which several types have been identified, including: 1) a normal-appearing type with gene expression patterns similar to normal breast; 2) a luminal type with expression of simple cytokeratins (CK8/18), and including subtypes that express estrogen receptor (ER+) and related genes such as the transcription factor GATA3, as well as two ER-negative subtypes; 3) one with enhanced expression of ErbB2; and 4) one with a basal subtype and expression of stratified keratins such as CK5/6, 14 and 17 [2-5]. These molecular classifications are associated with clinical characterizations based on histopathology as well as ER, progesterone receptor (PR), and HER2 status. In addition, these molecular classifications are correlated with relapse and disease-free survival [2-4, 6].

Current knowledge of the basic mechanisms underlying breast carcinogenesis and metastasis has largely been acquired through studies on cell lines derived from primary or metastatic breast cancers. These cancer cell lines mimic many aspects of clinical cancers and also fall into the molecular classifications of luminal ER+, ErbB2 enhanced, and basal [7]. In addition, a mesenchymal subtype is recognized [8]. Mesenchymal-like breast cancer cell lines express many of the genes typical of basal-like cell lines, but in addition express the mesenchymal intermediate filament protein vimentin. Importantly, different subtypes of breast cancer cell lines have different likelihoods of tumor formation upon transplantation into immunocompetent mice, with basal and mesenchymal types displaying a higher tumor incidence and shorter latency than other types, especially those cell lines classified as luminal. Furthermore, subsets of basal and mesenchymal cell lines are known to be metastatic. These breast cancer cell line characteristics have proven utility for *in vivo* modeling of cancer biology and for providing a preclinical assay system for therapeutic screening.

Cancer cell lines of the mesenchymal type are thought to be epithelial in origin, but reflect an epithelial-to-mesenchymal transition (EMT). The EMT represents a key developmental process in which epithelial cells lose polarity and adapt a more mesenchymal phenotype. A similar process has been proposed to occur with metastatic cancer cells, where EMT is needed to prepare transformed epithelial cells to locally invade surrounding tissues and metastasize to distant sites [1]. The EMT results ultimately in the loss of cytokeratins and E-cadherin intercellular adhesions between epithelial cells, along with an increased expression of vimentin. These alterations appear to facilitate cellular detachment and movement across the basement membrane and into the surrounding stroma and beyond. These characteristics appear to be important clinically, as breast cancers with EMT features have a poorer prognosis than those with more typical epithelial characteristics.

The influence of MesSCs on breast tumorigenesis and metastasis is actively being investigated by a number of laboratories, and there is a growing appreciation of the importance of this interaction in disease progression. Thus far these studies have yielded somewhat conflicting results in preclinical mouse models. Co-transplantation of breast cancer cell lines with MesSCs was reported to promote metastasis [9], but MesSCs injected into the tail vein shortly after seeding lungs with breast cancer cells was found to reduce tumor size [10]. Interpretation of these seemingly conflicting data requires a thorough understanding of the transplantation models, and are limited by the use of immunocompromised mice. Experiments evaluating the *in vivo* influence of MesSCs on tumorigenesis using syngeneic transplantation into an immune competent FVB/N mouse model system are underway in our laboratories.

In this system, we utilize the novel UMD227 cell line, which was isolated from a mammary tumor in an NRL-TGFα transgenic mouse. NRL-TGFα mice develop ER+, PR-negative) tumors that are refractory to the selective estrogen receptor modulators (SERMs) tamoxifen and fluvestrant. However, mammary tumors can be prevented in this model when SERMs are administered prior to hyperplasia development [11, 12]. UMD227 cells express ErbB1 and low levels of ER, are PR-negative, and nonresponsive to tamoxifen and fluvestrant but responsive to the ErbB1 inhibitor AG1478 *in vitro*. In addition, these cells are tumorigenic; syngeneic transplantation of $0.5 - 1.0 \times 10^6$ UMD227 cells subcutaneously or in mammary glands of FVB/N mice results in tumor formation with high incidence (about 80%) and short latency (about 8-10 weeks; unpublished data). We currently are evaluating the metastatic potential of UMD227 cells and the influence that MesSCs have on the UMD227 tumorigenesis process.

Mesenchymal Stem Cell Motility

Tumor establishment and progression is dependent upon tumor cell properties and interactions between cells encompassing the tumor stromal microenvironment. A multitude of bone marrow-derived cell types of both hematopoietic and non-hematopoietic lineages contribute to the tumor microenvironment and influence tumor development. Hemangioblasts, endothelial progenitor cells, pericyte progenitor cells, and vascular endothelial growth factor-1 expressing progenitor cells constitute a bone marrow-derived reservoir of stem and progenitor cells that migrate and modulate the tumor microenvironment [13-18]. In addition to these cell types, MesSCs have been identified as a bone marrow-derived stem cell population that contributes to establishing a supportive tumor microenvironment and promoting tumor neovascularization.

The ability of MesSCs to migrate and incorporate preferentially into the tumor stromal architecture was initially demonstrated in a mouse xenograft model [19]. The basis for this type of experiment is derived from initial observations that: 1) MesSCs migrate to target sites under conditions of tissue remodeling, such as after injury or inflammation (reviewed in [20]); 2) developing tumor stroma resembles wound healing [21, 22]; and 3) tumor growth requires a supportive mesenchymal-derived stroma [23]. Thus, development of the tumor stroma and wound healing most likely share many similar and overlapping properties, including cell migration signaling mechanisms [24]. Active recruitment of MesSCs to developing tumor sites and incorporation into the tumor microenvironment leads to endocrine and paracrine-mediated signaling between tumor cells and MesSCs and the promotion of metastatic spread [9]. For example, in a breast cancer xenograft model, injection of MesSC with weakly metastatic human breast carcinoma cells resulted in a greater metastatic potency of the tumor cells [9]. These results suggest that pharmacologically targeting MesSC/tumor cell migration and interaction is potentially a novel means of impacting the development of the tumor microenvironment and, hence, tumorigenesis.

As the underlying tumor-homing mechanisms of MesSCs are beginning to emerge, it has been suggested that the microenvironment of solid tumors provides a permissive environment for engraftment of MesSCs *via* chemoattractant cytokines released by the tumor [9, 19, 25-31]. Human MesSCs migrate towards the chemokine stromal derived factor-1 (SDF-1) suggesting that MesSCs, akin to hematopoietic stem/progenitor cells, upregulate the SDF-1 chemoattractant receptor CXCR4 [32-35]. Interestingly, in evaluating this type of MesSC cell migration experiment, careful attention must be made to the *in vitro* cultivation of primary MesSCs. Low passage MesSCs demonstrate enhanced migration ability as compared to high passage MesSCs and continuous passaging is associated with loss of CXCR4 [32, 36]. Augmentation of MesSC with increased levels of CXCR4 can increase migration of MesSCs to SDF-1 *in vitro* [25] or homing in irradiated animals [29]. Likewise, pretreatment of MesSCs under hypoxia, resulting in elevated CXCR4 expression, can lead to more efficient MesSC migration [37, 38]. SDF-1 stimulated MesSCs activate downstream signaling pathways *via* signal transducer and activator of transcription 3 (STAT3), extracellular signal-regulated kinases (ERKs) and mitogen-activated protein kinases (MAPKs). In turn, these downstream pathways activate focal adhesion kinases and paxillin, which leads to a reorganization of F-actin filaments. Several excellent reviews describing MesSC chemokine and chemokine receptors and their role in migration and homing in greater detail are available [18, 28, 31, 39, 40].

The fate of MesSCs that have migrated to the developing tumor is beginning to emerge. It has been proposed, and evidence suggests, that recruited MesSCs contribute to the formation of the fibroblast population in the tumor stroma [41-45]. MesSCs, exposed to tumor-conditioned media over time, express a tumor-associated fibroblast (TAF)/carcinoma-associated fibroblast phenotype [45]. *In vitro*, MesSCs acquire a TAF phenotype upon recruitment into adenocarcinoma xenograft models including breast, pancreatic and ovarian cancers. In addition, they express phenotypic markers associated with fibroblasts, including production of tumor promoting growth factors, factors for neovascularization, and markers associated with aggressive tumors [43].

With the ease of clinical isolation of autologous MesSCs as compared to other bone marrow-derived stem/progentior cell populations, and their demonstrated robust tropism for a variety of tumors *in vitro* and *in vivo*, engineered MesSCs have been proposed as therapeutic anticancer vehicles. Engineered autologous adult-derived stem cells represent a new and unique therapeutic approach to deliver localized tumoricidal factors to inhibit cancer growth and proliferation. While in its technological infancy, the use of bioengineered adult-derived MesSCs shows early promise as a delivery system of therapeutic cytokines in a variety of clinical applications. Previously, it has been demonstrated that human MesSCs transduced with interferon beta (MesSC/IFN) inhibited the proliferation of a breast carcinoma cell line *in vitro* [46]. MesSC/IFN cells injected into a mouse with established melanoma or breast cancer cell line-derived pulmonary metastases led to infiltration of the engineered MesSCs into the tumor architecture and prolonged mouse survival [46]. MesSC/IFN cells appear to suppress the growth and proliferation of glioma cells in *in vitro* and in human xenograft models [19, 47], and have also demonstrated therapeutic potential in mouse melanoma and prostate lung metastasis models [48, 49]. As further evidence supporting this therapeutic strategy, intratumoral inoculation of rat MesSCs expressing interleukin-2 significantly prolonged survival of rats with established intracranial 9L cell gliomas [50, 51]. Umbilical cord blood-derived MesSCs engineered to express tumor necrosis factor-related apoptosis-inducing ligand (TRAIL) inhibited tumor growth in glioma-bearing mice [52]. Intracranially injected neural progenitor-like cells isolated from bone marrow and engineered to express interleukin-23 exhibited protective effects in implanted intracranial tumor-bearing mice [6]. Anti-tumor activity of MesSCs expressing interleukin-12 has also been demonstrated in a mouse melanoma model [53]. MesSCs have been engineered to express a decoy receptor to inhibit growth of Burkitt's lymphoma, as well as for the delivery of oncolytic adenoviruses leading to increased survival in a mouse model of ovarian carcinoma [54, 55]. MesSCs have also been engineered to produce CX3CL1 (for mobilization of T-cells and NK-cells) or natural killer transcript-4 (an antagonist of hepatocyte growth factor) to inhibit lung metastasis and promote survival in a mouse metastasis model [56-58]. Taken together, these results suggest that bone marrow-derived stem cells hold exceptional utility as a novel weapon against cancers for which effective therapies are lacking. Given the pharmacological limitations associated with systemic delivery of anticancer cytokines (*e.g.* toxicity), localized cellular production *via* MesSCs is a promising delivery route of these tumoricidal agents. Importantly, a more complete understanding of MesSC migration and motility will open additional MesSC engineering approaches to increase their therapeutic efficacy.

Selected Methods to Study Cell Motility

A wide variety of approaches have been developed to study motility. In addition to a few very popular methods such as transwell and wound-healing assays, considerable ingenuity has been used in the development of numerous specialized assays by many laboratories.

Following is a description of some of these types of assays, along with examples from our own studies examining reciprocal interactions influencing MesSC and tumor cell motility. For this work, we have used the UMD227 breast cancer cell line described above, and syngeneic MesSC cells isolated from the femurs of FVB/N mice by standard protocols. Most of our studies to date have been conducted with an FVB/N MesSC cell line called A500.

Transwell Assays

Transwell, or filter, assays are among the most widely-used methods to study cell motility, and are adaptable to a large number of specific purposes, including studies of chemokinesis, chemotaxis, and invasion. This method stems from the studies of Boyden, who in 1962 published the details of the fabrication of a chamber that incorporated a Millipore filter membrane as a substrate to quantify cell migration [59]. The conceptual underpinnings are quite simple, and involve measuring the ability of cells placed on one side of a porous membrane to move to the other side of the membrane. The strength and flexibility of the method arise from the ability to manipulate the chemical makeup of the media on either side of the membrane, as well as apply different coatings, such as particular extracellular matrix proteins, or even cell layers, to the membrane itself. The pore size and chemical features of the membrane can also be varied to suit the cell types employed. Medium is placed in the lower chamber, and medium plus cells are placed in the upper chamber. The transwell device is maintained in a cell culture incubator for the desired length of time, during which cells settle on the membrane and subsequently migrate through the pores, if they are able and so inclined. Random motility can be measured if the media in both upper and lower chambers is the same, and directed motility can be measured if chemotactic compounds are added to the lower chamber. Invasion, or the ability of cells to penetrate some type of physical barrier, can be measured by coating the membrane with materials such as extracellular matrix proteins, or by establishing a continuous monolayer of cells across the upper surface of the membrane.

Two basic types of devices are usually used in transwell assays: single use multiwell plates where the membranes are bonded to cup-like inserts, and re-usable rigs where membranes are placed between two milled pieces that are clamped or screwed together. Single use plates and inserts are available from a number of vendors (e.g., Corning, BD-Biosciences), and a commercially available re-usable device is available from Neuro Probe Inc. (Gaithersburg, MD). Further information about the various kinds of single use devices can be found in [60]. In our studies, we have primarily used the AP48 device from Neuro Probe, using 5 and 8 µM-pore PCTE (polycarbonate track-etch) membranes.

A number of different methods have been developed to detect and quantify the numbers of cells that have migrated through the membrane. Colorimetric staining methods have long been in use, whereas fluorescence staining methods are rapidly gaining in popularity. Techniques to measure the numbers of migrated cells spectrophotometrically (using either absorbtion, transmittance, or fluorescence) have been described, but the most common method is to place the membrane on a microscope and count cells in multiple fields of view. Whether transwell multiwell plates, inserts, or re-usable rigs with membrane sheets are used, cells are usually removed from the upper (non-migrated) surface to aid in more clearly visualizing the cells that have migrated through the membrane. Typically, this is done by either rubbing with a cotton applicator (multiwell plates and inserts) or scraping with a razor blade, cell scraper, or other sharp surface (membranes from re-usable devices; accessories to do this are available from Neuro Probe).

Hematoxylin and crystal violet are popular stains to visualize cells on membranes, and can be used after fixing cells with 4% paraformaldehyde. A number of different types of fluorescence labeling methods have also been developed to visualize migrated cells. Cells lines expressing fluorescent reporters such as GFP can be well suited for transwell studies. Stably transfected cells, along with transient transfection methods combined with cell sorting, have been used [61]. Apart from transfection, cells can be fluorescently labeled using vital dyes such as calcein AM or CellTracker (Invitrogen) reagents, or after fixation and staining with a variety of fluorescent compounds. Nuclear fluorescence staining is helpful to distinguish migrated cells in close contact with each other, with the caveat that preparations containing a substantial number of multinucleated cells can lead to an overestimation of cell number. Nuclei can be fluorescently stained with Hoechst, SYTOX Green, YO-PRO-1, or a number of other dyes. In practice, whole-cell staining, whether colorimetric or fluorescent, has the advantage of facilitating cell identification and enumeration by showing the whole cell body; on the other hand, it can be difficult to differentiate cells that are in contact with each other. Colorimetric or fluorescent nuclear staining can help in quantifying cells in contact with each other, but some cell lines contain significant numbers of multinucleate cells, and it can be difficult to distinguish nuclei from similar sized particles of fluorescent, non-cellular material and debris. If either of these factors are present to a significant extent (cell clusters, debris, or multinucleate cells), it may be advisable to try a double-labeling method where both overall cytoplasm and nuclear staining are carried out. For example, paraformaldehyde-fixed cells can be permeabilized with 0.2% Triton X-100, and double-labeled with rhodamine phalloidin (which binds to filamentous actin and thus labels cytoplasm) and SYTOX Green (which labels nuclei).

If fluorescent labeling methods are used, two approaches can be employed to avoid having to remove cells from the upper (non-migrated) membrane surface prior to counting. Membranes can be examined using a confocal microscope, which blocks the collection of fluorescence from both above and below the plane of focus; alternatively, membranes that block fluorescence can be used. The confocal appoach has the advantage of furnishing data on both surfaces of the membrane to assess the motility and behavior of cells (Figure 1). On the other hand, fluorescence-blocking membranes obviate the need for a confocal microscope. Two sources for these membranes are FluoroBlok membranes from BD Biosciences (http://www.bdbiosciences.com/home/), and PCTE black membrane filters from GE Osmonics (http://www.osmolabstore.com/default.htm).

When conducting chemotaxis studies, it may be advisable to try to gain some appreciation of the contribution of both unstimulated cell migration and chemokinesis to the results. This can be accomplished by setting up replicate wells that have the same medium (containing the putative chemotactic compound) in both upper and lower chambers. A discussion of the resulting calculations can be found in [62]. Another consideration in both chemokinesis and chemotaxis studies is that the fetal bovine serum commonly used in cell culture media can have a pronounced effect on cell motility. Fetal bovine serum normally contains fibronectin and a variety of growth factors, which can strongly influence cell adhesion, spreading, and motility. Because of this consideration, many researchers grow cells in serum-free medium for a period of time prior to, and during, the motility assay.

We have used transwell assays to test the ability of UMD227 breast cancer cells and A500 MesSCs to regulate each other's motility via factors secreted into, and thus conditioning, the culture media. For this purpose, UMD227 or A500 cells were seeded into the upper wells of an AP48 transwell chamber fitted with a 5-micrometer-pore PCTE membrane (Neuro Probe Inc., http://www.neuroprobe.com) in regular maintenance medium (CEM medium, consisting of Iscove's modified MEM containing 9% Fetal Clone III and 9% horse serum). Conditioned or control media was added to the lower chamber. The medium was conditioned by seeding dishes with 2.5×10^4/ml UMD227 cells or 4×10^4/ml A500 cells, exchanging the medium 24 hours later with fresh medium, and further culturing for 48 hours. These cell densities resulted in cultures that were reaching 100% confluence without cell injury due to overcrowding at the end of the conditioning period. Medium was then removed from each dish, centrifuged to remove non-adherent cells, and used in the lower wells of the chamber. Control media included fresh CEM medium, as well as CEM medium that had been placed in a cell culture incubator for 48 hours without cells. These experiments demonstrate that the only treatment with a significant effect on UMD227 motility was an autocrine effect of UMD227 conditioned medium, and that A500 conditioned medium had little effect on motility (Figure 1). These assays were conducted in the presence of fetal bovine serum, which might have masked chemotactic factors in the A500 conditioned medium that were weaker than serum. Furthermore, there is evidence that cross-talk between tumor cells and MesSCs is critical in altering cytokine and chemokine secretion patterns, and this design primarily tested a one-way communication event. Therefore, further studies examining conditioned medium from co-cultures of UMD227s and MesSCs, both in the presence and absence of fetal bovine serum, have been initiated.

Wound Healing Assay

This method measures cell motility as a function of the ability of cells in a monolayer culture to migrate into an area cleared of cells by scraping or chemical desquamation [63, 64]. One widely used approach involves growing cells in multiwell plates until they form a confluent layer, and then dragging a micropipette tip across the surface of each well to form linear scratchs that are free of cells. Cell motility is measured as a function of the area initially cleared of cells that is filled in over time (Figure 2). In this format, chemokinesis, and not chemotaxis, is measured. Strengths include the fact that this is a very low-cost assay, and amenable to testing multiple samples at once. In fact, a high-throughput method has been developed to screen perturbants of cell motility by this method [65]. One shortcoming is that measurements from longer timepoints may reflect not only cell motility but also cell proliferation. This can be addressed by treating cultures with mitotic inhibitors. Another consideration is that cells are normally grown to confluence prior to wounding in order to produce a clear demarcation between the cellular and cell-free areas. Some types of cells can establish cell-cell junctions and alter certain features of their metabolism when confluent, and thus the behavior of a cell from a monolayer suddenly confronted with a free surface may be different from that of an individual cell from a low-density culture that has not been part of a continuous monolayer.

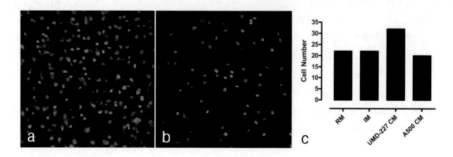

Figure 1. *Transwell migration assay.* (a) and (b), laser-scanning confocal micrographs of MesSCs on the top (unmigrated, a) and bottom (migrated, b) surfaces of a PCTE membrane. The membrane was coated with vitronectin, and as a chemoattractant, conditioned culture medium from MDA-MB-231 breast cancer cells was placed in the lower chamber. After six hours of culture, the membrane was removed from the transwell apparatus, and the cells fixed in 4% paraformaldehyde, permeabilized with 0.2% Triton X-100, stained with SYTOX Green, and photographed using a Nikon C1 confocal microscope. (a), upper surface of the membrane, showing non-migrated cells; (b), lower surface of the transwell membrane, showing migrated cells. A similar experiment was conducted to investigate whether conditioned media from A500 MesSCs influences the motility of UMD227 breast cancer cells. 2×10^4 UMD227 cells were added to the upper chamber in CEM medium, and conditioned or control media added to the lower chambers (see text for details). After a 16 hour incubation, the membranes were removed, the upper surfaces scraped to remove cells, and cells on the lower (migrated) surface fixed with 4% paraformaldehyde, stained with SYTOX Green, and examined with an inverted epifluorescence microscope. Migrated cells in five random fields of view were counted for each well; shown are the results for UMD227 cell migration from one of the experiments (c). Interestingly, A500 conditioned medium (A500CM) has little effect on the migration of UMD227 cells; however, there appears to be an autocrine effect of UMD227 conditioned medium (UMD227CM) that enhances their own motility. It should be noted that these experiments were conducted in the presence of serum, which itself influences cell motility and can blunt or mask the effects of other chemoattractive or chemorepellent substances.

Cell Scatter Assay

In this method, cells are grown at relatively low density under conditions that restrict motility and promote cell clustering. Subsequently, putative motility inducers are added and the ability of the cells to break free of the cluster and scatter is analyzed [68, 69]. This method is generally used for epithelial cells that are able to form well-defined clusters under certain conditions, such as in the absence of serum. A positive response to stimuli (such as EGF) involves detachment of cells from the clusters and migration away from the cluster, which has been reported to resemble the epithelial-mesenchymal transitions that occur during embryogenesis and some types of oncogenic transformations. An interesting aspect of this approach is the observation that the propensity of cell lines to cluster may reflect their invasive characteristics more accurately than their rate of travel [64, 70, 71].

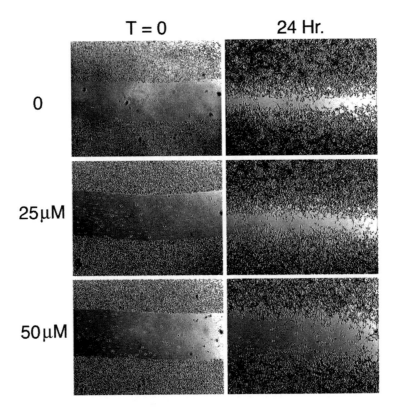

Figure 2. *Wound healing assay.* In this experiment, MDA-MB-231 breast cancer cells were seeded at high density in 24-well plates, allowed to grow to confluence, and then a linear area cleared of cells by dragging a 200 µl plastic pipette tip across the bottom of each well. The wells were then photographed, and either 25 or 50 µM curcumin added to some wells. After an overnight incubation, the wells were re-photographed and the extent of cell migration into the cleared areas examined. Curcumin has been shown to suppress cell motility in a number of different cell types [52, 66, 67], and a dose-related inhibitory effect on the migratory behavior of MDA-MB-231 cells is evident in this assay.

Phagokinesis Assay

The 2D motility of cells across a surface can be readily visualized using phagokinesis assays. This method takes advantage of the ability of cells to internalize small particles coating the surface they are moving over, leaving a cleared trail that can be measured for a number of parameters, such as area, pattern, and directionality. Initially, colloidal gold particles were used [72, 73]; more recently, fluorescent beads and quantum dots have also been adapted for this purpose [74, 75]. Shortcomings include the fact that as cells become loaded with the particles, their overall functioning can be affected. We have found that with time, cells cultured on a relatively dense layer (to better image cleared trails) of FluoSpheres fill with beads, become moribund, and detach from the coverslip. This problem can be addressed by limiting the assay time, as well as by reducing the FluoSphere coating density and measuring cell fluorescence by flow cytometry instead of trail dimensions. Also, significant care must be taken when coating the coverslips with substrate materials and fluorescent particles, as regional variation in motility can be observed in coverslips that have uneven coatings. Advantages of this assay include the fact that it is a sensitive reporter of multiple features of cell motility, and has the ability to provide unbiased data on the motility of all cells in a culture, rather than selectively detecting the most mobile fraction, as in a transwell assay [74].

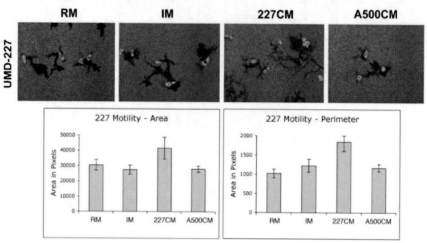

Figure 3. *Phagokinesis assay.* Epifluorescence microscopy images showing UMD-227 cells seeded at low density on glass coverslips pre-coated with polylysine and 0.5μm diameter green fluorescent FluoSpheres, generally following the protocol described in [74]. The cells were seeded in the same types of conditioned and control media described for the transwell assay in Figure 1 (RM, regular medium; IM, medium held in a cell culture incubator for 48 hours without cells; 227CM, UMD227 conditioned medium; A500CM, A500 MesSC conditioned medium). The non-fluorescent trails result from phagocytosis of the fluorescent microspheres by cells during their migration. Consequently, the cells themselves become fluorescent as they internalize the microspheres. For this experiment, cells were incubated for 16 hours in the different types of media, and then fixed with 4% paraformaldehyde in PBS and photographed with an epifluorescence microscope. Multiple random fields of view were photographed for each treatment, and the phagokinetic trails outlined in each digitized image using ImageJ and a Bamboo Fun (Wacom) drawing pad. Motility was evaluated by measuring both the total area and perimeter of the cleared trails. The graphs show the results from one experiment, in which the trails of between 12 and 17 cells from each treatment were outlined and measured (error bars represent standard error of the mean). Both visual inspection and the quantitative data indicate that motility of UMD227 cells is enhanced by UMD227 conditioned medium, but not control or A500 conditioned media. This finding agrees with the transwell result shown in Figure 1. Furthermore, other behavioral differences can be detected with the phagokinetic assay. The phagokinetic trails in UMD227 conditioned medium are generally narrower, more convoluted, and less completely cleared of beads than in the other types of media. This suggests that autocrine signals result in an alteration in the nature of UMD227 cell-substrate interactions and perhaps filopodial and/or lamellipodial activity, as well as distance traveled.

We have used this assay to test whether substances secreted into the culture medium from either UMD227 tumor cells or A500 MesSCs are able to influence UMD227 motility. For this purpose, UMD227 cells were seeded at low density (2×10^3/ml) on FluoSphere-coated coverslips in the presence of the same conditioned and control media described in the transwell assay experiment, above. Similar to the transwell results, the only effect on motility was an autocrine effect of UMD227-conditioned medium (Figure 3).

Under Agarose Assay

This method, initially described by Nelson et al. [76, 77], involves cutting wells in a layer of agarose in a cell culture dish, and adding cells to some wells and putative chemotactic compounds to adjacent wells. Responsive cells move between the surface of the culture dish and the overlying agarose, along the gradient formed by a chemotactic compound diffusing from a neighboring well. Although initially used to study leukocyte motility, this method has been used with a number of types of cells, including *Dictyostelium* amoebae, endothelial cells, osteoblasts, fibroblasts, and stem cells [78-82]. Compared to transwell assays, this method has the advantage of testing multiple chemotactic agents at once, with the ability to manipulate inter-well distance to form broader gradients [83].

Video Microscopy

There is a long and rich history behind the use of microscopy to study cell motility, and an entertaining review of this subject has been written by Dunn and Jones [84]. A wide range of methods have been developed for visualizing 2D and 3D cell motility by video microscopy [64, 85, 86]. Basically, this approach can be viewed as being composed of two components: an acquisition element, and an analysis element. Acquisition includes protocols and instrumentation to visualize and photograph living cells *in vitro*, and can range from relatively simple brightfield microscopy time-lapse methods to multiple fluorophore labeling and collection of 3D data sets over time. Similarly, analysis methods range from manual tracking of cell movements along X and Y coordinates, to automated analyses using detailed image processing and vector algorithms. A number of freeware, shareware, and commercially available software programs are available for these purposes, such as NIH Image/ImageJ, CellProfiler, Metamorph, and ImagePro Plus.

An example of a simple approach using video microscopy to study cell motility is shown in Figure 4. This experiment was conducted using teleost fish keratocytes, which display a high degree of motility *in vitro* [87]. *Medaka* keratocytes in 35 mm glass-bottom dishes (MatTek; http://www.glass-bottom-dishes.com) were cultured at room temperature in Leibovitz's L-15 medium containing 10% fetal calf serum, and vitally double-labeled with Hoechst 33342 (which labels nuclei blue) and tetramethylrhodamine methyl ester (TMRM) to label polarized mitochondria (red). Just prior to the start of filming, 10 µM carbonylcyanide-4-(trifluoromethoxy)-phenylhydrazone (FCCP) was added to the culture.

Immediately after the addition of FCCP, a time-lapse movie was started on a Nikon C1 laser-scanning confocal microscope, with one frame collected every 15 seconds for 100 frames. For the first 35 frames, motility and mitochondrial staining were normal for these cells; however, at about frame 40, TMRM labeling rapidly diminished as the FCCP depolarized the mitochondria (Figure 4). This experiment demonstrates that the motility of *Medaka* keratocytes slows after FCCP-induced mitochondrial depolarization.

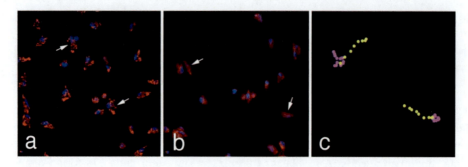

Figure 4. *Time-lapse video microscopy*. In this experiment, *Medaka* keratocytes were double-labeled with Hoechst (to label nuclei, blue) and TMRM (to label polarized mitochondria, red) and a time-lapse movie made using confocal microscopy, as described in the text. (a) shows the double-labeled keratocytes immediately after the addition of FCCP (see text), and at the start of the time-lapse movie. The arrows identify two cells that were tracked throughout the recording period. (b) shows frame 40 of the time-lapse sequence, at which point the TMRM signal was rapidly becoming lost from the mitochondria. The arrows identify the same cells marked in (a). The 100 frame sequence was saved as an AVI movie using Nikon C1 software, and opened on a MacBook Pro laptop running ImageJ (v1.41). A mark was placed over the nuclei of the two identified representative cells at 5-frame (75 second) intervals throughout the sequence; a yellow mark was used prior to mitochondrial depolarization, and a magenta mark was used after mitochondrial depolarization. (c) shows the position of the cells at five-frame (75 second) intervals. These tracks indicate that not only does motility slow after mitochondrial depolarization, but the direction traveled appears to shift from linear to random.

This is but one example of a plethora of different approaches toward visualizing cell motility *in vitro* by video microscopy methods. It should also be mentioned that in addition to *in vitro* methods, exciting advancements are being made using video microscopy to visualize cell behavior *in vivo* [88-92].

Use of Multicellular Spheroids in Motility Assays

Abundant evidence demonstrates that the behavior of both untransformed and tumorigenic cells is significantly different in two-dimensional (2D) and three-dimensional (3D) conditions. One of the most simple and straightforward methods of growing cells in 3D cultures is to simply culture them under non-adherent conditions. Depending on the cell line and specific culture medium used, cells in suspension can either remain dispersed, form clusters from either aggregation, proliferation, or a combination of both, or die through a form of apoptosis called anoikis. Cell clusters can range from loose aggregates to tightly packed spherical, elongate, or polymorphic structures, with wide variations in the presence or types of cell-cell junctions and extracellular matrix material produced, depending on the cell line. The different types of organization are reflected by different patterns of gene expression [93], and these changes include proteins associated with adhesion and motility [56, 94, 95]. Many types of cells produce compacted spherical structures called multicellular spheroids (MulCSs). Of relevance for cancer chemotherapy testing, the behavior of cells in MulCSs more closely resembles that of tumor cells *in situ* than that of cells in a monolayer 2D culture, and there is a growing realization that *in vitro* drug testing should be conducted primarily using MulCSs. In addition, there is clear evidence that cell motility in 3D is significantly different from that occurring on a 2D surface, and an increasing number of laboratories are investigating basic questions in cell motility and metastasis in 3D model systems. With respect to MulCSs, cell motility can be studied a) within MulCSs, b) between MulCSs, or between MulCSs and excised tissue or organ fragments (confrontation cultures), c) as MulCSs attach and spread on a culture surface, or d) as cells from MulCSs embedded in some type of support material (e.g., collagen) migrate out in a 3D matrix.

Production of Multicellular Spheroids

A number of methods have been used to generate MulCSs from a variety of cell types, but most involve culturing cells under non-adherent conditions. Not all cell lines are able to form MulCSs under non-adherent conditions due to the fact that some will die by via anoikis if deprived of contact with a substrate, or growth surface. Furthermore, some types of cells do not adhere well to each other in suspension (e.g., PC-3 prostate cancer cells). Of the cell lines that are able to form MulCSs in suspension culture, a range of morphologies, sizes, and organization can be observed. In small MulCSs, all cells may remain viable, but in larger MulCSs (in the range of hundreds of micrometers), a central necrotic core is usually produced, surrounded by a middle layer of quiescent cells and an outer layer of active, dividing cells [96, 97]. Methods used to produce MulCSs include culturing cells in low-adhesion or bacteriological grade plastic dishes, culturing cells on a layer of agarose, use of spinner flasks, and hanging drops. The hanging drop method is a very simple method to produce MulCSs of uniform size and cell number, and is the method we usually use to produce MulCSs for motility studies. For descriptions of this method, see [98, 99].

MulCSs can be generated from a single cell line, or from combinations of multiple cell lines. As part of our studies examining the reciprocal interactions between mesenchymal stem cells and tumor cells, we have generated both pure and mixed MulCSs from the UMD227 tumor cell and A500 MesSC lines. MulCSs composed of either cell line, or mixtures of the two, are made by using normal trypsinization methods to obtain a cell suspension, and then seeding 1×10^4 cells per 20 µl drop on the inside surface of the top of a sterile bacteriological grade petri dish. After filling the cover with drops, the cover is lowered, drop-side-down, onto the bottom part of the plate, which contains 10 ml of sterile distilled water to minimize evaporation of the drops. For mixed MulCSs, 0.5×10^4 A500 cells are combined with 0.5×10^4 UMD227 cells per 20 microliter drop. Plates containing the hanging drops are placed in a cell culture incubator for 3 days, by which time well-formed MulCSs are apparent. The MulCSs are then pooled and used for the motility assays.

Cells used to make MulCSs can be labeled by a number of methods prior to use in motility assays. Of course, stable transfectants expressing GFP or a related reporter are very useful for these purposes. Alternatively, cells can be labeled by a variety of commercially available products, such as the CellTracker, Qtracker, and FluoSphere probes (Invitrogen), and PKH reagents (Sigma). We have found that the same FluoSphere beads used for the phagokinesis assays work very well to label cells in culture prior to use for MulCS generation. A500 and UMD227 cells are grown to approximately 50% confluence in 5 ml of medium per 60 mm cell culture dish, and 5 µl of either the 0.5 µm diameter green or 1 µm diameter red fluorspheres added to each dish. Cultures with fluorospheres are incubated overnight, and the cells washed and trypsinized for use in MulCS production the following morning. The intensity of the labeling can be controlled by varying the amount of beads added to the overnight cultures, but care must be taken not to overload cells, which can damage or kill them.

Multicellular Spheroid Spreading Assays

One measure of the motility capabilities of cells resident in MulCSs involves allowing MulCSs to attach to cell culture dishes, after which they will usually flatten and spread out over the surface of the dish. The extent, rate, and morphological features of cell spreading can be used as an indication of the motility characteristics of the cells (Figure 5). The surface over which the spheroids spread can be manipulated, and can even consist of a cellular layer. For example, MulCS spreading has been studied using untreated cell culture plates [100], a layer of fibroblasts [101], and a layer of endothelial cells lying on collagen gels [102].

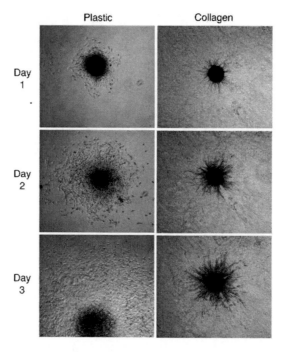

Figure 5. *2D and 3D MulCS Outgrowth*. The hanging drop method (see text) was used to construct MulCSs over three days from an initial seeding of 1 x 10^4 UMD227 cells. MulCSs were then either transferred to multiwell plates in culture medium for 2D culture, or suspended in type I rat tail collagen gels for 3D culture. Plates were briefly removed from the cell culture incubator and photographed at 24 hour intervals for three days to compare MulCS outgrowth on a plastic substrate with invasion into a collagen matrix. Note the difference in outgrowth patterns between the two preparations.

Collagen Invasion Assays

The motility of cells through 3D matrices can be studied *in vitro* by a number of methods. A number of different types of matrix materials have been developed to support cell growth and differentiation, and this is an ongoing effort in tissue engineering laboratories.

One of the oldest materials used for this purpose is type I collagen isolated from rat tail tendons. This type of collagen is commercially available, and also quite easily prepared in the laboratory [103]. In our experiments, we combine either cell suspensions or MulCSs with a liquid collagen solution that has been neutralized and made isotonic by the addition of sodium hydroxide and 10X PBS, and the mixture rapidly placed in multiwell plates and allowed to gel. A thin layer of feeding solution is added over the gels, and the cells or MulCSs cultured for the desired length of time. Cell movements through the collagen can be followed with video microscopy, either manually or with the use of a number of software image analysis programs. Invasion can be followed by seeding cells on top of a layer of collagen, and measuring the numbers of invading cells and their depth of penetration. Migration of cells from MulCSs embedded in collagen can be measured by a number of methods, including measuring the increase in distance of cells from the center of the spheroid over time [104, 105].

Not surprisingly, invasion of MulCS cells into a 3D collagen matrix exhibits a number of differences from spreading on a 2D surface. Generally, cords of cells invade the collagen, giving rise to an astral-like structure, compared to the more homogenous sheet-like spreading observed on a 2D substrate (Figure 5). Radial arrays in 3D culture can be challenging to quantify, and some researchers simply measure the distance to the cells lying farthest from the MulCS as the measure of motility. Fluorescently labeling cells prior to MulCSs construction can be helpful in visualizing cell dynamics during collagen invasion. For many purposes, stably-transfected cells constitutively expressing a fluorescent reporter molecule (e.g., GFP) are very useful for this purpose, and mixed spheroids constructed from multiple cell lines expressing different fluorophores can allow cell-cell regulation of motility to be studied. In addition, use of transient labeling methods can be used to gain insights into the interplay of cell division and cell motility; transient labels are usually randomly apportioned between daughter cells, and thus a decrease in labeling intensity is a reflection of mitotic activity. Using a transient FluoSphere labeling method, we have found that there are significant differences in how UMD227 tumor cells and A500 MesSCs invade 3D collagen matrices (Figure 6). After three days in culture, UMD227 MulCSs maintain a recognizable peripheral surface, with radial arrays of cells extending out from this surface into the surrounding collagen. In contrast, A500 MulCSs lose their well-defined periphery, suggesting that the MulCSs dissociate as mass cell migration into the matrix occurs. FluoSphere labeling patterns support this interpretation for A500 migration; in contrast, labeling in UMD227 MulCSs is largely restricted to the central MulCS mass, and the radial arrays of cells are largely unlabeled. This indicates that the matrix-invading cells from UMD227 MulCSs primarily represent multiple generations of cells derived from cell division in the peripheral layer of the MulCS, whereas invading A500 cells originate throughout the volume of the MulCS. Interestingly, UMD227 cells can be induced to invade the collagen matrix in a pattern similar to the A500s in mixed MulCSs composed of both cell types (Figure 6). This could reflect at least two mechanical processes: UMD227 cells in mixed MulCSs may not form cell-cell junctions to the same extent as in monoculture, thus allowing them to move more freely; alternatively, their enhanced invasion could reflect their access to channels through the collagen created by invading A500 cells that facilitate their exit from the MulCS. Alternatively, the change in their invasion pattern could be due to cell-cell signaling between these two cell types, or a combination of all of the above factors. Clearly, this approach constitutes an intriguing model system with which to study reciprocal cell-cell motility interactions between MesSCs and tumor cells in a 3D environment.

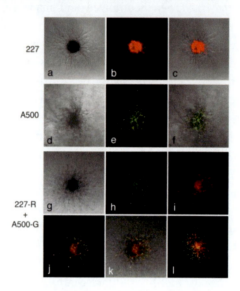

Figure 6. *Collagen Invasion Assay.* UMD227 and A500 cells in monolayer culture were incubated overnight in a 1:1000 dilution of 1 μm red (UMD227) or 0.5 μm green (A500) FluoSpheres. MulCSs were then allowed to assemble from 1×10^4 labeled cells in hanging drops for three days prior to being suspended in a collagen gel. Mixed MulCSs were made by combining 0.5×10^4 cells of each line per hanging drop. After three days of culture in collagen, MulCSs were photographed using both phase contrast and fluorescence optics, using a Nikon C1 confocal microscope. (a) and (b), a UMD227 spheroid shown by phase contrast (a) and fluorescence (b) optics. (c) shows an overlay of (a) and (b). Note that the fluorescence labeling is restricted to the central body of the MulCS, and to cells lying very close to the surface of the central body. The peripheral cells invading into the collagen exhibit little or no labeling, demonstrating that they are composed primarily of daughter generations of cells produced by mitotic division of the original MulCS cells. Their parental cells are presumed to be the peripheral MulCS cells, because the overall fluorescence of the central MulCS mass remains strong, and does not increase in size. (d) and (e), an A500 MulCS shown by phase contrast (d) and fluorescence (e) optics. (f) shows an overlay of (d) and (e). In contrast to UMD227 MulCSs, the central mass of A500 MulCSs becomes disaggregated as the cells invade the surrounding collagen. The extensive labeling throughout the invading cell population indicates that the invading cells originate from all areas of the original MulCS. Interestingly, the invasion pattern of UMD227 cells in mixed MulCSs changes, and more closely resembles the invasion pattern of A500 cells. (g-l), a mixed spheroid shown by phase contrast optics (g), and by fluorescence to reveal the distribution of labeled A500 (h, green) and UMD227 (i, red) cells. (j) shows an overlay of A500 and UMD227 fluorescence; (k) is an overlay of the phase contrast and fluorescence images, and (l) is a projection of a stack of image planes taken through the z-axis of the MulCS, showing the overall distribution of labeled cells.

Confrontation and Mixed MulCS Cultures

Interactions between different types of MulCSs, between MulCSs and tissue fragments, and between MulCSs and individual cells in suspension have been studied for a number of purposes. Methods have been developed to study the invasion of malignant cells into tissues *in vitro* using confrontation cultures of MulCSs and normal tissue fragments. Systems studied with these methods include glioma/brain [106], Melanoma/heart [107], bladder tumor cells/bladder mucosa [108], breast cancer/embryoid body [109], and lung carcinoma/bronchial mucosa [110]. Studies show that these systems can closely mimic the behavior of tumor cell invasion *in vivo* [111, 112]. Interactions between breast carcinoma MulCSs and MesSCs have been recently studied. Conditioned media from two different carcinoma cell lines (MCF7 and MDA-MB-231) attracted human MesSCs in transwell assays, and the MesSCs were also shown to invade MulCSs derived from these lines. Interestingly, the invading MesSCs disrupted the carcinoma MulCSs by activating ADAM-10 [113].

Conclusion

Cell motility has intrigued cell biologists since its discovery over three centuries ago, and the creative efforts of many laboratories over the years have resulted in a wealth of distinct approaches that can be used to gain insights into this complex phenomenon. Some methods are well suited for examining specific events related to motility, whereas others are designed to measure more general endpoints of the process. A characteristic common among studies of cell motility, cell division, and cell death is that each type of assay usually illuminates but one small facet of an intricate and highly regulated process. Therefore, a good first step in selecting a particular type of assay is to carefully consider what aspect of cell motility is of greatest relevance to the project at hand. Experimental approaches range from the involved, where, for example, teams composed of biomedical scientists, optical and software engineers, and mathematical modelers work with extremely expensive microscopes fitted with complex cell culture and manipulation devices, to the very simple, requiring only the efforts of a single person and perhaps a simple brightfield microscope or spectrophotometer. This flexibility, along with the importance of cell motility in health and disease, promises that the future of cell motility research will be at least as wide ranging and exciting as its history.

References

[1] Kalluri, R; Weinberg, RA. The basics of epithelial-mesenchymal transition. *J Clin Invest.*, 2009 Jun, 119(6), 1420-8.

[2] Perou, CM; Sorlie, T; Eisen, MB; van de Rijn, M; Jeffrey, SS; Rees, CA; et al. Molecular portraits of human breast tumours. *Nature*, 2000 Aug 17, 406(6797), 747-52.

[3] Sorlie, T; Perou, CM; Tibshirani, R; Aas, T; Geisler, S; Johnsen, H; et al. Gene expression patterns of breast carcinomas distinguish tumor subclasses with clinical implications. *Proc Natl Acad Sci*, U S A., 2001 Sep 11, 98(19), 10869-74.

[4] Sorlie, T; Tibshirani, R; Parker, J; Hastie, T; Marron, JS; Nobel, A; et al. Repeated observation of breast tumor subtypes in independent gene expression data sets. *Proc Natl Acad Sci*, U S A., 2003 Jul 8, 100(14), 8418-23.

[5] Sotiriou, C; Pusztai, L. Gene-expression signatures in breast cancer. *N Engl J Med.*, 2009 Feb 19, 360(8), 790-800.

[6] Hu, Z; Fan, C; Oh, DS; Marron, JS; He, X; Qaqish, BF; et al. The molecular portraits of breast tumors are conserved across microarray platforms. *BMC Genomics*, 2006, 7, 96.

[7] Kao, J; Salari, K; Bocanegra, M; Choi, YL; Girard, L; Gandhi, J; et al. Molecular profiling of breast cancer cell lines defines relevant tumor models and provides a resource for cancer gene discovery. *PLoS One.*, 2009, 4(7), e6146.

[8] Blick, T; Widodo, E; Hugo, H; Waltham, M; Lenburg, ME; Neve, RM; et al. Epithelial mesenchymal transition traits in human breast cancer cell lines. *Clin Exp Metastasis*, 2008, 25(6), 629-42.

[9] Karnoub, AE; Dash, AB; Vo, AP; Sullivan, A; Brooks, MW; Bell, GW; et al. Mesenchymal stem cells within tumour stroma promote breast cancer metastasis. *Nature*, 2007 Oct 4, 449(7162), 557-63.

[10] Loebinger, MR; Eddaoudi, A; Davies, D; Janes, SM. Mesenchymal stem cell delivery of TRAIL can eliminate metastatic cancer. *Cancer Res.*, 2009 May 15, 69(10), 4134-42.

[11] Rose-Hellekant, TA; Schroeder, MD; Brockman, JL; Zhdankin, O; Bolstad, R; Chen, KS; et al. Estrogen receptor-positive mammary tumorigenesis in TGFalpha transgenic mice progresses with progesterone receptor loss. *Oncogene*, 2007 Aug 9, 26(36), 5238-46.

[12] Rose-Hellekant, TA; Skildum, AJ; Zhdankin, O; Greene, AL; Regal, RR; Kundel, KD; et al. Short-term prophylactic tamoxifen reduces the incidence of antiestrogen-resistant/estrogen receptor-positive/ progesterone receptor-negative mammary tumors. *Cancer Prev Res (Phila Pa).*, 2009 May, 2(5), 496-502.

[13] Lyden, D; Hattori, K; Dias, S; Costa, C; Blaikie, P; Butros, L; et al. Impaired recruitment of bone-marrow-derived endothelial and hematopoietic precursor cells blocks tumor angiogenesis and growth. *Nat Med.*, 2001 Nov, 7(11), 1194-201.

[14] Rajantie, I; Ilmonen, M; Alminaite, A; Ozerdem, U; Alitalo, K; Salven, P. Adult bone marrow-derived cells recruited during angiogenesis comprise precursors for periendothelial vascular mural cells. *Blood*, 2004 Oct 1, 104(7), 2084-6.

[15] Song, S; Ewald, AJ; Stallcup, W; Werb, Z; Bergers, G. PDGFRbeta+ perivascular progenitor cells in tumours regulate pericyte differentiation and vascular survival. *Nat Cell Biol.*, 2005 Sep, 7(9), 870-9.

[16] Kaplan, RN; Riba, RD; Zacharoulis, S; Bramley, AH; Vincent, L; Costa, C; et al. VEGFR1-positive haematopoietic bone marrow progenitors initiate the pre-metastatic niche. *Nature*, 2005 Dec 8, 438(7069), 820-7.

[17] De Palma, M; Venneri, MA; Galli, R; Sergi Sergi, L; Politi, LS; Sampaolesi, M; et al. Tie2 identifies a hematopoietic lineage of proangiogenic monocytes required for tumor vessel formation and a mesenchymal population of pericyte progenitors. *Cancer Cell.*, 2005 Sep, 8(3), 211-26.

[18] Roorda, BD; ter Elst, A; Kamps, WA; de Bont, ES. Bone marrow-derived cells and tumor growth: contribution of bone marrow-derived cells to tumor micro-environments with special focus on mesenchymal stem cells. *Crit Rev Oncol Hematol.*, 2009 Mar, 69(3), 187-98.

[19] Studeny, M; Marini, FC; Champlin, RE; Zompetta, C; Fidler, IJ; Andreeff, M. Bone marrow-derived mesenchymal stem cells as vehicles for interferon-beta delivery into tumors. *Cancer Res.*, 2002 Jul 1, 62(13), 3603-8.

[20] Gregory, CA; Prockop, DJ; Spees, JL. Non-hematopoietic bone marrow stem cells: molecular control of expansion and differentiation. *Exp Cell Res.*, 2005 Jun 10, 306(2), 330-5.

[21] Dvorak, HF. Tumors: wounds that do not heal. Similarities between tumor stroma generation and wound healing. *N Engl J Med.*, 1986 Dec 25, 315(26), 1650-9.

[22] Park, CC; Bissell, MJ; Barcellos-Hoff, MH. The influence of the microenvironment on the malignant phenotype. *Mol Med Today*, 2000 Aug, 6(8), 324-9.
[23] Hanahan, D; Weinberg, RA. The hallmarks of cancer. *Cell.*, 2000 Jan 7, 100(1), 57-70.
[24] Spaeth, E; Klopp, A; Dembinski, J; Andreeff, M; Marini, F. Inflammation and tumor microenvironments: defining the migratory itinerary of mesenchymal stem cells. *Gene Ther.*, 2008 May, 15(10), 730-8.
[25] Ryser, MF; Ugarte, F; Thieme, S; Bornhauser, M; Roesen-Wolff, A; Brenner, S. mRNA Transfection of CXCR4-GFP Fusion-Simply Generated by PCR-Results in Efficient Migration of Primary Human Mesenchymal Stem Cells. *Tissue Eng Part C Methods.*, 2008 Sep, 14(3), 179-84.
[26] Chamberlain, G; Wright, K; Rot, A; Ashton, B; Middleton, J. Murine mesenchymal stem cells exhibit a restricted repertoire of functional chemokine receptors: comparison with human. *PLoS ONE.*, 2008, 3(8), e2934.
[27] Corcoran, KE; Trzaska, KA; Fernandes, H; Bryan, M; Taborga, M; Srinivas, V; et al. Mesenchymal stem cells in early entry of breast cancer into bone marrow. *PLoS ONE.*, 2008, 3(6), e2563.
[28] Fox, JM; Chamberlain, G; Ashton, BA; Middleton, J. Recent advances into the understanding of mesenchymal stem cell trafficking. *Br J Haematol.*, 2007 Jun, 137(6), 491-502.
[29] Kyriakou, C; Rabin, N; Pizzey, A; Nathwani, A; Yong, K. Factors that influence short-term homing of human bone marrow-derived mesenchymal stem cells in a xenogeneic animal model. *Haematologica.*, 2008 Oct, 93(10), 1457-65.
[30] Fritz, V; Jorgensen, C. Mesenchymal stem cells: an emerging tool for cancer targeting and therapy. *Curr Stem Cell Res Ther.*, 2008 Jan, 3(1), 32-42.
[31] Karp, JM; Leng Teo, GS. Mesenchymal stem cell homing: the devil is in the details. *Cell Stem Cell.*, 2009 Mar 6, 4(3), 206-16.
[32] Wynn, RF; Hart, CA; Corradi-Perini, C; O'Neill, L; Evans, CA; Wraith, JE; et al. A small proportion of mesenchymal stem cells strongly expresses functionally active CXCR4 receptor capable of promoting migration to bone marrow. *Blood*, 2004 Nov 1, 104(9), 2643-5.
[33] Sordi, V; Malosio, ML; Marchesi, F; Mercalli, A; Melzi, R; Giordano, T; et al. Bone marrow mesenchymal stem cells express a restricted set of functionally active chemokine receptors capable of promoting migration to pancreatic islets. *Blood*, 2005 Jul 15, 106(2), 419-27.
[34] Androutsellis-Theotokis, A; Leker, RR; Soldner, F; Hoeppner, DJ; Ravin, R; Poser, SW; et al. Notch signalling regulates stem cell numbers in vitro and in vivo. *Nature*, 2006 Aug 17, 442(7104), 823-6.
[35] Foshay, KM; Gallicano, GI. Regulation of Sox2 by STAT3 initiates commitment to the neural precursor cell fate. *Stem Cells Dev.*, 2008 Apr, 17(2), 269-78.
[36] Rombouts, WJ; Ploemacher, RE. Primary murine MSC show highly efficient homing to the bone marrow but lose homing ability following culture. *Leukemia.*, 2003 Jan, 17(1), 160-70.
[37] Annabi, B; Lee, YT; Turcotte, S; Naud, E; Desrosiers, RR; Champagne, M; et al. Hypoxia promotes murine bone-marrow-derived stromal cell migration and tube formation. *Stem Cells.*, 2003, 21(3), 337-47.
[38] Rosova, I; Dao, M; Capoccia, B; Link, D; Nolta, JA. Hypoxic preconditioning results in increased motility and improved therapeutic potential of human mesenchymal stem cells. *Stem Cells.*, 2008 Aug, 26(8), 2173-82.

[39] Sordi, V. Mesenchymal stem cell homing capacity. *Transplantation*, 2009 May 15, 87(9 Suppl), S42-5.
[40] Khaldoyanidi, S. Directing stem cell homing. *Cell Stem Cell.*, 2008 Mar 6, 2(3), 198-200.
[41] Sangai, T; Ishii, G; Kodama, K; Miyamoto, S; Aoyagi, Y; Ito, T; et al. Effect of differences in cancer cells and tumor growth sites on recruiting bone marrow-derived endothelial cells and myofibroblasts in cancer-induced stroma. *Int J Cancer.*, 2005 Jul 20, 115(6), 885-92.
[42] Direkze, NC; Hodivala-Dilke, K; Jeffery, R; Hunt, T; Poulsom, R; Oukrif, D; et al. Bone marrow contribution to tumor-associated myofibroblasts and fibroblasts. *Cancer Res.*, 2004 Dec 1, 64(23), 8492-5.
[43] Spaeth, EL; Dembinski, JL; Sasser, AK; Watson, K; Klopp, A; Hall, B; et al. Mesenchymal stem cell transition to tumor-associated fibroblasts contributes to fibrovascular network expansion and tumor progression. *PLoS ONE.*, 2009, 4(4), e4992.
[44] Mishra, PJ; Glod, JW; Banerjee, D. Mesenchymal stem cells: flip side of the coin. *Cancer Res.*, 2009 Feb 15, 69(4), 1255-8.
[45] Mishra, PJ; Humeniuk, R; Medina, DJ; Alexe, G; Mesirov, JP; Ganesan, S; et al. Carcinoma-associated fibroblast-like differentiation of human mesenchymal stem cells. *Cancer Res.*, 2008 Jun 1, 68(11), 4331-9.
[46] Studeny, M; Marini, FC; Dembinski, JL; Zompetta, C; Cabreira-Hansen, M; Bekele, BN; et al. Mesenchymal stem cells: potential precursors for tumor stroma and targeted-delivery vehicles for anticancer agents. *J Natl Cancer Inst.*, 2004 Nov 3, 96(21), 1593-603.
[47] Nakamizo, A; Marini, F; Amano, T; Khan, A; Studeny, M; Gumin, J; et al. Human bone marrow-derived mesenchymal stem cells in the treatment of gliomas. *Cancer Res.*, 2005 Apr 15, 65(8), 3307-18.
[48] Burdick, JA; Vunjak-Novakovic, G. Review: Engineered Microenvironments for Controlled Stem Cell Differentiation. *Tissue Eng Part A.*, 2008 Aug 11.
[49] Lowry, WE; Richter, L; Yachechko, R; Pyle, AD; Tchieu, J; Sridharan, R; et al. Generation of human induced pluripotent stem cells from dermal fibroblasts. *Proc Natl Acad Sci, U S A.*, 2008 Feb 26, 105(8), 2883-8.
[50] Hamada, H; Kobune, M; Nakamura, K; Kawano, Y; Kato, K; Honmou, O; et al. Mesenchymal stem cells (MSC) as therapeutic cytoreagents for gene therapy. *Cancer Sci.*, 2005 Mar, 96(3), 149-56.
[51] Nakamura, K; Ito, Y; Kawano, Y; Kurozumi, K; Kobune, M; Tsuda, H; et al. Antitumor effect of genetically engineered mesenchymal stem cells in a rat glioma model. *Gene Ther.*, 2004 Jul, 11(14), 1155-64.
[52] Kim, HI; Huang, H; Cheepala, S; Huang, S; Chung, J. Curcumin inhibition of integrin (alpha6beta4)-dependent breast cancer cell motility and invasion. *Cancer Prev Res (Phila Pa).*, 2008 Oct, 1(5), 385-91.
[53] Elzaouk, L; Moelling, K; Pavlovic, J. Anti-tumor activity of mesenchymal stem cells producing IL-12 in a mouse melanoma model. *Exp Dermatol.*, 2006 Nov, 15(11), 865-74.
[54] Komarova, S; Kawakami, Y; Stoff-Khalili, MA; Curiel, DT; Pereboeva, L. Mesenchymal progenitor cells as cellular vheicles for delivery of oncolytic andenoviruses. *Mol Cancer Ther.*, 2006, 5(3), 755-66.
[55] Kyriakou, CA; Yong, KL; Benjamin, R; Pizzey, A; Dogan, A; Singh, N; et al. Human mesenchymal stem cells (hMSCs) expressing truncated soluble vascular endothelial

growth factor receptor (tsFlk-1) following lentiviral-mediated gene transfer inhibit growth of Burkitt's lymphoma in a murine model. *J Gene Med.*, 2006, 8(3), 253-64.

[56] Grun, B; Benjamin, E; Sinclair, J; Timms, JF; Jacobs, IJ; Gayther, SA; et al. Three-dimensional in vitro cell biology models of ovarian and endometrial cancer. *Cell Prolif.*, 2009 Apr, 42(2), 219-28.

[57] Kanehira, M; Xin, H; Hoshino, K; Maemondo, M; Mizuguchi, H; Hayakawa, T; et al. Targeted delivery of NK4 to multiple lung tumors by bone marrow-derived mesenchymal stem cells. *Cancer Gene Ther.*, 2007 Nov, 14(11), 894-903.

[58] Inberg, A; Bogoch, Y; Bledi, Y; Linial, M. Cellular processes underlying maturation of P19 neurons: Changes in protein folding regimen and cytoskeleton organization. *Proteomics.*, 2007 Mar, 7(6), 910-20.

[59] Boyden, S. The chemotactic effect of mixtures of antibody and antigen on polymorphonuclear leucocytes. *J Exp Med.*, 1962 Mar 1, 115, 453-66.

[60] Eccles, SA; Box, C; Court, W. Cell migration/invasion assays and their application in cancer drug discovery. *Biotechnol Annu Rev.*, 2005, 11, 391-421.

[61] Wu, K; Katiyar, S; Li, A; Liu, M; Ju, X; Popov, VM; et al. Dachshund inhibits oncogene-induced breast cancer cellular migration and invasion through suppression of interleukin-8. *Proc Natl Acad Sci, U S A.*, 2008 May 13, 105(19), 6924-9.

[62] Zigmond, SH; Foxman, EF; Segall, JE. Chemotaxis assays for eukaryotic cells. *Curr Protoc Cell Biol.*, 2001 May, Chapter 12, Unit 12 1.

[63] Gotlieb, AI; Spector, W. Migration into an in vitro experimental wound: a comparison of porcine aortic endothelial and smooth muscle cells and the effect of culture irradiation. *Am J Pathol.*, 1981 May, 103(2), 271-82.

[64] Terryn, C; Bonnomet, A; Cutrona, J; Coraux, C; Tournier, JM; Nawrocki-Raby, B, et al. Video-microscopic imaging of cell spatio-temporal dispersion; and migration. *Crit Rev Oncol Hematol.*, 2009 Feb, 69(2), 144-52.

[65] Yarrow, JC; Perlman, ZE; Westwood, NJ; Mitchison, TJ. A high-throughput cell migration assay using scratch wound healing, a comparison of image-based readout methods. *BMC Biotechnol.*, 2004 Sep 9, 4, 21.

[66] Seo, JH; Jeong, KJ; Oh, WJ; Sul, HJ; Sohn, JS; Kim, YK; et al. Lysophosphatidic acid induces STAT3 phosphorylation and ovarian cancer cell motility: Their inhibition by curcumin. *Cancer Lett.*, 2009, Jul 30.

[67] Holy, J. Curcumin inhibits cell motility and alters microfilament organization and function in prostate cancer cells. *Cell Motil Cytoskeleton.*, 2004 Aug, 58(4), 253-68.

[68] Pope, MD; Graham, NA; Huang, BK; Asthagiri, AR. Automated quantitative analysis of epithelial cell scatter. *Cell Adh Migr.*, 2008 Apr, 2(2), 110-6.

[69] Chen, HC. Cell-scatter assay. *Methods Mol Biol.*, 2005, 294, 69-77.

[70] Matos, M; Raby, BN; Zahm, JM; Polette, M; Birembaut, P; Bonnet, N. Cell migration and proliferation are not discriminatory factors in the in vitro sociologic behavior of bronchial epithelial cell lines. *Cell Motil Cytoskeleton.*, 2002 Sep, 53(1), 53-65.

[71] Nawrocki Raby, B; Polette, M; Gilles, C; Clavel, C; Strumane, K; Matos, M; et al. Quantitative cell dispersion analysis: new test to measure tumor cell aggressiveness. *Int J Cancer.*, 2001 Sep 1, 93(5), 644-52.

[72] Albrecht-Buehler, G. Phagokinetic tracks of 3T3 cells: parallels between the orientation of track segments and of cellular structures which contain actin or tubulin. *Cell.*, 1977 Oct, 12(2), 333-9.

[73] Albrecht-Buehler, G. The phagokinetic tracks of 3T3 cells. *Cell.*, 1977 Jun, 11(2), 395-404.

[74] Windler-Hart, SL; Chen, KY; Chenn, A. A cell behavior screen: identification, sorting, and enrichment of cells based on motility. *BMC Cell Biol.*, 2005, 6(1), 14.
[75] Gu, W; Pellegrino, T; Parak, WJ; Boudreau, R; Le Gros, MA; Alivisatos, AP; et al. Measuring cell motility using quantum dot probes. *Methods Mol Biol.*, 2007, 374, 125-31.
[76] Nelson, RD; Quie, PG; Simmons, RL. Chemotaxis under agarose: a new and simple method for measuring chemotaxis and spontaneous migration of human polymorphonuclear leukocytes and monocytes. *J Immunol.*, 1975 Dec, 115(6), 1650-6.
[77] Nelson, RD; Herron, MJ. Agarose method for human neutrophil chemotaxis. *Methods Enzymol.*, 1988, 162, 50-9.
[78] Woznica, D; Knecht, DA. Under-agarose chemotaxis of Dictyostelium discoideum. *Methods Mol Biol.*, 2006, 346, 311-25.
[79] Trapp, T; Kogler, G; El-Khattouti, A; Sorg, RV; Besselmann, M; Focking, M; et al. Hepatocyte growth factor/c-MET axis-mediated tropism of cord blood-derived unrestricted somatic stem cells for neuronal injury. *J Biol Chem.*, 2008 Nov 21, 283(47), 32244-53.
[80] Dee, KC; Anderson, TT; Bizios, R. Osteoblast population migration characteristics on substrates modified with immobilized adhesive peptides. *Biomaterials.*, 1999 Feb, 20(3), 221-7.
[81] Rupnick, MA; Stokes, CL; Williams, SK; Lauffenburger, DA. Quantitative analysis of random motility of human microvessel endothelial cells using a linear under-agarose assay. *Lab Invest.*, 1988 Sep, 59(3), 363-72.
[82] Orredson, SU; Knighton, DR; Scheuenstuhl, H; Hunt, TK. A quantitative in vitro study of fibroblast and endothelial cell migration in response to serum and wound fluid. *J Surg Res.*, 1983 Sep, 35(3), 249-58.
[83] Heit, B; Kubes, P. Measuring chemotaxis and chemokinesis: the under-agarose cell migration assay. *Sci STKE.*, 2003 Feb 18, 2003(170), PL5.
[84] Dunn, GA; Jones, GE. Cell motility under the microscope: Vorsprung durch Technik. *Nat Rev Mol Cell Biol.*, 2004 Aug, 5(8), 667-72.
[85] Bahnson, A; Athanassiou, C; Koebler, D; Qian, L; Shun, T; Shields, D, et al. Automated measurement of cell motility and proliferation. *BMC Cell Biol.*, 2005, 6(1), 19.
[86] Soon, L; Braet, F; Condeelis, J. Moving in the right direction-nanoimaging in cancer cell motility and metastasis. *Microsc Res Tech.*, 2007 Mar, 70(3), 252-7.
[87] Lee, J; Ishihara, A; Jacobson, K. The fish epidermal keratocyte as a model system for the study of cell locomotion. *Symp Soc Exp Biol.*, 1993, 47, 73-89.
[88] Kedrin, D; Wyckoff, J; Sahai, E; Condeelis, J; Segall, JE. Imaging tumor cell movement in vivo. *Curr Protoc Cell Biol.*, 2007 Jun, Chapter 19, Unit 19 7.
[89] Gligorijevic, B; Kedrin, D; Segall, JE; Condeelis, J; van Rheenen, J. Dendra2 photoswitching through the Mammary Imaging Window. *J Vis Exp.*, 2009(28).
[90] Kedrin, D; Gligorijevic, B; Wyckoff, J; Verkhusha, VV; Condeelis, J; Segall, JE; et al. Intravital imaging of metastatic behavior through a mammary imaging window. *Nat Methods.*, 2008 Dec, 5(12), 1019-21.
[91] Cooper, MS; D'Amico, LA; Henry, CA. Confocal microscopic analysis of morphogenetic movements. *Methods Cell Biol.*, 1999, 59, 179-204.
[92] Hardman, RC; Kullman, SW; Hinton, DE. Non invasive in vivo investigation of hepatobiliary structure and function in STII medaka (Oryzias latipes): methodology and applications. *Comp Hepatol.*, 2008, 7, 7.

[93] Kenny, PA; Lee, GY; Myers, CA; Neve, RM; Semeiks, JR; Spellman, PT; et al. The morphologies of breast cancer cell lines in three-dimensional assays correlate with their profiles of gene expression. *Mol Oncol.*, 2007 Jun, 1(1), 84-96.

[94] Gaedtke, L; Thoenes, L; Culmsee, C; Mayer, B; Wagner, E. Proteomic analysis reveals differences in protein expression in spheroid versus monolayer cultures of low-passage colon carcinoma cells. *J Proteome Res.*, 2007 Nov, 6(11), 4111-8.

[95] Timmins, NE; Maguire, TL; Grimmond, SM; Nielsen, LK. Identification of three gene candidates for multicellular resistance in colon carcinoma. *Cytotechnology*, 2004 Sep, 46(1), 9-18.

[96] Kunz-Schughart, LA; Kreutz, M; Knuechel, R. Multicellular spheroids: a three-dimensional in vitro culture system to study tumour biology. *Int J Exp Pathol.*, 1998 Feb, 79(1), 1-23.

[97] Mueller-Klieser, W. Three-dimensional cell cultures: from molecular mechanisms to clinical applications. *Am J Physiol.*, 1997 Oct, 273(4 Pt 1), C1109-23.

[98] Kelm, JM; Timmins, NE; Brown, CJ; Fussenegger, M; Nielsen, LK. Method for generation of homogeneous multicellular tumor spheroids applicable to a wide variety of cell types. *Biotechnol Bioeng.*, 2003 Jul 20, 83(2), 173-80.

[99] Timmins, NE; Nielsen, LK. Generation of multicellular tumor spheroids by the hanging-drop method. *Methods Mol Med.*, 2007, 140, 141-51.

[100] Xu, J; Ma, M; Purcell, WM. Characterisation of some cytotoxic endpoints using rat liver and HepG2 spheroids as in vitro models and their application in hepatotoxicity studies. II. Spheroid cell spreading inhibition as a new cytotoxic marker. *Toxicol Appl Pharmacol.*, 2003 Jun 1, 189(2), 112-9.

[101] Indovina, P; Rainaldi, G; Santini, MT. Hypoxia increases adhesion and spreading of MG-63 three-dimensional tumor spheroids. *Anticancer Res.*, 2008 Mar-Apr, 28(2A), 1013-22.

[102] Zamora, PO; Danielson, KG; Hosick, HL. Invasion of endothelial cell monolayers on collagen gels by cells from mammary tumor spheroids. *Cancer Res.*, 1980 Dec, 40(12), 4631-9.

[103] Price, PJ. Preparation and use fo rat-tail collagen. 1975.

[104] Del Duca, D; Werbowetski, T; Del Maestro, RF. Spheroid preparation from hanging drops: characterization of a model of brain tumor invasion. *J Neurooncol.*, 2004 May, 67(3), 295-303.

[105] Tamaki, M; McDonald, W; Amberger, VR; Moore, E; Del Maestro, RF. Implantation of C6 astrocytoma spheroid into collagen type I gels: invasive, proliferative, and enzymatic characterizations. *J Neurosurg.*, 1997 Oct, 87(4), 602-9.

[106] Steinsvag, SK; Laerum, OD; Bjerkvig, R. Interaction between rat glioma cells and normal rat brain tissue in organ culture. *J Natl Cancer Inst.*, 1985, 74, 1095-104.

[107] Helige, C; Smolle, J; Zellnig, G; Hartmann, E; Fink-Puches, R; Kerl, H; et al. Inhibition of K1735-M2 melanoma cell invasion in vitro by retinoic acid. *Clin Exp Metastasis*, 1993 Sep, 11(5), 409-18.

[108] Vatne, V; Fjellbirkeland, L; Litlekalsoey, J; Hoestmark, J. A human in vitro model of bladder tumor cell invasion. *Anticancer Res.*, 1998, 18, 3985-9.

[109] Gunther, S; Ruhe, C; Derikito, MG; Bose, G; Sauer, H; Wartenberg, M. Polyphenols prevent cell shedding from mouse mammary cancer spheroids and inhibit cancer cell invasion in confrontation cultures derived from embryonic stem cells. *Cancer Lett.*, 2007 May 18, 250(1), 25-35.

[110] Fjellbirkeland, L; Bjerkvig, R; Laerum, OD. Non-small-cell lung carcinoma cells invade human bronchial mucosa in vitro. *In Vitro Cell Dev Biol Anim.*, 1998 Apr, 34(4), 333-40.
[111] Bjerkvig, R; Laerum, OD; Mella, O. Glioma cell interactions with fetal rat brain aggregates in vitro and with brain tissue in vivo. *Cancer Res.*, 1986 Aug, 46(8), 4071-9.
[112] Mork, S; De Ridder, L; Laerum, OD. Invasive pattern and phenotypic properties of malignant neurogenic rats cells in vivo and in vitro. *Anticancer Res.*, 1982 Jan-Apr, 2(1-2), 1-9.
[113] Dittmer, A; Hohlfeld, K; Lutzkendorf, J; Muller, LP; Dittmer, J. Human mesenchymal stem cells induce E-cadherin degradation in breast carcinoma spheroids by activating ADAM10. *Cell Mol Life Sci.*, 2009, Jul 15.

In: Cytoskeleton: Cell Movement...
Editors: S. Lansing et al., pp. 127-137

ISBN: 978-1-60876-559-1
© 2010 Nova Science Publishers, Inc.

Chapter V

Centriole Duplication or DNA Replication - What Starts Earlier?

R. E. Uzbekov[1,2*] *and I. B. Alieva*[3**]

[1]Laboratory of Cell Biology and Electron Microscopy,
Faculty of Medicine, François Rabelais University,
2 Boulevard Tonnnelé, BP 3223, 37032 Tours, France.
[2]Faculty of Bioengineering and Bioinformatics, Moscow State University.
[3] Electron Microscopy Department, A.N. Belozersky Institute of Physical and Chemical Biology, Moscow State University, 119992 Moscow, Russia.

Abstract

Animal centrosome an organelle consists of centrioles and associated structures surrounded by pericentriolar material, is the major microtubule organizing center in interphase cell and spindle pole component in mitosis and indispensable organelle for cilia and flagella formation.

In diploid cells, the centrosome usually includes not more then two centrioles and since the number of centrosomes in the cell is determined by the number of centrioles, cells have developed effective mechanisms to control centriole formation and to tightly coordinate this process with DNA replication. Duplication of this organelle and chromosomes redoubling during DNA replication are two principal events of cell cycle in the course of cell division progression. The principal question is what starts earlier, the duplication of centrioles or DNA replication? During last five years, some proteins, which participate in the process of procentriole formation, were found, but temporal sequences of cell cycle events are not still fully investigated. Traditionally the time of centriole replication beginning denote like G_1/S or even S, although precise analysis was not ever undertaken.

In present study, the ultrastructural analysis of centrosomes from cells that were previously in one's lifetime observed after mitosis was used in combination with

---

[*] Corresponding authors: Email: rustuzbekov@aol.com
[**] E-mail: irina_alieva@belozersky.msu.ru

autoradiography of the same cells. PE cells were individually monitored after mitosis and procentriole appearance was detected by electron microscopy as soon as 5–6 h after mitosis. This period was 1–2 h shorter than minimal duration of G_1-phase in PE cell line. Ultrastructural serial sections analysis of centrosomes in the cells with known "cell cycle age" in combination with ^{3}H-thimidine autoradiography study of the same cells directly confirmed that centrioles duplication started earlier than cells entered in S-phase of cell cycle, i.e., preceded the DNA replication. The data were obtained showed that centriole duplication started before the beginning of DNA replication.

Keywords: Proteins, centrosome, centriole, centriole duplication, cell cycle, DNA replication.

Introduction

The centrioles are the basic structural components of the centrosome, which is the principal microtubule-organizing center in animal interphase and mitotic cells, organizing microtubule network and mitotic spindles during cell division. Although the centrioles are not directly involved in the microtubule nucleation centrosomal activity, they play an important role in determining the number of spindle poles during mitosis. It is principal function of centrioles because the spindle bipolarity needs precise quantity of centrioles, it's quantity is under the strong intercellular control. Process of centriole duplication by analogy to the process of DNA doubling is often called "replication", because the new copy of this organelle is usually formed close to already existing centriole. As it has been shown earlier for DNA [2, 3], "replication" of centrioles is semi-conservative; experiments with biotinilated tubulin injection in cells have shown that each daughter cell gets one "old" centriole and one newly formed centriole [4]. However, the mechanisms of DNA replication and "replication" of centrioles are essentially different so we will use the term "centriole duplication" instead of "centriole replication".

Centriolar cylinders can appear in the cell in two ways. First, new centriolar cylinders can arise *de novo* without direct connection with already existing centriole [5–8]. Alternatively, they appear near the surface of pre-existing centrioles or basal bodies, that is characteristic for the majority of cell types. Process of centriole duplication has no analogous mechanisms; the new copy is created not along with the old one, but perpendicular to it. Moreover, a small distance filled by fine fibrillar material is always present between the mother and daughter centriolar cylinders [9].

Near each parent centrioles only one new centriolar cylinder usually appears (Figure. 1); Gall proposed to name it the "procentriole" [9]. In the majority of cells, the number of centriolar cylinders corresponds to the number of genome copies (ploidy): in diploid cell in G_1 phase of cell cycle there are two centrioles, and in tetraploid cell in G_2-phase, four centrioles [10]. This accordance maintains to a certain extent for polyploid cells, too [11]. In contrast to DNA, whose doubling can be revealed by the inclusion of labelled precursors, just the beginning of centrioles doubling can be shown reliably only by electron microscopy but not immunofluorescence which can recognize more advanced stages of procentriole formation. The data about centriole ultrastructure in cells of different stages of a cell cycle allowed correlating events of the cell cycle and of the centriolar cycle [10, 12]. Stubblefield proposed to subdivide the centriolar cycle into the phases of maturation, reproduction and separation of centrioles [12]. Robbins with co-authors [10] for the first time described the basic events of centriolar cycle of somatic cells and found that the first structural reorganization of centrosome structure occurred in early G_1-phase, when centrioles loose the typical for mitotic cells mutual-perpendicular orientation. These authors added the phase of "disorientation" in description of centrosome cycle. Unlike the phases of a nuclear cycle replacing each other, the phases of centriolar cycle are usually overlapped. In particular, in significant part of cell types the centrioles separate simultaneously or just after the disorientation phase in early G_1-phase [13]; in other cell types, the separation occurs after the beginning of duplication centrioles, i.e. during the phase of maturation [14].

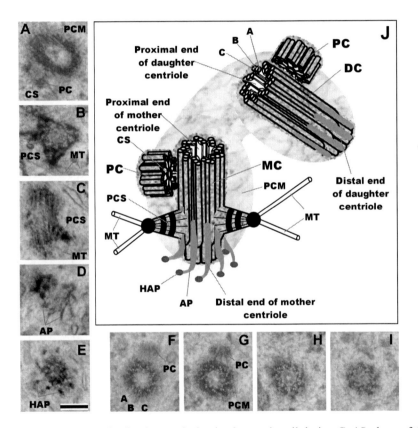

Figure 1. The centrosome organization in a typical animal somatic cell during G_1 / S-phase of the cell cycle. **A-I** – Centrosome ultrastructure (electron microscopy images); **J** – simplified scheme (the primary cilium and striated rootlets are not shown). **A-E** – selected sections through the maternal centrioles; **F-I** – serial sections through the daughter centriole. *Scale bar, 0.2 µm.* Mothers (maternal) (**MC**) and daughter (**DC**) centrioles are surrounded by a pericentriolar material (=pericentriolar matrix) (**PCM**); procentriole (**PC**) with catrtwheel structure (axis with spokes) (**CS**) is forming near the proximal end of the maternal centriole. Pericentriolar satellites (=sub-distal appendages) (**PCS**) with attached microtubules (**MT**) and appendages (=distal appendages) (**AP**) are localized on the maternal centriole; **HAP** – head of appendage. The wall of centrioles are built of nine microtubule blades, and in high animals each blade is formed by a microtubule triplet; **A** – microtubule of triplet; **B** – microtubule of triplet; **C** – microtubule of triplet. © Reproduced with permission Elsevier B.V., from [1] with modifications.

The principal question of nuclear and centriolar cycles is what starts earlier, the duplication of centrioles or DNA replication? Different authors do not have the common opinion. Robbins with co-authors showed that in synchronized HeLa cell fraction with 20% cells in S-phase, centriole duplication at the early stages was detected in 65–70% of cells [10]. It means that at least in part of the cells, centriole duplication started in G_1. On the other hand, in one of the classical works on the ultrastructural analysis of centriolar cycle in PE cells, procentrioles were found only during S-phase of cell cycle [15].

Independence of the beginning of centrioles duplication from DNA synthesis was shown experimentally [16, 17]. The principal mechanism of cellular regulation of centrioles doubling was described in [18–20]. However, no detailed studies of the succession of nuclear and centriolar events in cells with known "age" in a cell cycle have been performed yet. In the present study, the ultrastructural analysis of centrosomes on serial sections of cells that were previously observed after mitosis was used in combination with autoradiography study of the same cells; the data show that centriole duplication in PE cells can start before the beginning of DNA duplication.

Material and Methods

Cell culture. Cell line PE (SPEV; pig kidney of embryonic age) was obtained from the Russian collection of cell cultures (RCCC, St. Petersburg). Cells were cultured at 37°C in 5% of CO_2 atmosphere in cell culture "Medium 199" supplemented with 10% embryonic calf serum (Vector, Russia) and antibiotics. For experiments, cells were plated on coverslips and cultured in Petri dishes.

Live cells observation. For live-cell observation a special camera was constructed. The camera volume was 1.25 ml; 25-mm coverslips forming top and bottom of the camera were strictly parallel, to allow for high-quality phase contrast (objective Plan-Neofluar 40/0.9, Opton, Germany). During the observations and recordings, orange filter was used, and the temperature of the microscope stage was kept constant at 37°C. Cells were photographed using MFN-12 photo equipment 2–3 times during mitosis, and subsequently once an hour until fixation.

Autoradiography and electron microscopy. For autoradiography, cells were cultured in the full medium containing [^{3}H] thymidine (400 kBq/ml) during one hour before fixation. Then cells were fixed in 2.5% glutaraldehyde (Fluka, Germany) in phosphate buffer (pH 7.4), postfixed with OsO_4 (Agar Scientific LTD, UK), dehydrated in ethanol and acetone, and embedded in EPON-812 resin according to a standard technique. After polymerization of the resin, coverslips were removed from the blocks in liquid nitrogen and the surfaces of blocks were covered (under a weak red light) with photo emulsion of type "M" (NIIKhIMFOTOPROEKT, Russia). Several control samples of the same block containing individually monitored cells were covered by photo emulsion simultaneously with the sample, for determination an optimal time of exposition, which was found to be 10 days. In developed autographs, experimental cells were then located and photographed by means of the light microscope equipped by phase-contrast system. Serial ultra thin sections (70 nm) of these cells were obtained using ultramicrotomes LKB-III and LKB-V (LKB, Sweden).

Sections were mounted on single slot grids with Formwar film and were additionally contrasted by incubation in aqueous solution of 4% uranyl acetate and in lead citrate. Samples were investigated and photographed using electron microscope HU-11, HU-12 (Hitachi, Japan) or Philips CM-12 (Netherlands).

Results

The detailed ultrastructural analysis of the cells monitored after mitosis has shown that centriole duplication starts much earlier than it could be expected on the basis of results of the previous study of PE cells [15], even if the duration of a G_1-phase in these cells was minimal. The present work was initiated by the previous study, which showed an unusually early beginning of the centriole duplication (6 h after mitosis) in control sister cells with intact centrosomes [21]. A detailed monitoring of cells after the end of mitosis performed in the present study has confirmed the results obtained in [21]. In the first series of experiments, 19 cells were monitored individually and used for the ultrastructural analysis. In cells fixed at 3–4 h (5 cells) and 4 h–4 h 40 min (5 cells) after the beginning of anaphase, replicated centrioles were never found.

For the first time the beginning of procentriole growth near the proximal ends of mother centrioles was detected in the cell fixed 5 h 6 min after the beginning of anaphase, i.e., less than 5 h after the end of mitosis. In all investigated cells fixed 5–6 h (4 cells) and 6 h–7 h 10 min after mitosis (5 cells) the short procentrioles were found. Thus, according to these experiments, duplication of centrioles starts at least 1–2 h prior to the beginning of DNA replication, which for PE cells begins not earlier than 7 h (10 h in the average) after mitosis [22].

However, all these results, as well as the data of previous works, are indirect. Theoretically, it cannot be excluded that investigated cells had an abnormally short G_1-phase. For the direct verification of the obtained data, the experiments with parallel evaluation of the "age in cell cycle" by means of vital monitoring, the assessment of the phase of a cell cycle by autoradiography, and the ultrastructural analysis of centrosome in the same cells were carried out. Live cells were monitored and fixed at 5 h 48 min to 8 h 50 min (9 cells) after mitosis. None of the nine individually monitored cells incorporated ^{3}H-thymidine in their nucleus, i.e., all of them were in G_1-phase at the moment of fixation. Three out of these cells were used for the ultrastructural analysis. In all of them procentrioles were found near the parent centrioles (Figure. 2). Thus, the data of direct experiment have confirmed a hypothesis that duplication centrioles in cells PE can precede DNA replication.

Interestingly, the length of procentrioles in all investigated cells did not exceed 100 nm, i.e., noticeable lengthening of procentrioles did not occur during G_1-phase. We did not found any clear correlation between the cell age and the length of procentrioles; procentrioles in more "advanced" (within a cell cycle) cells often were shorter than in "younger" cells. At the same time, in spite of the fact that the majority of procentrioles were 75–95 nm in length, in three cells the procentrioles were shorter than 50 nm. Analisys of ultrastrucure can possibility to describe three phases of initial events of centriole replication (Figure. 3). During first phase dense disc appeared near surface of mother centriole, later this disc moved away from the surface of centriole, during this phase the central hub of catrtwheel structure was clearly visible, and the process of procentriole elongation was started later. During all phases young newborn procentriole connected with mother centriole by filamentous material (Figure. 3).

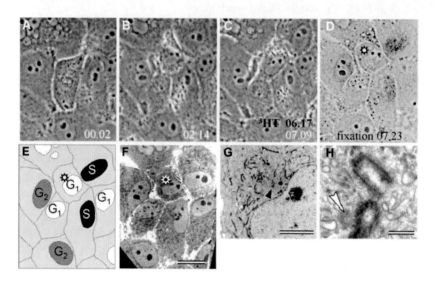

Figure 2. Autoradiography study of cells and centrosome ultrastructure 7 h 23 min after the beginning of anaphase. **A–C** - Live cells observation; time after anaphase of mitosis is shown on the photos and the time of [^{3}H] thymidine addition to the culture medium is also indicated on **C**. **D** - Cells after fixation and autoradiography development, time period from anaphase of mitosis to fixation is shown. **E** - Scheme of cells contours corresponding to phase contrast (**D**) and low magnification EM (**F**); letters on cell nuclei designate a phase of a cell cycle. **G, H** - The centrosome region at intermediate and high magnification. Asterisk (**D-F**) designates the cell whose centrosome was further studied; the arrowhead (**G**) shows a centrosome region, and the arrow (**H**) points to a young procentriole. *Scale bar, 20 μm* (**A-F**), *4 μm* (**G**), *and 0.2 μm* (**H**). © Reproduced with permission Pleiades Publishing, Ltd, from [23] with modifications.

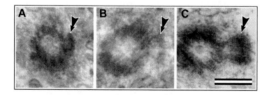

Figure 3. Ultrastructure of centrosome during the second half of G$_1$-phase of a cell cycle. Early stages of centriole duplication. A-C – stages of procentriole (arrow) formation near the proximal end of parent centriole. *Scale bar, 0.2 μm.* © Reproduced with permission Pleiades Publishing, Ltd, from [23] with modifications.

Discussion

For a better understanding of centrosomal cycle and other intracellular processes, a combination of morphological and biochemical approaches is necessary. Biochemical mechanisms of the regulation of centrioles duplication were discovered independently in three laboratories [18–20]. The basic stages of this process are the following. In the second half of G_1 restriction point (R-point) a cell "decides" whether to enter the next mitosis or not. At that moment, a complex of the biochemical reactions starts. These reactions depend on a number of factors, such as cell size, the presence of external growth factors and other conditions of cell growth, and on the cell interactions with surrounding cells. The complex of Cyclin D/CDK 4/6 phosphorylates the protein pRB. This protein loses the ability to connect with factors of activation of transcription EF2. Released factor EF2 activates the synthesis of cyclins E and A that leads to the beginning of centriole duplication [18–20]. As these signal cyclins molecules which are responsible for centriole duplication appear in the cell cycle near R-point, that is prior to the beginning of replication, it is possible to assume that procentriole formation occurs in G_1 too. Another direction of modern investigations is search of initial structures and key proteins involved in centriole assembly [24-32]. Recently, it has been shown that in *C. elegans* centriole formation is triggered by a signal mediated by several key molecules, including ZYG-1 causes the recruitment of SAS5 and SAS6, resulting in the assembly of an intermediate precursor form of the centriole [24]. Then, nine sets of microtubules are organized onto the precursor to organize the centriolar barrel in a SAS4-dependent manner [25, 26]. Despite some morphological variations of the centriole, functional homologs of most of these molecules have been identified in some other species, suggesting that the basic mechanism of centriole biogenesis is common among diverse organisms [27-32].

Location of key regulators in centrosome gives the reason to believe that centrosome is the site of the cell "decision" to pass restriction point and to continue cell cycle. In the present work, a comparative study of nuclear and centrosomal cycles in PE cells has been carried out. The obtained results are in a good agreement with the data obtained on HeLa cells [10] and L929 cells [16], but differ from the data obtained on PE cells earlier [15]. However, in last cited paper cell cycle stages of analysed cells were determined exclusively on the basis of autoradiography without monitoring live cells after mitosis. Therefore, cells in late G_1-phase could be excluded from the analyzed group in this work [15]. At the earliest stages the procentrioles are clearly visible only on sections that have well turned orientation; the length of early procentrioles we found out was even shorter then 50 µm (Figure. 3), which could be invisible at other orientation of the section. The first description of the earliest stages of procentriole formation was made by Sorokin in chick duodenal epithelial cells [6]. The morphology of second phase of procentrioles formation in PE cells is practically identical to this description (Figure. 3 in [6] and Figure. 3b in the present paper). On the other hand, we found more early initial stage, when an electron-dense "primiry disc" formed near the surface of the parent centrioles, which is precursor of catrtwheel structure of procentriole (Figure. 3a).

Further, the newborn procentriole formed at the distance about 50 nm from surface of parent centriole with annular structure accompanied with visible "antrum" appearance in the central part of centriole (Figure. 4 in [6] and Figure. 3b in the present paper). In summary, there are grounds to assume that once a cell reaches a restriction point, the centriole duplication process can be activated at a certain period of cell cycle, starting from the second half of G_1-phase. PE cell line is not an exception in this regard, and the dynamics of the procentriole occurrence generally coincides with that in HeLa [10] and L929 cells [16].

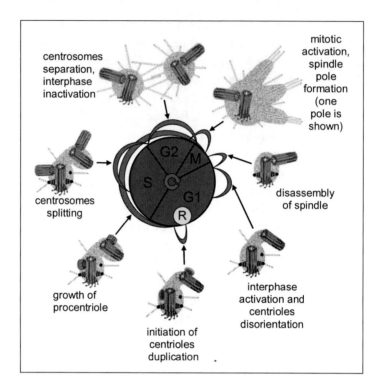

Figure 4. Centrosomal and nuclear cycles correlation in mammalian cell. **G1, S, G2** and **M** (mitosis) — cell cycle phases, **R** — restriction point (R-point). Reproduced with permission, © *Tsitologiia* from [40] with modifications.

It should be noted that centrosome intactness plays a key role in the cell cycle progression. A damage or removal of centrioles at various phases of cell cycle may have various consequences. If centrioles were damaged by a microirradiation in anaphase of mitosis, cells could finish division [33] but never reached S-phase [34]. However, if centrioles were destroyed by a laser microirradiation after transition of a restriction point (synchronization by hydroxyurea between G_1-and S-phase during the time period equivalent to 1.5 cell cycles), new centrioles formed *de novo* similarly to their formation in mouse blastomers [35]. Such cells were capable to continue cell cycle and to enter mitosis. The results of the present work can explain, why cells synchronized by hydroxyurea (or aphidicolin) were capable to continue centriolar cycle [17] and even to re-establish the destroyed centriolar cylinders [35]. As these cells have already passed a restriction point, cytoplasm of these cells already possessed the factors necessary for centriole duplication, irrespective of whether replication DNA proceeds or not. Restoration of centrioles after microirradiation [35] is one of the proofs that reproductive ability of centrioles is not directly correlated with their triplet structure. Transfer of the information about triplet structure can occur not only through the deuterosomes (ciliogenesis), but also through other cytoplasm precursors that have no centriolar structure, as it takes place during oogenesis and embryogenesis. We reported here that lengthening of procentrioles over 100 nm did not occur during G_1-phase. This corresponds to the results of Gorgidze and Vorobjev [36] who found that in cytoplasts, i.e., in cells with removed nuclei, new procentrioles could appear, but their lengthening was not detected. On the contrary, if cell cycle was experimentally blocked in mitosis, the lengthening of centrioles did occur so that their length exceeded their normal size [37, 38]. According to our data the scheme of mutual relation between centriolar and nuclear cycles looks as follows (Figure. 4). As opposed to cell (nuclear) cycle, the centrosome cycle phases can be overlapped and even can be absent. For example, the centrosome splitting phases are absent if centrioles are separated on the long distance in G_1, and the centrosomes separation phase is replaced by phase of centrosomes rapprochement, if centrioles are separated on the distance excees the size of mitotic spindle [39].

Thus, it may be concluded that restriction point is the point of coordination of cell (nuclear) and centrosome cycles. The complex of external and internal signals triggers centriole duplication that serve a morphological criterion of cell transition through the restriction point from the G_1-post-mitotical (G_1-pm) to the G_1-presynthetical (G_1-ps) phases [41]. However, the procentriole growth stops at a certain stage, since the cell enters S-phase. If DNA replication is normal, cell "allows" the continuation of centriole elongation process. Further on, after the end of DNA replication, centrosomes receive a signal for the separation and formation of the poles of mitotic spindle.

Acknowledgments

The authors are grateful to I.I. Kireev and S.V. Uzbekova for helpful discussion, and to Yu.A. Komarova, for valuable technical advice concerning autoradiography analysis.

This work was supported by the Russian Foundation for Basic Research (grants No. 06-04-49233 and 09-04-00363).

References

[1] Uzbekov, R. E. & Prigent C. (2007). Clockwise or anticlockwise? Turning the centriole triplets in the right direction! *FEBS Lett.*, *581*, 1251-1254.

[2] Taylor, J. H., Woods, P. S. & Hughes, W. L. (1957). The Organization and Duplication of Chromosomes As Revealed by Autoradiographic Studies Using Tritium-Labeled Thymidine. *Proc. Nat. Acad. Sci. USA*, *43*, 122-128.

[3] Meselson, M. & Stahl, F. W. (1958). The Replication of DNA in *Escherichia coli*. *Proc. Nat. Acad. Sci.*, USA, *44*, 671-682.

[4] Kochanski, R. S. & Borisy, G. G. (1990). Mode of Centriole Duplication and Distribution. *J. Cell Biol.*, *110*, 1599-1605.

[5] Dirksen, E. R. (1961). The Presence of Centrioles in Artificially Activated Sea Urchin Eggs. *J. Biophys. Biochem. Cytol.*, *11*, 244-247.

[6] Sorokin, S. P. (1968). Reconstructions of Centriole Formation and Ciliogenesis in Mammalian Lungs. *J. Cell Sci.*, *3*, 207-230.

[7] Szollosi, D. (1964). The Structure and Function of Centrioles and Their Satellites in the Jellyfish *Phialidium gregarium*. *J. Cell Biol.*, *21*, 465-479.

[8] Krioutchkova, M. M. & Onishchenko, G. E. (1999). Structural and Functional Characteristics of the Centrosome in Gametogenesis and Early Embryogenesis of Animals. *Int. Rev. Cytol., 185*, 107-156.

[9] Gall, J. G. (1961). Centriole Replication. A Study of Spermatogenesis in the Snail *Viviparus. J. Biophys. Biochem. Cytol., 10*, 163-193.

[10] Robbins, E., Jentzsch, G. & Micali, A. (1968). The Centriole Cycle in Synchronized Hela Cells *J. Cell Biol., 36*, 329-339.

[11] Onishchenko, G. E. (1978). Correlation between the Number of Centrioles and Ploidy of Mouse Liver Hepatocytes. *Tsitologiya, 20(4)*, 395-399.

[12] Stubblefield, E. (1968). Centriole Replication in a Mammalian Cell, The Proliferation and Spread of Neoplastic Cells. A Collection of Papers Presented at the 21 Annual (1967) Symposium on Fundamental Cancer Reseach, Baltimore: The Williams and Wilkins Co., 175-193.

[13] Komarova, Yu. A., Ryabov, E. V., Alieva, I. B., Uzbekov, R. E., Uzbekova, S. V. and Vorobjev, I. A. (1997). Polyclonal Antibodies against Human Gamma-Tubulin Stain Centrioles in Mammalian Cells from Different Tissues. *Membr. Cell Biol., 10*(5), 503-513.

[14] Uzbekov, R., Kireev, I. & Prigent, C. (2002). Centrosome Separation: Respective Role of Microtubules and Actin Filaments. *Biol. Cell., 9(4-5)*, 275-288.

[15] Vorobjev, I. A. & Chentsov, Yu.S. (1982). Centrioles in the Cell Cycle. I. Epithelial Cells, *J. Cell Biol., 98*, 938-949.

[16] Rattner, J. B. & Phillips, G. (1973). Independence of Centriole Formation and DNA Synthesis. *J. Cell Biol., 57*, 359-372.

[17] Balczon, B., Bao, L., Zimmer, W. E., Brown, K., Zinkowski, R. P. & Brinkley, B. R. (1995). Dissociation of Centrosome Replication Events from Cycles of DNA Synthesis and Mitotic Division in Hydroxyurea-Arrested Chinese Hamster Ovary Cells. *J. Cell. Biol., 130*, 105-115.

[18] Hinchcliffe, E. H., Li C., Thompson, E. A., Maller, J. L. & Sluder, G. (1999). Requirement of Cdk2-Cyclin E Activity for Repeated Centrosome Reproduction in *Xenopus* Egg Extracts, *Science, 283*, 851-854.

[19] Lacey, K. R., Jackson, P. K. & Stearns, T. (1999). Cyclin-Dependent Kinase Control of Centrosome Duplication, *Proc. Natl. Acad. Sci. USA, 96(6)*, 2817-2822.

[20] Meraldi, P., Lukas, J., Fry, A. M., Bartek, J. & Nigg, E. A. (1999). Centrosome Duplication in Mammalian Somatic Cells Requires E2F and Cdk2-Cyclin A. *Nat. Cell Biol., 1*, 88-93.

[21] Uzbekov, R. E. & Vorob'ev, I. A. (1992). The Effect of the UV Microirradiation of the Centrosome on Cell Behavior. III. The Ultrastructure of the Centrosome after Irradiation. *Tsitologiya, 34(2)*, 62-67.

[22] Sakharov, V. N. & Voronkova, L. N. (1993). The Kinetics of the Transition to DNA Synthesis in the Cell Cycle of Sister Cells of the ESK Line in Culture. *Tsitologiya, 35(6-7)*, 79-85.

[23] Uzbekov, R. E. (2007). Centriole Duplication in PE (SPEV) cells starts before the beginning of the DNA replication. *Biochemistry (Moscow) Supplement Series A: Membranes and cell Biology, 1(3)*, 206-211.

[24] O'Connell, K. F., Caron, C., Kopish, K. R., Hurd, D. D., Kemphues, K. J. & White, J. G. (2001). The C. elegans zyg-1 gene encodes a regulator of centrosome duplication with distinct maternal and paternal roles in the embryo. *Cell, 10*, 547-558.

[25] Delattre, M., Canard, C. & Gonczy, P. (2006). Sequential protein recruitment in C. elegans centriole formation. *Curr Biol., 16*, 1844-1849.

[26] Pelletier, L., O'Toole, E., Schwager, A., Hyman, A. A. & Muller-Reichert, T. (2006). Centriole assembly in Caenorhabditis elegans. *Nature, 444*, 619-623.

[27] Bettencourt-Dias, M. & Glover, D. M. (2007). Centrosome biogenesis and function: centrosomics brings new understanding. *Nat Rev Mol Cell Biol, 8*, 451-463.

[28] Azimzadeh, J. & Bornens, M. (2007). Structure and duplication of the centrosome. *J Cell Sci., 120(Pt 13)*, 2139-2142.

[29] Bornens, M. & Azimzadeh, J. (2007). Origin and evolution of the centrosome. *Adv Exp Med Biol., 607*, 119-129.

[30] Strnad, P. & Gonczy, P. (2008). Mechanisms of procentriole formation. *Trends Cell Biol., 18*, 389-396.

[31] Loncarek, J., Hergert, P., Magidson, V. & Khodjakov, A. (2008). Control of daughter centriole formation by the pericentriolar material. *Nat Cell Biol., 10(3)*, 322-328.

[32] Loncarek, J. & Khodjakov, A. (2009). Ab ovo or de novo *Mol Cells, 27(2)*, 135-142.

[33] Uzbekov, R. E., Votchal, M. S. & Vorobjev, I. A. (1995). Role of the Centrosome in Mitosis: UV Microirradiation Study. *J. Photochem. Photobiol. B., 29*, 163-170.

[34] Neverova, A. L., Uzbekov, R. E., Votchal, M. S. & Vorob'ev, I. A. (1996). The Effect of Ultraviolet Microbeam Irradiation of the Centrosome on Cellular Behavior. IV. Synthetic Activity, Cell Spreading and Growth with an Inactivated Centrosome. *Tsytologiya, 38(2)*, 145-154.

[35] Khodjakov, A., Rieder, C. L., Sluder, G., Cassels, G., Sibon, O. & Wang, C. L. (2002). De novo Formation of Centrosomes in Vertebrate Cells Arrested during S Phase. *J. Cell Biol., 158*, 1171-1181.

[36] Gorgidze, L. A. & Vorobjev, I. A. (1994). Centrioles Can Replicate in Cultured Cells in the Absence of a Nucleus. *Tsitologiya, 36(8)*, 837-843.

[37] Alieva, I. B. & Vorobjev, I. A. (1991). Induction of Multipolar Mitoses in Cultured Cells: Decay and Restructuring of the Mitotic Apparatus and Distribution of Centrioles, *Chromosoma, 100(8)*, 532-542.

[38] Azimzadeh, J., Hergert, P., Delouvée, A., Euteneuer, U., Formstecher, E., Khodjakov, A. & Bornens, M. (2009). hPOC5 is a centrin-binding protein required for assembly of full-length centrioles. *J Cell Biol., 185(1)*, 101-114.

[39] Uzbekov, R., Kireev, I. & Prigent, C. (2002). Centrosome separation: respective role of microtubules and actin filaments. *Biol.Cell., 94(4-5)*, 275-288.

[40] Uzbekov, R. E. & Alieva, I. B. (2008). The Centrosome - a riddle of the "Cell Processor". *Tsitologiya, 50(2)*, 91-112.

[41] Zetterberg, A. & Larsson, O. (1995). Cell Cycle Progression and Cell Growth in Mammalian Cells: Kinetic Aspects of Transition Events. In C. Hutchison, & D. M. Glover, (Eds.), *Cell Cycle Control*, (206-227). Oxford: IRL Press at Oxford Univpress.

In: Cytoskeleton: Cell Movement...
Editors: S. Lansing et al., pp. 139-147

ISBN: 978-1-60876-559-1
© 2010 Nova Science Publishers, Inc.

Chapter VI

The Myosin Light Chain-IQGAP Interaction: What is its Function?

David J Timson[*]
School of Biological Sciences, Queen's University Belfast,
Medical Biology Centre, 97 Lisburn Road, Belfast, BT9 7BL. UK.

Abstract

The first members of the IQGAP family of proteins were characterised over 15 years ago. It is now known that these molecules act at the interface between cellular signalling pathways and the actin cytoskeleton. They bind to a diverse range of signalling molecules – including those involved in calcium, GTPase, kinase and growth factor signalling. One intriguing interaction is that between mammalian IQGAP1 and the myosin essential light chain isoform, Mlc1sa. Although this has been demonstrated *in vitro*, its *in vivo* role is not known. Indeed, it would be tempting to dismiss it as an experimental artefact, except for the existence of a parallel interaction in the budding yeast, *Saccharomyces cerevisae*. In this organism, the IQGAP-like protein (Iqg1p) interacts with a myosin essential light chain (Mlc1p). This interaction is critical for the correct execution of cytokinesis. IQGAP-like proteins also play key roles in cytokinesis in other fungi. Recent work implicating mammalian IQGAP1 in cytokinesis may help explain the role of the interaction in higher eukaryotes.

Introduction: The IQGAP Family of Proteins

The first member of this family of proteins to be identified was human IQGAP1 [1,2]. The protein was named due to the presence of two types of sequence motif – calmodulin binding IQ-motifs and a CDC42 binding RasGAP-like domain [1,2]. Although most GAPs (<u>G</u>TPase <u>a</u>ccelerating <u>p</u>roteins) enhance the rate of GTP hydrolysis by their respective

---

[*]Corresponding author: Email: d.timson@qub.ac.uk, Telephone: +44(0)28 9097 5875, Fax: +44(0)28 9097 5877.

GTPase protein partners, IQGAP1 has been shown, experimentally, to inhibit the GTPase activity of CDC42, Rac1 and Rap1 [1-4]. Following the discovery of human IQGAP1, two more human isoforms have been identified – IQGAP2 [5] and IQGAP3 [6,7]. Proteins with similar sequences have been identified in various fungi including the budding yeast, *Saccharomyces cerevisiae* [8-10], the fission yeast, *Schitzosaccharomyces pombe* [11], the pathogen *Candida albicans* [12] and the filamentous fungus *Ashbya gossypii* [13]. In addition similar proteins have been characterised in a range of eukaryotic organisms, including *Hydra vulgaris* [14], the sea urchin *Hemicentrotus pulcherrimus* [15], the slime mould *Dictyostelium discoideum* [16] and the amphibian *Xenopus laevis* [17].

The main function of the IQGAP family is to act as an interface between cellular signalling pathways and the cytoskeleton [18-21]. A diverse range of signalling molecules have been shown to interact with human IQGAPs. These include small GTPases (CDC42, Rac1, Rap1) [1-4,22,23], kinases (ERK1, MEK1, MEK2 and B-Raf) [24-26], a kinase scaffold (AKAP79) [27], a growth factor receptor (VEGFR2) [28] and calcium sensors (calmodulin, S100B) [29-33]. IQGAPs influence the actin cytoskeleton directly through a calponin homology domain (CHD) at the N-terminus of the molecules. Interaction with actin at this site promotes actin filament bundling [34-37]. In addition, indirect interactions may be mediated *via* another protein which acts at the signalling-cytoskeleton interface, N-WASP [38] and there is also evidence that IQGAP1 plays a role in the regulation of microtubules through the proteins CLIP-170 and APC [39,40]. IQGAPs also influence cell-cell adhesion in multicellular eukaryotes through calcium-calmodulin dependent interactions with E-cadherin [41-44]. The proteins' involvement in cytoskeletal reorganisation, cell movement and cell adhesion mean that they are key players in tumour cell development and metastasis [45-49].

Calmodulin and S100B are believed to interact with IQGAP1, primarily through four IQ-motifs which occur approximately in the middle of the primary sequence [31-33]. IQ-motifs are found in a wide range of eukaryotic proteins, including most myosins. The consensus sequence is IQXXXRGXXXR, although there is considerable variation possible [50]. The motif adopts an α-helical conformation and mediates interaction with calmodulin and closely related proteins such as myosin light chains [51]. The presence of four IQ-motifs in IQGAP1 means that there is the possibility of binding four calmodulin molecules at once. This calmodulin:IQGAP1 stoichiometry is believed to be controlled by the concentration of calcium ions – although the precise details of this are the subject of debate [31,32].

Myosin light chains were first identified as components of muscle myosins and are divided into two groups – the essential light chains (ELC) and the regulatory light chains (RLC). These proteins bind to the myosin heavy chain, wrapping themselves around two IQ-motifs in an extended, α-helical region of the molecule [51]. Their role is to strengthen this region of the molecule and to provide sites for the regulation and modulation of the activity of the myosin motor [52-55].

The IQGAP-Myosin Light Chain Interaction

For many years, it was believed that the ELC was restricted to interacting only with myosin heavy chains and actin. However, one particular isoform of the ELC, Mlc1sa, has been shown to interact with IQGAP1 [56,57]. The interaction was predicted on the basis of the similarity of the first IQ-motif in IQGAP1 to the ELC binding site in skeletal muscle myosin [56]. This interaction has been demonstrated *in vitro* by yeast two hydrid experiments, pull downs and gel shift assays [56,57]. These gel shift assays, using peptides corresponding to the four IQ-motifs of human IQGAP1 demonstrate that only the first IQ-motif is the binding site for Mlc1sa [57]. To date, the interaction has not been demonstrated *in vivo* nor has any functional role been assigned to it in mammals.

The Iqg1p-Mlc1p Interaction in Budding Yeast and its Role in Cytokinesis

Saccharomyces cerevisae has proteins which show similarity to IQGAP1 and Mlc1sa. These are Iqg1p and Mlc1p, respectively. Consequently, this model organism has been used to study the *in vivo* roles of the IQGAP family of proteins. It has been shown, in this organism, that Iqg1p and Mlc1p interact both *in vitro* and *in vivo* [10,58-64]. Disruption of this interaction (eg by deletion of the IQ-motifs of Iqg1p) results in defects in cytokinesis [10,64]. Cytokinesis requires a precise stoichiometric ratio of Iqg1p and Mlc1p: while overexpression of Iqg1p results in failure of cytokinesis, this can be rescued by overexpression of Mlc1p [64]. The role of Mlc1p is to target Iqg1p to the bud neck and then to recruit a myosin II (Myo1p) [59,65]. This myosin provides the contractile force which results in the separation of the bud from the mother cell [66]. Following completion of cytokinesis, Iqg1p undergoes ubquitin-mediated proteolysis [67].

The Role of IQGAP-like Proteins in Cytokinesis in Other Fungi

In *S. pombe* a myosin light chain, Cdc4p, interacts with an IQGAP-like protein, Rng2p [68]. Rng2p is required for cytokinesis in this organism and this process, like in *S. cerevisiae* involves precise, sequential interactions between this IQGAP-like protein and various partners, including Cdc4p [11,69,70]. Direct interaction between Cdc4p and Rng4p has been demonstrated by co-immunoprecipitation experiments [68]. However, the precise sequence of events is different to *S. cerevisiae* and Cdc4p-Rng2p co-localisation appears to persist throughout cytokinesis [70]. Of course, co-localisation does not necessarily mean that the proteins are interacting directly and, given that a myosin II also co-localises with Rng2p [70], alternative binding partners are also present.

In *C. albicans*, phosphorylation of the IQGAP-like protein, Iqg1, at multiple serine and threonine residues by cyclin dependent kinases is critical for the correct regulation of cytokinesis [12]. In *A. gossipii*, the IQGAP-like protein Cyk1 is present at the site of septation and forms part of the contractile ring [13,71].

The Role of the IQGAP-Mlc1sa Interaction in Mammals

No equivalent, functional role for the IQGAP-ELC interaction has been established in mammals. Indeed for many years it was not certain whether, or not, IQGAP played a role in cytokinesis in these organisms. However, recent work has shown conclusively that mammalian IQGAP1 is implicated in cytokinesis. Examination of the localisation of IQGAP1 in mouse oocytes showed that the protein has a cytoplasmic localisation in maturing cells, but is concentrated at the contractile ring in dividing ones [72]. Experiments with toxin B (which irreversibly inactivates CDC42 by glycosylating it and preventing exchange of GDP for GTP [73]) disrupted this relocalisation of IQGAP1, suggesting that CDC42 acts upstream of IQGAP1 in this process [72]. Our understanding of the role of IQGAP proteins in mammalian cytokinesis is still at an early stage. Whether, or not, a myosin light chain- IQGAP interaction is involved has yet to be determined. However, given its role in budding yeast, it would be worthwhile determining if such an interaction occurs in mammalian cells and, assuming it does, how disruption of the interaction affects cytokinesis. If such an interaction is shown to be important it would help unify the studies in yeast and mammals, thus increasing the utility of yeast as a model organism in this area of research. If, however, the interaction is shown not to occur (or not to be important in cytokinesis) it would raise interesting evolutionary questions about the loss and gain of functions by the IQGAP family of proteins.

In addition to a role in cytokinesis, human IQGAP1 has also been implicated in phagocytosis. Interactions with the diaphanous-related formin protein, Dia1, are required for the colocalisation of both proteins to the phagocytoic cup [74]. Interestingly, the founder member of this family of proteins, the *Drosophila melanogaster* protein diaphanous, is required for cytokinesis in this organism [75]. This suggests that the interaction between human IQGAP1 and Dia1 may be important in cytokinesis as well as phagocytosis.

Conclusion

The role of the Mlc1sa-IQGAP1 interaction in mammals is unclear. However the requirement for the homologous interaction in budding yeast cytokinesis combined with recent work showing that mammalian IQGAP1 is involved in cytokinesis, makes it reasonable to hypothesise that the interaction has a similar role in mammals. We await experimental evidence for (or against) this proposition.

Acknowledgments

Work in my laboratory on IQGAP proteins has been funded by BBSRC (BB/D000394/1) and Action Cancer, Northern Ireland (PG2 2005).

References

[1] Weissbach, L., Settleman, J., Kalady, M. F., Snijders, A. J., Murthy, A. E., Yan, Y. X. & Bernards, A. (1994). Identification of a human rasGAP-related protein containing calmodulin-binding motifs. *J Biol Chem.*, *269*, 20517-20521.

[2] Hart, M. J., Callow, M. G., Souza, B. & Polakis, P. (1996). IQGAP1, a calmodulin-binding protein with a rasGAP-related domain, is a potential effector for cdc42Hs. *EMBO J.*, *15*, 2997-3005.

[3] McCallum, S. J., Wu, W. J. & Cerione, R. A. (1996). Identification of a putative effector for Cdc42Hs with high sequence similarity to the RasGAP-related protein IQGAP1 and a Cdc42Hs binding partner with similarity to IQGAP2. *J Biol Chem.*, *271*, 21732-21737.

[4] Jeong, H. W., Li, Z., Brown, M. D. & Sacks, D. B. (2007). IQGAP1 binds Rap1 and modulates its activity. *J Biol Chem.*, *282*, 20752-20762.

[5] Brill, S., Li, S., Lyman, C. W., Church, D. M., Wasmuth, J. J., Weissbach, L., Bernards, A. & Snijders, A. J. (1996). The Ras GTPase-activating-protein-related human protein IQGAP2 harbors a potential actin binding domain and interacts with calmodulin and Rho family GTPases. *Mol Cell Biol.*, *16*, 4869-4878.

[6] Bernards, A. (2003). GAPs galore! A survey of putative Ras superfamily GTPase activating proteins in man and *Drosophila*. *Biochim Biophys Acta.*, *1603*, 47-82.

[7] Wang, S., Watanabe, T., Noritake, J., Fukata, M., Yoshimura, T., Itoh, N., Harada, T., Nakagawa, M., Matsuura, Y., Arimura, N. & Kaibuchi, K. (2007). IQGAP3, a novel effector of Rac1 and Cdc42, regulates neurite outgrowth. *J Cell Sci.*, *120*, 567-577.

[8] Osman, M. A. & Cerione, R. A. (1998). Iqg1p, a yeast homologue of the mammalian IQGAPs, mediates cdc42p effects on the actin cytoskeleton. *J Cell Biol.*, *142*, 443-455.

[9] Epp, J. A. & Chant, J. (1997). An IQGAP-related protein controls actin-ring formation and cytokinesis in yeast. *Curr Biol.*, *7*, 921-929.

[10] Shannon, K. B. & Li, R. (1999). The multiple roles of Cyk1p in the assembly and function of the actomyosin ring in budding yeast. *Mol Biol Cell.*, *10*, 283-296.

[11] Eng, K., Naqvi, N. I., Wong, K. C. & Balasubramanian, M. K. (1998). Rng2p, a protein required for cytokinesis in fission yeast, is a component of the actomyosin ring and the spindle pole body. *Curr Biol.*, *8*, 611-621.

[12] Li, C. R., Wang, Y. M. & Wang, Y. (2008). The IQGAP Iqg1 is a regulatory target of CDK for cytokinesis in *Candida albicans*. *EMBO J.*, *27*, 2998-3010.

[13] Wendland, J. & Philippsen, P. (2002). An IQGAP-related protein, encoded by AgCYK1, is required for septation in the filamentous fungus *Ashbya gossypii*. *Fungal Genet Biol.*, *37*, 81-88.

[14] Venturelli, C. R., Kuznetsov, S., Salgado, L. M. & Bosch, T. C. (2000). An IQGAP-related gene is activated during tentacle formation in the simple metazoan Hydra. *Dev Genes Evol.*, *210*, 458-463.

[15] Nishimura, Y. & Mabuchi, I. (2003). An IQGAP-like protein is involved in actin assembly together with Cdc42 in the sea urchin egg. *Cell Motil Cytoskeleton.*, *56*, 207-218.

[16] Faix, J., Clougherty, C., Konzok, A., Mintert, U., Murphy, J., Albrecht, R., Muhlbauer, B. & Kuhlmann, J. (1998). The IQGAP-related protein DGAP1 interacts with Rac and is involved in the modulation of the F-actin cytoskeleton and control of cell motility. *J Cell Sci.*, *111*, 3059-3071.
[17] Yamashiro, S., Noguchi, T. & Mabuchi, I. (2003). Localization of two IQGAPs in cultured cells and early embryos of *Xenopus laevis*. *Cell Motil Cytoskeleton.*, *55*, 36-50.
[18] Briggs, M. W. & Sacks, D. B. (2003). IQGAP1 as signal integrator: Ca^{2+}, calmodulin, Cdc42 and the cytoskeleton. *FEBS Lett.*, *542*, 7-11.
[19] Briggs, M. W. & Sacks, D. B. (2003). IQGAP proteins are integral components of cytoskeletal regulation. *EMBO Rep.*, *4*, 571-574.
[20] Machesky, L. M. (1998). Cytokinesis: IQGAPs find a function. *Curr Biol.*, *8*, R202-5.
[21] Mateer, S. C., Wang, N. & Bloom, G. S. (2003). IQGAPs: integrators of the cytoskeleton, cell adhesion machinery, and signaling networks. *Cell Motil Cytoskeleton.*, *55*, 147-155.
[22] Mataraza, J. M., Briggs, M. W., Li, Z., Frank, R. & Sacks, D. B. (2003). Identification and characterization of the Cdc42-binding site of IQGAP1. *Biochem Biophys Res Commun.*, *305*, 315-321.
[23] Owen, D., Campbell, L. J., Littlefield, K., Evetts, K. A., Li, Z., Sacks, D. B., Lowe, P. N. & Mott, H. R. (2008). The IQGAP1-Rac1 and IQGAP1-Cdc42 interactions: interfaces differ between the complexes. *J Biol Chem.*, *283*, 1692-1704.
[24] Ren, J. G., Li, Z. & Sacks, D. B. (2007). IQGAP1 modulates activation of B-Raf. *Proc Natl Acad Sci, U S A.*, *104*, 10465-10469.
[25] Roy, M., Li, Z. & Sacks, D. B. (2004). IQGAP1 binds ERK2 and modulates its activity. *J Biol Chem.*
[26] Roy, M., Li, Z. & Sacks, D. B. (2005). IQGAP1 is a scaffold for mitogen-activated protein kinase signaling. *Mol Cell Biol.*, *25*, 7940-7952.
[27] Nauert, J. B., Rigas, J. D. & Lester, L. B. (2003). Identification of an IQGAP1/AKAP79 complex in beta-cells. *J Cell Biochem.*, *90*, 97-108.
[28] Yamaoka-Tojo, M., Ushio-Fukai, M., Hilenski, L., Dikalov, S. I., Chen, Y. E., Tojo, T., Fukai, T., Fujimoto, M., Patrushev, N. A., Wang, N., Kontos, C. D., Bloom, G. S. & Alexander, R. W. (2004). IQGAP1, a novel vascular endothelial growth factor receptor binding protein, is involved in reactive oxygen species—dependent endothelial migration and proliferation. *Circ Res.*, *95*, 276-283.
[29] Ho, Y. D., Joyal, J. L., Li, Z. & Sacks, D. B. (1999). IQGAP1 integrates Ca^{2+}/calmodulin and Cdc42 signaling. *J Biol Chem.*, *274*, 464-470.
[30] Joyal, J. L., Annan, R. S., Ho, Y. D., Huddleston, M. E., Carr, S. A., Hart, M. J. & Sacks, D. B. (1997). Calmodulin modulates the interaction between IQGAP1 and Cdc42. Identification of IQGAP1 by nanoelectrospray tandem mass spectrometry. *J Biol Chem.*, *272*, 15419-15425.
[31] Li, Q. & Stuenkel, E. L. (2004). Calcium negatively modulates calmodulin interaction with IQGAP1. *Biochem Biophys Res Commun.*, *317*, 787-795.
[32] Li, Z. & Sacks, D. B. (2003). Elucidation of the interaction of calmodulin with the IQ motifs of IQGAP1. *J Biol Chem.*, *278*, 4347-4352.

[33] Mbele, G. O., Deloulme, J. C., Gentil, B. J., Delphin, C., Ferro, M., Garin, J., Takahashi, M. & Baudier, J. (2002). The zinc- and calcium-binding S100B interacts and co-localizes with IQGAP1 during dynamic rearrangement of cell membranes. *J Biol Chem.*, *277*, 49998-50007.

[34] Bashour, A. M., Fullerton, A. T., Hart, M. J. & Bloom, G. S. (1997). IQGAP1, a Rac- and Cdc42-binding protein, directly binds and cross-links microfilaments. *J Cell Biol.*, *137*, 1555-1566.

[35] Erickson, J. W., Cerione, R. A. & Hart, M. J. (1997). Identification of an actin cytoskeletal complex that includes IQGAP and the Cdc42 GTPase. *J Biol Chem.*, *272*, 24443-24447.

[36] Mateer, S. C., McDaniel, A. E., Nicolas, V., Habermacher, G. M., Lin, M. J., Cromer, D. A., King, M. E. & Bloom, G. S. (2002). The mechanism for regulation of the F-actin binding activity of IQGAP1 by calcium/calmodulin. *J Biol Chem.*, *277*, 12324-12333.

[37] Mateer, S. C., Morris, L. E., Cromer, D. A., Bensenor, L. B. & Bloom, G. S. (2004). Actin filament binding by a monomeric IQGAP1 fragment with a single calponin homology domain. *Cell Motil Cytoskeleton.*, *58*, 231-241.

[38] Le Clainche, C., Schlaepfer, D., Ferrari, A., Klingauf, M., Grohmanova, K., Veligodskiy, A., Didry, D., Le, D., Egile, C., Carlier, M. F. & Kroschewski, R. (2007). IQGAP1 stimulates actin assembly through the N-WASP-Arp2/3 pathway. *J Biol Chem.*, *282*, 426-435.

[39] Watanabe, T., Wang, S., Noritake, J., Sato, K., Fukata, M., Takefuji, M., Nakagawa, M., Izumi, N., Akiyama, T. & Kaibuchi, K. (2004). Interaction with IQGAP1 links APC to Rac1, Cdc42, and actin filaments during cell polarization and migration. *Dev Cell.*, *7*, 871-883.

[40] Fukata, M., Watanabe, T., Noritake, J., Nakagawa, M., Yamaga, M., Kuroda, S., Matsuura, Y., Iwamatsu, A., Perez, F. & Kaibuchi, K. (2002). Rac1 and Cdc42 capture microtubules through IQGAP1 and CLIP-170. *Cell.*, *109*, 873-885.

[41] Kuroda, S., Fukata, M., Nakagawa, M., Fujii, K., Nakamura, T., Ookubo, T., Izawa, I., Nagase, T., Nomura, N., Tani, H., Shoji, I., Matsuura, Y., Yonehara, S. & Kaibuchi, K. (1998). Role of IQGAP1, a target of the small GTPases Cdc42 and Rac1, in regulation of E-cadherin- mediated cell-cell adhesion. *Science.*, *281*, 832-835.

[42] Kuroda, S., Fukata, M., Nakagawa, M. & Kaibuchi, K. (1999). Cdc42, Rac1, and their effector IQGAP1 as molecular switches for cadherin-mediated cell-cell adhesion. *Biochem Biophys Res Commun.*, *262*, 1-6.

[43] Li, Z., Kim, S. H., Higgins, J. M., Brenner, M. B. & Sacks, D. B. (1999). IQGAP1 and calmodulin modulate E-cadherin function. *J Biol Chem.*, *274*, 37885-37892.

[44] Noritake, J., Watanabe, T., Sato, K., Wang, S. & Kaibuchi, K. (2005). IQGAP1: a key regulator of adhesion and migration. *J Cell Sci.*, *118*, 2085-2092.

[45] Miyamoto, S., Baba, H., Kuroda, S., Kaibuchi, K., Fukuda, T., Maehara, Y. & Saito, T. (2000). Changes in E-cadherin associated with cytoplasmic molecules in well and poorly differentiated endometrial cancer. *Br J Cancer.*, *83*, 1168-1175.

[46] Mataraza, J. M., Briggs, M. W., Li, Z., Entwistle, A., Ridley, A. J. & Sacks, D. B. (2003). IQGAP1 promotes cell motility and invasion. *J Biol Chem.*

[47] Nabeshima, K., Shimao, Y., Inoue, T. & Koono, M. (2002). Immunohistochemical analysis of IQGAP1 expression in human colorectal carcinomas: its overexpression in carcinomas and association with invasion fronts. *Cancer Lett.*, *176*, 101-109.

[48] Nakamura, H., Fujita, K., Nakagawa, H., Kishi, F., Takeuchi, A., Aute, I. & Kato, H. (2005). Expression pattern of the scaffold protein IQGAP1 in lung cancer. *Oncol Rep.*, *13*, 427-431.

[49] Morris, L. E., Bloom, G. S., Frierson, H. F.,Jr & Powell, S. M. (2005). Nucleotide variants within the IQGAP1 gene in diffuse-type gastric cancers. *Genes Chromosomes Cancer.*, *42*, 280-286.

[50] Mooseker, M. S. & Cheney, R. E. (1995). Unconventional myosins. *Annu Rev Cell Dev Biol.*, *11*, 633-675.

[51] Rayment, I., Rypniewski, W. R., Schmidt-Base, K., Smith, R., Tomchick, D. R., Benning, M. M., Winkelmann, D. A., Wesenberg, G. & Holden, H. M. (1993). Three-dimensional structure of myosin subfragment-1: a molecular motor. *Science.*, *261*, 50-58.

[52] Gulick, A. M. & Rayment, I. (1997). Structural studies on myosin II: communication between distant protein domains. *Bioessays.*, *19*, 561-569.

[53] Timson, D. J. (2003). Fine tuning the myosin motor: the role of the essential light chain in striated muscle myosin. *Biochimie.*, *85*, 639-645.

[54] Trybus, K. M. (1994). Role of myosin light chains. *J Muscle Res Cell Motil.*, *15*, 587-594.

[55] Stepkowski, D. & Kakol, I. (1993). The significance of myosin light chains in mechanochemical coupling in skeletal muscle. *Acta Biochim Pol.*, *40*, 345-351.

[56] Weissbach, L., Bernards, A. & Herion, D. W. (1998). Binding of myosin essential light chain to the cytoskeleton-associated protein IQGAP1. *Biochem Biophys Res Commun.*, *251*, 269-276.

[57] Pathmanathan, S., Elliott, S. F., McSwiggen, S., Greer, B., Harriott, P., Irvine, G. B. & Timson, D. J. (2008). IQ motif selectivity in human IQGAP1: binding of myosin essential light chain and S100B. *Mol Cell Biochem.*, *318*, 43-51.

[58] Pathmanathan, S., Barnard, E. & Timson, D. J. (2008). Interactions between the budding yeast IQGAP homologue Iqg1p and its targets revealed by a split-EGFP bimolecular fluorescence complementation assay. *Cell Biol Int.*, *32*, 1318-1322.

[59] Lippincott, J. & Li, R. (1998). Sequential assembly of myosin II, an IQGAP-like protein, and filamentous actin to a ring structure involved in budding yeast cytokinesis. *J Cell Biol.*, *140*, 355-366.

[60] Corbett, M., Xiong, Y., Boyne, J. R., Wright, D. J., Munro, E. & Price, C. (2006). IQGAP and mitotic exit network (MEN) proteins are required for cytokinesis and re-polarization of the actin cytoskeleton in the budding yeast, *Saccharomyces cerevisiae*. *Eur J Cell Biol.*, *85*, 1201-1215.

[61] Boyne, J. R., Yosuf, H. M., Bieganowski, P., Brenner, C. & Price, C. (2000). Yeast myosin light chain, Mlc1p, interacts with both IQGAP and class II myosin to effect cytokinesis. *J Cell Sci.*, *113 Pt 24*, 4533-4543.

[62] Osman, M. A., Konopka, J. B. & Cerione, R. A. (2002). Iqg1p links spatial and secretion landmarks to polarity and cytokinesis. *J Cell Biol.*, *159*, 601-611.

[63] Korinek, W. S., Bi, E., Epp, J. A., Wang, L., Ho, J. & Chant, J. (2000). Cyk3, a novel SH3-domain protein, affects cytokinesis in yeast. *Curr Biol., 10*, 947-950.

[64] Shannon, K. B. & Li, R. (2000). A myosin light chain mediates the localization of the budding yeast IQGAP-like protein during contractile ring formation. *Curr Biol., 10*, 727-730.

[65] Luo, J., Vallen, E. A., Dravis, C., Tcheperegine, S. E., Drees, B. & Bi, E. (2004). Identification and functional analysis of the essential and regulatory light chains of the only type II myosin Myo1p in Saccharomyces cerevisiae. *J Cell Biol., 165*, 843-855.

[66] Brown, S. S. (1997). Myosins in yeast. *Curr Opin Cell Biol., 9*, 44-48.

[67] Ko, N., Nishihama, R., Tully, G. H., Ostapenko, D., Solomon, M. J., Morgan, D. O. & Pringle, J. R. (2007). Identification of yeast IQGAP (Iqg1p) as an anaphase-promoting-complex substrate and its role in actomyosin-ring-independent cytokinesis. *Mol Biol Cell., 18*, 5139-5153.

[68] D'souza, V. M., Naqvi, N. I., Wang, H. & Balasubramanian, M. K. (2001). Interactions of Cdc4p, a myosin light chain, with IQ-domain containing proteins in *Schizosaccharomyces pombe*. *Cell Struct Funct., 26*, 555-565.

[69] Wu, J. Q., Sirotkin, V., Kovar, D. R., Lord, M., Beltzner, C. C., Kuhn, J. R. & Pollard, T. D. (2006). Assembly of the cytokinetic contractile ring from a broad band of nodes in fission yeast. *J Cell Biol., 174*, 391-402.

[70] Wu, J. Q., Kuhn, J. R., Kovar, D. R. & Pollard, T. D. (2003). Spatial and temporal pathway for assembly and constriction of the contractile ring in fission yeast cytokinesis. *Dev Cell., 5*, 723-734.

[71] Kaufmann, A. & Philippsen, P. (2009). Of bars and rings: Hof1-dependent cytokinesis in multiseptated hyphae of *Ashbya gossypii*. *Mol Cell Biol., 29*, 771-783.

[72] Bielak-Zmijewska, A., Kolano, A., Szczepanska, K., Maleszewski, M. & Borsuk, E. (2008). Cdc42 protein acts upstream of IQGAP1 and regulates cytokinesis in mouse oocytes and embryos. *Dev Biol., 322*, 21-32.

[73] Just, I., Selzer, J., Wilm, M., von Eichel-Streiber, C., Mann, M. & Aktories, K. (1995). Glucosylation of Rho proteins by *Clostridium difficile* toxin B. *Nature, 375*, 500-503.

[74] Brandt, D. T., Marion, S., Griffiths, G., Watanabe, T., Kaibuchi, K. & Grosse, R. (2007). Dia1 and IQGAP1 interact in cell migration and phagocytic cup formation. *J Cell Biol., 178*, 193-200.

[75] Castrillon, D. H. & Wasserman, S. A. (1994). Diaphanous is required for cytokinesis in *Drosophila* and shares domains of similarity with the products of the limb deformity gene. *Development., 120*, 3367-3377.

Chapter VII

Migrating Plant Cell: F-Actin Asymmetry Directed by Phosphoinositide Signaling

Koji Mikami[*]
Faculty of Fisheries Sciences, Hokkaido University,
3-1-1 Minato-cho, Hakodate 041-8611, Japan.

Abstract

Polarity is a fundamental cell property essential for differentiation, proliferation and morphogenesis in unicellular and multicellular organisms. It is well known that polarized distribution of F-actin is important in providing the driving force for directional migration in mammalian leukocytes and *Dictyostelium* cells. Phosphoinositide (PI) signaling, including phosphatidylinositol kinases and phospholipases, is also critical for the formation of cell polarity in these cells. A monospore from the marine red alga *Porphyra yezoensis* is well known as a migrating plant cell and thus is a unique and useful material for investigating polarity determination in plant cells. As in leukocytes and *Dictyostelium* cells, monospore migration requires asymmetrical distribution of F-actin, whose establishment is regulated by the phosphatidylinositol 3-kinase and phospholipase C, whereas phospholipase D is involved in the maintenance of F-actin distribution. These findings indicate that the regulation of F-actin asymmetry by PI signaling cascades is evolutionarily conserved in terms of the establishment of cell polarity in migrating eukaryotic cells.

---

[*]Corresponding author: Tel/Fax: +81-138-40-8899; E-mail: komikami@fish.hokudai.ac.jp

Introduction

The initial establishment of cell polarity, exhibited as asymmetrical cell division and directional migration, depends on asymmetrical cues that lead to reorganization of the cytoskeleton and polarized distribution of cortical proteins and membrane lipids (Iglesias and Devreotes, 2008; Janetopoulos and Firtel, 2008). When *Dictyostelium* cells and leukocytes respond to external stimuli such as cAMP and cytokines, cells in the axialized form can rapidly change their body shape along with the formation of cell polarity in response to the chemoattractant, following the rapid formation of a leading edge on the side of the cell exposed to the highest concentration of the chemoattractant with a trailing edge appearing on the opposite side (Iglesias and Devreotes, 2008; Janetopoulos and Firtel, 2008). Formation of the leading edge occurs in parallel with the polarized localization of F-actin, whereas assembled myosin II is enriched at the trailing edge. Thus, the polarized distribution of cytoskeletal components provides the driving and contractile forces required for directional cell migration during chemotaxis. Involvement of the cytoskeleton in the establishment of cell polarity has also been reported in land plants (Staiger, 2000; Hepler *et al.*, 2001; Smith, 2003). F-actin and microtubules (MTs) have also been shown to play important roles in the establishment of polarity during tip growth of pollen tubes and root hairs (Fu *et al.*, 2001; Sieberer *et al.*, 2005). These findings show that the polarized accumulation of cytoskeletal elements, particularly F-actin, is important for the establishment of cell polarity in both animals and land plants.

The marine red alga *Porphyra yezoensis* has been proposed as a model marine plant for physiological and genetic studies in seaweed because of its biological and economic importance (Saga and Kitade, 2002). The life cycle of *P. yezoensis* is characterized as a heteromorphic haplodiploid type, in which the haploid and diploid phases are large leafy gametophyte and microscopic filamentous sporophyte, conchocelis, respectively (Klinger, 1993; Coelho *et al.*, 2007). In addition to the sexual life cycle, *P. yezoensis* can propagate asexually using monospores, which are produced in the marginal region of gametophytic blades (see Figure 1). It is noteworthy that the monospore is an example of a moving plant cell (Pickett-Heaps *et al.*, 2001; Ackland *et al.*, 2007); therefore, these cells have been employed to elucidate the regulatory mechanisms in the establishment of cell polarity required for cell migration in plant cells (Li *et al.*, 2008; Li *et al.*, 2009). This chapter will highlight the involvement of asymmetrical distribution of F-actin and phosphoinositide signaling in the formation of cell polarity required for monospore migration.

Asymmetrical Distribution of F-Actin in Migrating Monospores

Gametophytes of *P. yezoensis* are flat sheets composed of one layer of cells (Figure 1A). From the edge of these flat sheets, monospores are released as round somatic cells (Figure 1B). Because of the lack of a flagellum, retractile and amoeboid migration of monospores is found in cells that have undergone morphological change, exhibiting a tapered tail after release (Figure 1C). Pharmacological studies have shown that motility of monospores was completely inhibited by the disruption of local F-actin accumulation by Cyt B and Lat B. This indicates that generating the force for directed migration is dependent on the organization of F-actin in monospores (Li et al., 2008). These findings are similar to those in the red alga *P. pulchella* (Ackland et al., 2007).

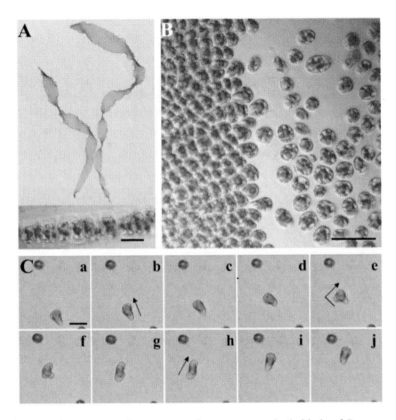

Figure 1. Discharge and movement of monospores from a gametophytic blade of *P. yezoensis*. (A) Leafy gametophyte of laboratory cultured *P. yezoensis* (strain TU-1); the image below shows a transverse section of a single layered gametophyte. Scale bar = 10 µm. (B) Release of monospores from the marginal region of a gametophyte. Scale bar = 50 µm. (C) Sequential images of monospore migration after release. Monospores usually showed directional migration (a-d, h-j); however, a change in the direction of polarized migration was sometimes observed (e -g). Eight minutes elapsed from panels a- j. Scale bar = 15 µm

Staining the cells with Alex Flour 488 phalloidin provided evidence of the clear relationship between F-actin accumulation and cell movement in monospores (Li et al., 2008; Li et al., 2009). In freshly released monospores, actin filaments were observed as bundles in the cell (Figure 2A); however, once the monospores moved, F-actin became densely assembled at the leading edge (Figure 2B). Since F-actin is generally involved in cytoskeleton arrangement, which is crucial for the establishment and maintenance of cell polarity (Samaj et al., 2000; Jedd and Chua, 2002), localized accumulation of F-actin at the leading edge during movement is thought to play roles in the establishment and/or maintenance of cell polarity in monospores.

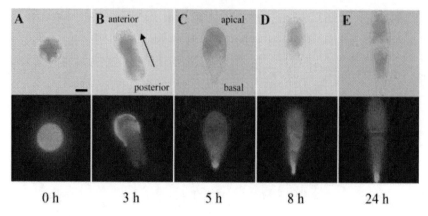

Figure 2. F-actin distribution during the early development of monospores.
F-actin was stained with Alex Flour 488 phalloidin. Upper and lower photos in each panel show brightfield and fluorescent images, respectively. The times below the panels indicate the time elapsed after monospore release. (A) Newly released monospore. (B) Migrating monospore with the arrow indicating the direction of migration. (C) Adhering monospore. (D) Elongating monospore. (E) First asymmetric cell division. Scale bar = 5 µm.

Asymmetrical localization of F-actin in monospores was also observed after conversion of cell axis from anterior-posterior to apical-basal during early development (Li *et al.*, 2008). Monospores observed five hours after release were seen to adhere to the substratum, establishing the apical-basal axis and becoming upright by elongation of the bottom part of the cell (Figures 1C and D). After elongation, the first asymmetric cell division occurred perpendicular to the apical-basal axis (Figure 1E). Since F-actin highly accumulated at the bottom of cells during these stages (Figures 2C-E), it is thought to be necessary for germlings to grow upright, and for the maintenance of cell axis.

Involvement of Phosphatidylinositol Signaling in the Establishment and Maintenance of Cell Polarity in Monospores

Phosphoinositides (PIs) are derivatives of phosphatidylinositol (PtdIns) and are involved in a wide variety of physiological regulation of the cytoskeleton, vesicle trafficking, ion channels and ion pumps (Zonia and Munnik, 2006). Many works have accumulated evidence regarding the role of PtdIns kinases and phospholipases in the distribution of PI derivatives (e.g., phosphatidylinositol-4,5-bisphosphate [PtdIns(4,5)P$_2$] and phosphatidylinositol-3,4,5-trisphosphate [PtdIns(3,4,5)P$_3$]) in migrating cells. This section highlights the involvement of PI signaling in the formation of cell polarity in monospores, and provides brief summaries of those in *Dictyostelium* and mammalian cells.

Phosphatidylinositol 3-Kinase (PI3K)

The response of *Dictyostelium* cells to chemoattractants results in he formation of a new leading edge in which preferential activation of PI 3-kinase (PI3K) to produce PtdIns(3,4,5)P$_3$ on the side facing the chemoattractant gradient is necessary for polarized F-actin localization and directional movement (Janetopoulos and Firtel, 2008). In contrast, phosphatase and Tensin homolog (PTEN) and Src homology 2 domain-containing inositol-5-phosphatase 1 (SHIP1), both of which dephosphorylate PtdIns(3,4,5)P$_3$, are localized on the trailing edge where they act as negative regulators of PI3K signaling in *Dictyostelium* cells and neutrophils (Funamoto et al., 2000; Nishio et al., 2007). Localized distributions of PI3K and PtdIns(3,4,5)P$_3$ phosphatase therefore help cells define their polarity by organizing polarized localization of F-actin. In plants, the importance of PI3K was also demonstrated in polar tip growth of root hairs (Lee et al., 2008). However, little is known about the kinds of D-3 PIs involved in tip growth.

It has recently been demonstrated that PI3K activity is required for the establishment of cell polarity, leading to asymmetrical localization of F-actin in migrating monospores (Li et al., 2008). Since the use of LY294002, a PI3K inhibitor, prevented monospore migration, it was concluded that the PI3K activity is essential for the establishment of cell polarity and asymmetric distribution of F-actin for migration. These results are similar to those observed in *Dictyostelium* cells and leukocytes.

Of the three types of PI3Ks, the type I PI3K is responsible for the production of PtdIns(3,4,5)P$_3$ in *Dictyostelium* and mammalian cells (Funamoto et al., 2002). Although the PtdIns3P-producing type III PI3K is found in plants (Michell, 2008), plant genomes have no gene encoding the type I PI3K. This is consistent with the fact that PtdIns(3,4,5)P$_3$ have not yet been detected in any plant cell (Mueller-Roeber and Pical, 2002). Interestingly, yeast cells, which also lack PtdIns(3,4,5)P$_3$, can produce PtdIns(3,4,5)P$_3$ in a type III PI3K-dependent manner, when their PTEN-homologue was inactivated by gene disruption (Mitra et al., 2004). It is still unclear whether PtdIns(3,4,5)P$_3$ exists and corresponds to the LY29400-sensitive D3-phosphorylated PtdIns in *P. yezoensis*.

Phospholipase C (PLC) Signaling Cascade

Phospholipase C (PLC) hydrolyzes PtdIns(4,5)P$_2$ to produce two second messengers, diacylglycerol (DG) and inositol-1,4,5-trisphoshphate (IP$_3$). These messengers in turn activate protein kinase C and facilitate the release of Ca^{2+} from intracellular stores via the IP$_3$ receptor (IP3R) (Berridge and Irvine, 1984). PLC is involved in chemotaxis in T cells via an increase in Ca^{2+} from intracellular stores by IP3R (Bach et al., 2007). In addition, during cAMP-dependent chemotaxis in *Dictyostelium* cells, PLC is thought to control the concentration of PtdIns(4,5)P$_2$ that is phosphorylated by PI3K to produce PtdIns(3,4,5)P$_3$, which is involved in chemotaxis (Kortholt et al., 2007). Thus, PLC has two different roles: the regulation of Ca^{2+}-dependent downstream signaling via IP3R, and determination of the PtdIns(4,5)P$_2$ concentration involved in the activation of PI3K signaling.

Li et al. (2009) have demonstrated the involvement of PLC in the establishment of cell polarity in monospores. In the presence of U73122, a specific inhibitor of PLC, monospores did not start moving when the asymmetrical distribution of F-actin (Figure 3B) was inhibited. This was further confirmed by the use of the inactive analog U73343, which did not affect monospore motility. These results indicate that PLC is involved in the establishment of cell polarity to direct the asymmetrical localization of the F-actin of monospores.

In plants, DG produced by PLC is immediately converted by diacylglycerol kinase (DGK) to phosphatidic acid (PA), an important second messenger involved in various physiological processes in plant cells (Zonia and Munnik, 2006). When the role of DGK in the polarity formation of monospores was tested using a DGK inhibitor R59022, migration and asymmetrical distribution of F-actin in monospores were inhibited (Figure 3C). Moreover, the requirement for IP3R-like activity in monospore migration was examined using an IP3R antagonist, 2-APB. This antagonist inhibits IP3R activity on the ER membrane in animal cells. In the presence of this antagonist, both monospore migration and asymmetrical distribution of F-actin were prevented (Figure 3D). Thus, DGK and IP3R-like protein are possibly involved in the establishment of cell polarity in monospores (Li et al., 2009), which is consistent with the effects of PLC. DGK involvement was also demonstrated in polarization and polar growth of zygotes in the brown alga *Silvetia compressa* (Peters et al., 2008).

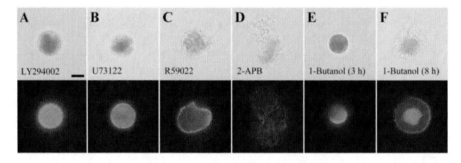

Figure 3. Effects of inhibitors on polarized F-actin accumulation during early development of monospores.
F-actin was stained with Alex Flour 488 phalloidin after incubation with inhibitors for 3 hours and with 1-Butanol for 8 hours. Upper and lower photos in each panel show bright and fluorescent field images, respectively. Monospores treated with chemicals became too weak to bear the weight of the glass cover slip. Changes in the color of chloroplasts and/or enhanced fluorescence signal from chloroplasts sometimes occurred as the monospores were crushed by the cover slips (Li et al., 2008; Li et al., 2009). (a) Monospore treated with 0.2 mM Cyt B, which cleaves actin filaments. (b) Monospore treated with 25 µM Lat B, which impairs polymerization of G-actin. (c) Monospore treated with 15 µM LY294002, which inhibits PI3K. (d) Monospore treated with 1 µM U73122, which inhibits PLC. (e) Monospore treated with 15 µM R59022, which inhibits DGK. (f) Monospore treated with 20 µM 2-APB, which inhibits IP3R. (g) Monospore treated for 3 hours with 0.4% 1-Butanol, which inhibits PLD (h) Monospore treated with 0.4% 1-Butanol for 8 hours. Scale bar = 5 µm.

In land plants, the presence and nature of IP3R, which acts as an IP_3-dependent Ca^{2+} channel on vacuolar and/or ER membranes, have yet to be determined. Indeed, no IP3R genes bearing a homology to animal genes have so far been found in the genomes of *Arabidopsis thaliana*, rice and *Physcomitrella patens*. In contrast, IP3R homologues have been identified in green algae *Chlamydomonas reinhardtii* and *Volvox carterii*, suggesting the loss of IP3R by land plants when they diverged (Wheeler and Brownlee, 2008). Thus, it is possible that red algae also have orthotic IP3R, since green and red algae originated from the same single ancestor (Palmer, 2000; McFadden and van Dooren, 2004). Identification of IP3R in *P. yezoensis* will be of further importance in understanding the PI signaling system in migrating monospores.

Phospholipase D (PLD)

Phospholipase D (PLD) catalyzes the production of PA from phosphatidylcholine (PC) in a PtdIns(4,5)P$_2$-dependent manner (Hodgkin *et al.*, 2000). PLD inhibition resulted in a rapid decrease in PtdIns(4,5)P$_2$ synthesis, leading to defects in actin-based motility in *Dictyostelium* cells (Zouwail *et al.*, 2005). PLD activity has also been shown to regulate microtubule organization for cell polarity determination in Fucoid zygotes (Peters *et al.*, 2007). Moreover, PtdIns(4,5)P$_2$-dependent PLD activity is involved in tip growth of pollen tubes (Potocký *et al.*, 2003). These findings suggest that the PtdIns(4,5)P$_2$-dependent activation of PLD is important for motility regulation.

Involvement of PLD in the formation of cell polarity has also been demonstrated in monospores (Li *et al.*, 2009). Treatment of monospores with 1-butanol for three hours decreased migration, whereas F-actin was asymmetrically localized (Figure 3E). However, treatment of monospores for eight hours with 1-butanol resulted in symmetrically distributed F-actin without migration (Figure 3F). This observation indicates that inhibition of PLD activity did not disrupt the formation of F-actin asymmetry but prevented its maintenance. Thus, PLD participates in the maintenance, but not in the establishment, of cell polarity in monospores.

Conclusion

The establishment and maintenance of cell polarity during migration of monospores is under complex regulation. As discussed above, inhibition of the establishment of cell polarity, as judged by the ability of F-actin to localize asymmetrically, occurred when monospores were treated with inhibitors of PI3K, PLC, DGK and IP3R (Figure 3). In contrast, PLD inhibition prevented monospore migration but not asymmetrical localization of F-actin (Figure 3). Therefore, there is functional diversity between the PLC and PLD signaling systems in terms of the formation of cell polarity; the former being critical for the establishment of cell polarity and the latter playing a role in the maintenance of established cell polarity (Figure 4). Recently, it has been demonstrated that Ca^{2+} influx is indispensable for asymmetric localization of F-actin and migration in monospores (Li *et al.*, 2009). These results indicate the involvement of Ca^{2+}-dependent activation of PI3K and PLC to establish cell polarity (Figure 4). In light of these findings and related literature, it appears that the mechanisms mediating the formation of cell polarity in migrating eukaryotic cells converge into conserved PI signaling pathways. Therefore, dissecting these molecular mechanisms could help in further understanding the interrelationship between PI signaling and F-actin asymmetry, which can provide new insights into the machinery regulating the formation of cell polarity in eukaryotes.

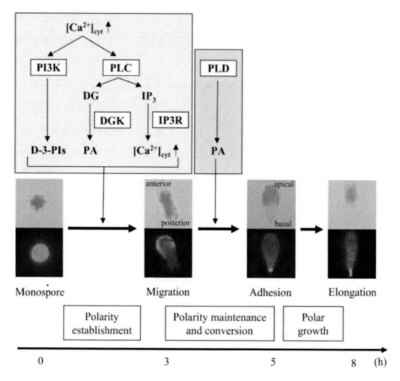

Figure 4. A model of the involvement of PI signaling in the formation of cell polarity in *P. yezoensis* monospores.
Ca^{2+}-dependent activation of PI3K and PLC directs the establishment of the anterior-posterior axis that leads to asymmetrical organization of F-actin, which is localized at the leading edge, thus providing the force for migration. PLD is required for the maintenance of established cell polarity. The anterior-posterior axis is converted to the apical-basal axis as the cell adheres to the substratum, causing localized accumulation of F-actin at the bottom of the monospore; this is important for the maintenance of apical-basal polarity and succeeding polar growth.

Further studies are needed to elucidate the function of individual PIs in the formation of cell polarity in migrating monospores. The ability to visualize the subcellular localization of PI-binding protein domains fused to fluorescent proteins would be a powerful tool for understanding the physiological importance and roles of PIs. Recently, we have developed a system for the efficient expression of humanized fluorescent proteins in *P. yezoensis* cells. This system was successfully employed in visualizing the localization of human Pleckstrin homology domains in plasma membranes and the nuclear localization of transcription factors (Mikami *et al.*, 2009; Uji *et al.*, 2009). However, overexpression of humanized fluorescent proteins had an inhibitory effect on the development of monospores (Mikami *et al.*, 2009; Uji *et al.*, 2009), which prevented the analysis of the molecular mechanisms regulating the development of monospores. The visualization of asymmetrical distribution of PIs is critical for understanding how monospore migration is regulated by PI signaling systems. Therefore, it is necessary to remove the inhibitory effects of overexpressed fluorescent proteins on monospore development. Such an approach could reveal how PI-regulated F-actin asymmetry is conserved in migrating eukaryotic cells.

Acknowledgments

I would like to thank my colleagues for valuable discussions, and especially Lin Li and Megumu Takahashi for sharing their unpublished works and assistance in the preparation of figures.

References

Ackland, J. C., West, J. A. & Pickett-Heaps, J. (2007). Actin and myosin regulate pseudopodia of *Porphyra pulchella* (Rhodophyta) archeospores. *Journal of Phycology, 43*, 129-138.

Bach, T. L., Chen, Q. M., Kerr, W. T., Wang, Y., Lian, L., Choi, J. K., Wu, D., Kazanietz, M. G., Koretzky, G. A., Zigmond, S. & Abrams, C. S. (2007). Phospholipase Cβ is critical for T cell chemotaxis. *The Journal of Immunology, 179*, 2223-2227.

Berridge, M. J. & Irvine, R. F. (1984). Inositol trisphosphate, a novel second messenger in cellular signal transduction. *Nature, 312*, 315-321.

Coelho, S. M., Peters, A. F., Charrier, B., Roze, D., Destombe, C., Valero, M. & Cock, J. M. (2007). *Complex life cycles of multicellular eukaryotes: new approaches based* on the use of model organisms. *Gene, 406*, 152-170.

Fu, Y., Wu, G. & Yang, Z. (2001). Rop GTPase-dependent dynamics of tip-localized F-actin controls tip growth in pollen tube. *The Journal of Cell Biology, 152*, 1019-1032.

Funamoto, S., Meili, R., Lee, S., Parry, L. & Firtel, R. A. (2002). Spatial and temporal regulation of 3-phosphoinositides by PI 3-kinase and PTEN mediates chemotaxis. *Cell, 109*, 611-623.

Hepler, P. K., Vidali, L. & Cheung, A. Y. (2001). Polarized cell growth in higher plants. *Annual Review of Cell and Developmental Biology, 17*, 159-187.

Hodgkin, M. N., Masson, M. R., Powner, D., Saqib, K. M., Ponting, C. P. & Wakelam, M. J. O. (2000). Phospholipase D regulation and localisation is dependent upon a phosphatidylinositol 4,5-bisphosphate-specific PH domain. *Current Biology, 10*, 43-46

Iglesias, P. A. & Devreotes, P. N. (2008) Navigating through models of chemotaxis. *Current Opinion in Cell Biology, 20*, 35-40.

Janetopoulos, C. & Firtel, R. A. (2008) Directional sensing during chemotaxis. *FEBS Letters, 582*, 2075-2085.

Jedd, G. & Chua, N. H. (2002). Visualisation of peroxisomes in living plant cells reveals acto-myosin-dependent cytoplasmic streaming and peroxisome budding. *Plant and Cell Physiology, 43*, 384-392.

Klinger, T. (1993). The persistence of haplodiploidy in algae. *Trends in Ecology and Evolution, 8*, 256-258.

Kortholt, A., King, J. S., Keizer-Gunnink, I., Harwood, A. J. & van Haastert, P. J. M. (2007). Phospholipase C regulation of phosphatidylinositol 3,4,5-trisphosphate-mediated chemotaxis. *Molecular Biology of the Cell*, *18*, 4772-4779.

Lee, Y., Bak, G., Choi, Y., Chuang, W.I., Cho, H.T. & Lee, Y. (2008) Roles of phosphatidylinositol 3-kinase in root hair growth. *Plant Physiology*, *147*, 624-635.

Li, L., Saga, N. & Mikami, K. (2008). Phosphatidylinositol 3-kinase activity and asymmetrical accumulation of F-actin are necessary for establishment of cell polarity in the early development of monospores from the marine red alga *Porphyra yezoensis*. *Journal of Experimental Botany*, *59*, 3575-3586.

Li, L., Saga, N. & Mikami, K. (2009). Ca^{2+} influx and phosphoinositide signaling are essential for the establishment and maintenance of cell polarity in monospores from the red alga *Porphyra yezoensis*. *Journal of Experimental Botany*, *60*, 3477-3489.

McFadden, G. I. & van Dooren, G. G. (2004). Evolution: red algal genome affirms a common origin of all plastids. *Current Biology*, *14*, R514-R516.

Michell, R. H. (2008). Inositol derivatives *Nature Reviews Molecular Cell Biology*, *9*, 151-61.

Mikami, K., Uji, T., Li, L., Takahashi, M., Yasui, H. & Saga, N. (2009). Visualization of phosphoinositides via the development of the transient expression system of a cyan fluorescent protein in the red alga *Porphyra yezoensis*. *Marine Biotechnology*, *11*, 563-569.

Mitra, P., Zhang, Y., Rameh, L. E., Ivshina, M. P., McCollum, D., Nunnari, J. J., Hendricks, G. M., Kerr, M. L., Field, S. J., Cantley, L. C. & Ross, A. H. (2004). A novel phosphatidylinositol(3,4,5)P_3 pathway in fission yeast. *Journal of Cell Biology*, *166*, 205-211.

Mueller-Roeber, B. & Pical, C. (2002). Inositol phospholipid metabolism in *Arabidopsis*. Characterized and putative isoform of inositol phospholipid kinase and phosphoinositide-specific phospholipase C. *Plant Physiology*, *130*, 22-46.

Nishio, M., Watanabe, K., Sasaki, J., Taya, C., Takasuga, S., Iizuka, R., Balla, T., Yamazaki, M., Watanabe, H., Itoh, R., Kuroda, S., Horie, Y., Förster, I., Mak, T. W., Yonekawa, H., Penninger, J. M., Kanaho, Y., Suzuki, A. & Sasaki, T. (2007). Control of cell polarity and motility by the PtdIns(3,4,5)P_3 phosphatase SHIP1. *Nature Cell Biology*, *9*, 36-44.

Palmer, J. D. (2000). Molecular evolution: A single birth of all plastids? *Nature*, *405*, 32-33.

Peters, N. T., Logan, K. O., Miller, A. C. & Kropf, D. L. (2007). Phospholipase D signaling regulates microtubule organization in the fucoid alga *Silvetia compressa*. *Plant and Cell Physiology*, *48*, 1764-1774.

Peters, N. T., Pol, S. U. & Kropf, D. L. (2008). Phospholipid signaling during stramenopile development. *Plant Signaling & Behavior*, *3*, 398-400.

Pickett-Heaps, J. D., West, J. A., Wilson, S. M. & McBride, D. L. (2001). Time-lapse videomicroscopy of cell (spore) movement in red algae. *European Journal of Phycology*, *36*, 9-22.

Potocký, M., Eliáš, M., Profotová, B., Novotná, Z., Valentová, O. & Zárský, V. (2003). Phosphatidic acid produced by phospholipase D is required for tobacco pollen tube growth. *Planta*, *217*, 122-130.

Saga, N. & Kitade, Y. (2002). *Porphyra*: A model plant in marine science. *Fisheries Science, 68*, S1075-S1078.

Samaj, J., Peters, M., Volkmann, D. & Baluska, F. (2000). Effects of myosin ATPase inhibitor 2,3-butanedione 2-monoxime on distributions of myosins, F-actin, microtubules, and cortical endoplasmic reticulum in maize root apices. *Plant and Cell Physiology, 41*, 571-582.

Sieberer, B. J., Ketelaar, T., Esseling, J. J. & Emons, A. M. (2005). Microtubules guide root hair tip growth. *New Phytologist, 167*, 711-719.

Smith, L.G. (2003). Cytoskeletal control of plant cell shape: Getting the fine points. *Current Opinion in Plant Biology, 6*, 63-73.

Staiger, C. J. (2000). Signaling to the actin cytoskeleton in plants. *Annual Review of Plant Physiology and Plant Molecular Biology, 51*, 257-288.

Uji, T. Takahashi, M, Saga, N. & Mikami, K. (2009). Visualization of nuclear localization of transcription factors with cyan and green fluorescent proteins in the red alga *Porphyra yezoensis*. *Marine Biotechnology*, DOI 10/107/s10126-009-9210-5.

Wheeler, G. L. & Brownlee, C. (2008). Ca^{2+} signalling in plants and green algae-changing channels. *Trends in Plant Science, 13*, 506-514.

Zonia, L. & Munnik, T. (2006). Cracking the green paradigm: Functional coding of phosphoinositide signals in plant stress responses. *Subcellular Biochemistry, 39*, 207-237.

Zouwail, S., Pettitt, T. R., Dove, S. K., Chibalina, M. V., Powner, D. J., Haynes, L., Wakelam, M. J. & Insall, R. H. (2005). Phospholipase D activity is essential for actin localization and actin-based motility in *Dictyostelium*. *Biochemical Journal, 389*, 207-214.

In: Cytoskeleton: Cell Movement...
Editors: S. Lansing et al., pp. 161-177

ISBN: 978-1-60876-559-1
© 2010 Nova Science Publishers, Inc.

Chapter VIII

Membrane Microdomains and Neural Impulse Propagation: Field Effects in Cytoskeleton Corrals

Ron Wallace
Department of Anthropology, University of Central Florida,
Orlando, Florida, USA

The possibility that an ensemble of neural-membrane lipids could regulate the duration of the ion-channel "open" conformation may have direct implications for local gating of the action potential (AP). The control of channel dynamics is equivalent to controlling the transmembrane ion conductances responsible for neural depolarization and hyperpolarization. Accordingly, if a membrane region in an axon were to contain (for example) clusters of Na^+ channels with relatively longer open states, such a structure would be conducive to a local depolarization (spike) and the continuing propagation of the neural impulse. By contrast, if the Na^+ channels had brief open states, the structure would be conducive to impulse propagation failure. Modulation of the membrane state through other channel types would of course also be possible. A good example is the A-current delayed-rectifier K^+ channel (K_A), currently the object of intensive research because of its possible role in conduction failure. The K_A channel is gated by membrane hyperpolarization, which it increases and prolongs by rapidly conducting potassium ions out of the cytosol. A prolonged open time for this channel could hypothetically strengthen the delayed-rectifier effect and significantly increase the probability of conduction block.

This chapter examines the possible role of neural membrane microdomains in regulating the propagation of the action potential. These data are particularly important because they appear consistent with the concept that "local switches" regulate AP propagation (Scott, 1995). The chapter begins with an overview of the experimental evidence for AP conduction failure. It then examines the two major alternative models: one emphasizing the role of impedance mismatch due to neuron branching geometry; the other emphasizing the role of prolonged hyperpolarization due to the A-current potassium channel (K_A). A model emphasizing the possible interaction of a microdomain-cytoskeleton system with neuron branching geometry will then be presented (Wallace, 2004).. Because of the large number of studies bearing on the subject, the K_A channel will be used as the basic example, although the possible contributions of other channel types will be briefly discussed. The chapter concludes with a discussion of how microdomain regulation of AP propagation may explain a number of neuron features that strikingly depart from cable properties.

4.1. Conduction Failure in Neurons: Evidence and Models

The earliest evidence for AP propagation failure in neurons preceded by 17 years the patch-clamp experiments conducted on the squid axon by A.L. Hodgkin and A.F. Huxley that culminated in the standard model of neuron electrical signaling (1952a, 1952b, 1952c, 1952d). Thus it was evident nearly 70 years ago that a neural depolarization (spike) was not inevitably propagated from the point of its origin to the presynaptic terminal. D.H. Barron and B.H.C. Matthews (1935) applied electrical stimuli to a cat spinal cord axon and recorded the propagating signals at two locations. They found that signals recorded at the first point were intermittently not detectable at the second point, but the physical basis for the conduction failure was unclear.

Following the Barron-Matthews study, axonal propagation failure was experimentally demonstrated in a variety of vertebrate and invertebrate species: e.g., the molluscan central neuron, crayfish abdominal axons, the walking leg of the crayfish, leech sensory neurons, rat motoneurons, and the visual callosal axons of the rabbit (Tauc and Hughes, 1963; Parnas, 1972; Hatt and Smith, 1975; van Essen, 1973; Krnjevic and Miledi, 1959; Swadlow and Waxman, 1976). Similarly, dendritic conduction failure was identified in cochlear neurons of the monkey, hedgehog, owl, and bat, and in alligator Purkinje neurons (Bogoslovskaya et al., 1973; Llinas et al., 1969). As the data accumulated, it became evident that axonal and dendritic branch points frequently had a low "safety factor" for impulse conduction. However, there was (and is) no consensus explanation. Instead there has been the largely separate development of models emphasizing either branching geometry or local hyperpolarization driven by the A-current potassium channel. The possibility that a molecular ensemble of some type could "decide" whether or not AP propagation should continue has not been systematically explored.

In the former set of models, impulse failure is related to the degree of impedance mismatch associated with the diameters of mother and daughter neural branches. The optimal geometry is given by Goldstein and Rall (1974) as

$$d_0^{3/2} = d_1^{3/2} + d_2^{3/2} \tag{1}$$

where d_1 and d_2 are diameters of daughter branches and d_0 is the parent branch radius. Accordingly the Goldstein-Rall (GR) ratio is given by

$$GR = d_1^{3/2} + d_2^{3/2} / d_0^{3/2} \qquad (2)$$

When GR is 1, impedances are perfectly matched and the conduction probability is high.

For GR< 1, the AP propagates with slightly increased velocity, as if the axon were tapering (Koch, 1999). The most common situation is GR > 1, where the electrical load of the daughter branches exceeds that of the parent branch. For 1<GR<10, conduction past the branch point is still assured, with the failure rate increasing for GR>10. Applications of the GR ratio to actual neurons have encountered mixed success. Rall successfully applied it to the electrical behavior of cat α motoneurons in 1977 (see also Rall et al., 1992) inspiring a related study by Fleshman, Segev, and Burke (1988). However, as several researchers subsequently determined, real neurons seldom conform to the structural requirements of the GR model: e.g., the 3/2 diameter rule at branch points, and "the assumption that all dendrites terminate at the same distance from the cell body" (Koch, 1999).

Alternative models of AP conduction failure have emphasized the role of the A-current potassium channel (K_A). The K_A current is an outward transmembrane flow of K^+ ions activated by hyperpolarization following a depolarizing pulse (Levitan and Kaczmarek, 2002). The current is subsequently inactivated at the return of the resting potential (-60mV). The K_A channel, by prolonging hyperpolarization, slows the return of the transmembrane voltage difference toward the resting potential. Clusters of K_A channels at branch points theoretically maintain the interior of the neuron at a hyperpolarized potential for a sufficient period of time to block the propagation of an AP This possibility has been investigated through *in vitro* slice electrophysiological studies and computer simulations (Debanne et al., 1999; Kopysova and Debanne, 1998). It was found that a K_A current could be activated by a brief (150 msec) hyperpolarizing prepulse (where voltage command ranged between -50 and -110mV) followed by a somatic depolarization (+30mV) of 50 msec duration.

The geometric and K_A approaches effectively frame the issue: What are the relative contributions of neuron branching geometry and branch-point K_A channel clusters to AP conduction failure? The query raises a related---and more general---question: Do K_A and other types of channel clusters communicate with one another, thus constitituting a molecular network operating within geometric constraints?

4.2. Regulated Lipid Diffusion through Cytoskeleton Gates

Viewed from an adaptive standpoint, a neuron must be able to modify its AP propagation behavior with regard to fluctuating cognitive or behavioral requirements. This is perhaps the most plausible argument for a synthesis of the ionic and geometric approaches: microstructural changes in the ion-channel environment can alternately reinforce or overcome the effects of neuron geometry. For example, neocortical neurons are components of neural networks subserving integrative cognitive functions. Accordingly, these neurons are characterized by highly arborized axons (Destexhe et al., 2003). However, in terms of the GR model and related geometric approaches, the branching geometry, while necessary for integrating cognitive modules, is highly unfavorable for AP propagation success. Accordingly, a molecular-level system must overcome this structural problem by insuring high depolarizing spike amplitude (and propagation success) at the axonal branch points. Conversely, in hippocampal CA3 networks, which according to several models, simplify or "index" complex cortical inputs for cross-modal comparison and identification of novelty, the suppression of irrelevant information would be essential for adaptive function (Gray, 1982. Also see review of comparator models in Vinogradova, 2001). Axonal branch points of CA3 neurons should thus be enriched with molecular systems that selectively reinforce the effects of neuron branching geometry by generating prolonged membrane hyperpolarization.

The modulating effects suggested above would require stepwise adjustments in the concentration of membrane unsaturated lipids proposed in this study to regulate ion-channel dynamics. Of course, if the membrane were indeed a fluid mosaic, as originally suggested by Singer and Nicolson (1972), the stochastic mixing of lipids would make such a regulatory role impossible. For that reason, the possible existence of gated barriers regulating local membrane lipid composition was speculatively suggested by Kinnunen in 1991. At that time, however, there was little or no evidence that such barriers actually existed. This situation is rapidly changing as new evidence is being put forward indicating that the neuron cytoskeleton may be equipped with dynamic molecular gates.

The cytoskeleton is a dense protein matrix of microtubules, intermediate filaments, and actin filaments located immediately beneath (and to some extent, within) the membrane in all eukaryotic cells (Kirkpatrick and Brady, 1999). The structure is the basis for the unique morphology of cells comprising different types of tissue; without it, an animal cell would be an amorphous bag of fluid. In addition, the cytoskeleton defines metabolic compartments within the cytosol, and provides tracks for intracellular transport. Recent evidence suggests that cytoskeleton compartments ranging in diameter from 100-600 nm and with a thickness of ~6 nm enclose membrane lipids and regulate their inter-compartmental diffusion in a stepwise fashion (See Figure 4, Appendix). The earliest investigations suggesting regulated lateral membrane diffusion focused on proteins rather than lipids. The movement of protein band 3 within the erythrocyte membrane was the basis for computational models that utilized a Monte Carlo approach (Tomishige et al., 1998; Tomishige et al., 1999; Brown et al., 2000; Leitner et al., 2000). The Tomishige studies found that, on average, a Band 3 protein moves from one cytoskeleton compartment to another every 350 ms. The investigators proposed that intercompartmental diffusion may be regulated by spectrin, a component of the cytoskeleton. The spectrin molecule consists of two chains which are aligned in an anti-parallel arrangement and wound around each other to form a heterodimer. Two heterodimers then associate head-to-head to produce a tetramer ~200 Å in length. The spectrin network is attached to the membrane through binding with ankyrin and protein 4.1 (Vale et al. in Hall, 1992). In the "skeleton fence" or "picket fence" cytoskeleton model, the spectrin heterodimer dissociates into two dimers, and then re-associates into a tetramer, thereby creating a dynamic gate for intercompartmental molecular diffusion.

The dissociation of the protein tetramer can be "fast" or "slow". Average opening rates, as determined by the Monte Carlo studies, were 5, 10, and 20 s^{-1}, while closing rates ranged from 1 to 10^6 s^{-1}. Accoiding to the Tomishige model, the increasingly faster closing rates would confine lipids inside a compartment. However, the precise physical basis for spectrin dissociation-reassociation remains controversial. Separate studies identify chemical and electrical mechanisms, and it may be that both are required (Wallis et al., 1992; Wallis et al., 1993; Zagon et al., 1986; Vassilev et al., 1982; Vassilev et al., 1983; Vater et al., 1998). Brain spectrin conformational change in response to Ca^{2+} binding to four high-affinity sites has been demonstrated by flow dialysis and NMR studies. However, the process by which intracellular Ca^{2+} concentration is modulated during neuron signaling, i.e. capacitative calcium entry through the endoplasmic reticulum, is not well understood (Putney, 2003). Alternatively, microtubules, which directly cross-link with spectrin in vivo, have been observed in solution to become aligned in an electric field because of the microtubule internal dipole. It follows, at least hypothetically, that field-induced microtubule alignment during an AP could mechanically modify the conformation of bound spectrin.

Do lipids move through cytoskeleton gates in a manner comparable to protein Band 3? The Kusumi Membrane Organizer Project is presently investigating this process through single-particle tracking studies (Fujiwara et al., 2002; See review in Kusumi, 2005). In their 2002 study, the movement of the unsaturated (and *non-microdomain*) lipid, 1,2-dioleoyl-sn-glycero-3-phosphoethanolamine (DOPE), labeled with Cy3, a long-wavelength dye frequently used in fluorescence microscopy, was tracked in a normal rat kidney fibroblastic cell membrane. The study found that the labeled lipids moved between cytoskeleton compartments via hop diffusion. Compartment size was ~230 nm, and the mean residency time for the lipids was 11 ms. Although these findings appear to be consistent with the present model, they must be viewed with caution. DOPE, as noted, is a non-microdomain lipid. Thus, the hop diffusion rate for microdomains is unknown. Also, the NRK membrane contains double (or nested) compartments; i.e. it is compartmentalized into 750-nm and then into 230-nm compartments. This type of compartmentalization has not been found in other cell types, including neurons. However, shortly after this study, lipid diffusion was investigated in the neuron utilizing both fluorescently-labeled phospholipids and lipids attached to gold particles (Nakada et al., 2003). As Boiko and Winckler (2003) note in their commentary, each technique has its limitations. Weak and short-lived fluorescence signals generate a low signal-to-noise ratio, and consequent low spatial and temporal resolution. On the other hand, the results of single particle tracking studies may reflect the interaction of the attached bead with extra-cellular components. Nonetheless, in the Nakada study, similar results were obtained through both techniques. Diffusion of membrane lipids out of the axon initial segment (AIS) was blocked; lipids were immobilized in the AIS region. Importantly, ankyrin binding proteins (proposed components of cytoskeleton fences) are enriched in the AIS, consistent with the picket fence model.

4.3. The K_A Potassium Channel and Neural Impulse Regulation

The evidence presented above appears consistent with a molecular regulatory system comprised of corralled microdomains and the K_A channel operating in concert with branching neuron geometry to control the propagation of the action potential (See Figure 5, Appendix). The basic properties of the proposed molecular system are the following: 1) K_A channels are distributed in clusters at neuron branch points and axonal swellings, for which there is a low safety factor for AP propagation. 2) An individual K_A channel or subset of channels within a cluster can be activated by an electric field conducted in the plane of the membrane. 3) Individual K_A channels are surrounded and stabilized by microdomains. 4) Microdomains vary in saturated/unsaturated lipid ratios. 5) K_A channel clusters and lipid microdomains are enclosed by a cytoskeleton corral. 6) Cytoskeleton corrals are dynamically gated by spectrin tetramer dissociation and reassociation. 7) Average gating rates vary between corrals, with faster gating rates confining lipids within the enclosure. Together these features may comprise a molecular regulatory system capable of rapid on-line modulation of the AP neural code.

As an example of how this system may operate, we may first consider a K_A channel cluster associated with a high rate of conduction failure, as in hippocampal CA3 neurons discussed above. In this type of molecular system, K_A channel clusters would be associated with unsaturated-lipid microdomains and slow cytoskeleton gates. The applied electric field associated with K_A channel gating would induce intra- and intercompartmental diffusion of unsaturated lipids toward the source of the field. As a result, the concentration of unsaturated lipids would increase in the immediate vicinity of the channel. The adjacent unsaturated bonds, both proximate to the head group and at the kink in the diacyl chains, would become aligned and polarized in the applied electric field. The folding of the gated K_A channels to the closed α-helix conformation would be "timed" by electrostatic interactions between charge groups in the unfolded (random-coil) channel and dipoles in the surrounding membrane. The relatively large number of electrostatic interactions involved would constitute a form of complex problem, requiring a protracted search for a solution (the lower-energy closed-channel conformation). In this manner, an elevated concentration of unsaturated lipids would prolong the open time of the gated K_A channels. Prolonged K_A channel open time would in turn generate strong local hyperpolarization, increasing the probability of AP propagation failure.

Alternatively, we may consider the function of corralled K_A channels in branching neocortical neurons, where AP propagation through branch points (i.e. low failure rate) is essential for normal network activity. The present model predicts that branch points in neocortical neurons would be enriched with K_A channel clusters associated with saturated-lipid microdomains and fast-gated cytoskeleton corrals. In this type of system, relatively brief K_A channel open times would result from the reduced complexity of the electrostatic interactions. This feature would reduce local hyperpolarization and thus increase the probability of AP propagation success. It might be argued that AP propagation success at neocortical neuron branch points could be more directly achieved by the absence of K_A channels altogether. Although this argument has an intuitive appeal, the complete absence of K_A channels would likely not be adaptive. In many systems of neurons, and neocortical neurons in particular, it would be physiologically essential to have an "emergency" system to dampen uncontrolled activity (e.g. epilepsy). This aspect of K_A channel behavior will be examined in some detail in the following chapter.

4.4. Implications of the Model: Molecular Networks in the Neuron

It has been recently suggested that the existence of cytoskeleton corrals enclosing membrane lipids may constitute a "paradigm shift" in cell biology (Kusumi et al., 2005). The present study would extend that claim by proposing that the new viewpoint may introduce a similar shift in our understanding of nervous systems as well. The K_A channel is the best-studied example of several types of ion-channel clusters which could communicate with one another and thereby regulate neuron signaling in complex and subtle ways. It is a commonplace that neurons are organized into networks. But are molecular networks operating within each neuron? Whatley and Harris (1996) have reviewed a large number of studies indicating that several types of ion channels interact directly with the cytoskeleton and are distributed in clusters. Examples include the ligand-gated channels such as nicotinic acetylcholine receptors, glycine receptors, glutamate receptors and $GABA_A$ receptors. In addition, Rasband and Schrager (2000) observed Na^+ channel clustering at nodes of Ranvier, and Shaker-type K^+ channel clustering near axoglial junctions. If subsequent studies reveal that these clusters are part of a larger compartmentalized structure similar to K_A channel cluster organization, the "network" concept would apply to coding within the neuron.

It is intriguing to consider the operation of hypothetical sub-neural molecular networks in relation to neural activity that appears to depart markedly from cable properties. Possibly the most striking example of this departure is an experiment conducted by Magee and Cook (2000) in which excitatory postsynaptic potentials (EPSPs) recorded in dendrites of the hippocampal CA1 region grew "progressively stronger with distance from the cell body, almost exactly counteracting the distance-dependent signal attrition one would expect to find" (Mel, 2002). As Mel notes, this finding is at variance with electrical conduction in a standard cable, where signals typically decay with distance from the source ("voltage drop"). Magee and Cook state that although the mechanism underlying increased EPSP amplitude is presently uncertain, an increased number of AMPA receptors or quanta of released glutamate (or both factors) may be responsible. Either mechanism would appear consistent with the present model. In a related investigation, Hering et al. (2003) demonstrated that AMPA receptors are associated with cholesterol/sphingolipid microdomains, which are necessary for their stability and hence for the maintenance of synapses. Sphingolipid clustering, followed by unsaturated-bond alignment and polarization could regulate the duration of the AMPA receptor channel "open" state. Synchronized "open" states of several AMPA channels would generate a pronounced dendritic spike amplitude at a distal site from the soma. Microdomains may also regulate distal spike amplitude through their possible role in transmitter exocytosis. Salaun et al. (2004) have recently reviewed a growing body of studies suggesting that the SNARE protein complex, essential for vesicle fusion with the neuron plasma membrane, is associated with sphingolipid-rich microdomains. The latter spatially concentrate the SNARE proteins at defined sites, a mechanism which could plausibly function to increase the quanta of released transmitter. Together these examples provide tantalizing glimpses of communicating membrane modules which may regulate AP propagation as well as the strength of the signal itself.

References

Alfsen, A., 1989. Membrane dynamics and molecular traffic and sorting in mammalian cells. *Prog. Biophys. Mol. Biol.* 54, 145-157.

Antonucci, D., Lim, S., Vassanelli, S., Trimmer, J., 2001. Dynamic localization and clustering of dendritic Kv2.1 voltage-dependent potassium channels in developing hippocampal neurons. *Neuroscience* 108, 69-81.

Atmar, W., 1994. Notes on the simulation of evolution. *IEEE Trans. Neural. Netw.* 5, 130-147.

Baroni, A., Paoletti, I., Silvestri, I., Buommino, E., Carriero, M., 2003. Early vitronectin downregulation in a melanoma cell line during all-trans retinoic acid-induced apoptosis. *Br. J.Dermatol.* 148(3), 424-433.

Barron, D., Matthews, B., 1935. Intermittent conduction in the spinal cord. *J. Physiol.* 85, 73-103.

Birnbaum, S., Varga, A., Yuan, L.-L., Anderson, A., Sweatt, J., Schrader, L., 2004. Structure and function of Kv4-family transient potassium channels. *Physiol. Rev.* 84, 803-833.

Biron, E., Otis, F., Meillon, J.-C., Robitaille, M., Lamothe, J., Van Hove, P., Cormier, M.-E., Voyer, N., 2004. Design, synthesis and characterization of peptide nanostructures having ion-channel activity. *Bioorg. Med. Chem.* 12, 1279-1290.

Bogoslovskaya, I., Lyubinskii, I., Pozin, N., Putsillo, Y., Shmelev, I., Shura-Bura, T., Spread of excitation along a fiber with local inhomogeneities. *Biophysics* 18, 944-948.

Boiko, T., Winckler, B., 2003. Picket and other fences in biological membranes. *Dev. Cell.* 5, 191-192.

Booth, P., Templer, R., Curran, A., Allen, S., 2001. Can we identify the forces that drive the folding of integral membrane proteins? *Biochem. Soc. Trans.* 29, 408-413.

Booth, P., Curran, A., 1999. Membrane protein folding. *Curr. Opin. Struc. Biol.* 9, 115-121.

Branton, D., Park, R. 1968a. Introduction. In: Branton, D., Park, R., (Eds.), *1968b Papers on Biological Membrane Structure.* Little, Brown, and Company, Boston.

Branton, D., Park, R., (Eds.), 1968b. *Papers on Biological Membrane Structure.* Little, Brown and Company, Boston.

Brown, R., 1998. Sphingolipid organization in biomembranes: what physical studies of model membranes reveal. *J. Cell Science* 111, 1-9.

Brown, F., Leitner, D., McCammon J., Wilson K., 2000. Lateral diffusion of membrane proteins in the presence of static and dynamic corral: suggestions for appropriate observables. *Biophys J.* 78, 2257-2269.

Buldum, A., Lu, J., 2003. Electron field emission properties of closed and open carbon nanotubes. In: *Technical Proceedings of the 2003 Nanotechnology Conference and Trade Show,* vol.3, Nanotech 2003, San Francisco, pp. 297-300.

Cantor, R., 1999. Lipid composition and the lateral pressure profile in bilayers. *Biophys. J.* 76, 2625-2639.

Catterall, W., 2002. Molecular mechanisms of gating and drug block of sodium channels. *Novartis Found. Symp.* 241, 206-218.

Churchland, P., Sejnowski, T., 1992. *The Computational Brain.* The MIT Press, Cambridge.

Cooper, G., 1997. *The Cell: A Molecular Approach.* Sinauer Associates, Sunderland.

Cornea, R., Thomas, D., 1994. Effects of membrane thickness on the molecular dynamics and enzymatic activity of reconstituted Ca-ATPase. *Biochemistry* 33(10), 2912-2920.

Cragg, P., 2002. Artificial transmembrane channels for sodium and potassium. *Sci. Progr.* 85, 219-241.

Dai, H., 2002. Carbon nanotubes: synthesis, integration, and properties. *Acc. Chem. Res.* 35, 1035-1044.

Danielli, J. and Davson, H., 1935. A contribution to the theory of permeability of thin films. *J. Cell Comp. Physiol*.5: 495-508.

Dawkins, R., 1986. *The Blind Watchmaker: Why the Evidence of Evolution Reveals a Universe Without Design*. W.W. Norton and Company, New York.

Dawkins, R. 1997. *Climbing Mount Improbable*. W.W. Norton and Company, New York.

Debanne, D., Kopysova, I., Bras, H., Ferrand, N., 1999. Gating of action potential propagation by an axonal A-like potassium conductance in the hippocampus: a new type of non-synaptic plasticity. *J. Physiol*. Paris 93, 285.

Delgado-Escueta, A., Wilson, W., Olsen, R., Porter, R., 1999. New waves of research in the epilepsies: Crossing into the third millennium. In: Delgado-Escueta, A., Wilson, W., Olsen, R., Porter, R., (Eds.), *Jasper's Basic Mechanisms of the Epilepsies*. Vol. 79. Lippincott Williams and Wilkins, Philadelphia.

De Planque, M., Goormaghtigh, E., Greathouse, D., Koeppe, R. 2nd, Kruijtzer, J., Liskamp, R., de Kruijff, B., Killian, J., 2001. Sensitivity of single membrane-spanning alpha-helical peptides to hydrophobic mismatch with a lipid bilayer: effects on backbone structure, orientation, and extent of membrane incorporation. *Biochemistry* 40(16), 5000-5010.

Destexhe, A., Rudolph, M., Pare, D., 2003. The high conductance state of neocortical neurons in vivo. *Nature Rev. Neurosci.* 4 (9), 739-751.

Dichter, M., 1994. Emerging insights into mechanisms of epilepsy: Implications for new antiepileptic drug development. *Epilepsia* 35, 551-557.

Dichter, M., 1997. Basic mechanisms of epilepsy: Targets for therapeutic intervention. *Epilepsia* 38, 52-56.

Doktycz, M., Zhang, L., Melechko, A., Klein, K., McKnight, T., Britt, P., Guillorn,M., Merkulov, V., Lowndes, D., Simpson, M., 2003. Nanofiber structures as mimics for cellular membranes. *Nanotechnology*, 420-423.

Dresselhaus, M., Dresselhaus, G., Ecklund, P., 1996. *Science of Fullerenes and Carbon Nanotubes*. Academic Press, New York.

Drexler, K., 1994. Molecular nanomachines: Physical principles and implementation strategies. In: Stroud, R., Cantor, C., and Pollard, T. (Eds.), *Annual Review of Biophysics and Biomolecular Structure*. Annual Reviews Inc., Palo Alto.

Dumas, F., Lebrun, M., Tocanne, J-F., 1999. Is the protein/lipid hydrophobic matching principle relevant to membrane organization and functions? *FEBS Letters* 458, 271-277.

Dumas F., Sperotto M., Lebrun M., Tocanne J., Mouritsen O., 1997. Molecular sorting of lipids by bacteriorhodopsin in dilauroylphosphatidylcholine/distearoylphosphatidylcholine lipid bilayers. *Biophys. J.* 73, 1940-1953.

Dykstra, C., 1997. *Physical Chemistry: A Modern Introduction*. Prentice Hall, Upper Saddle River.

Edidin, M., 1989. Fluorescent labeling of cell surfaces. In: Wang, Y-L., Taylor, D., (Eds.), *Fluorescent microscopy of living cells in culture: Part A*. Academic Press, New York.

Emilien, G., Maloteaux, M., 1998. Pharmacological management of epilepsy. Mechanism of action, pharmacokinetic drug interactions, and new discovery possibilities. *Int. J. Clin. Pharmacol. Ther.* 36, 181-194.

Fleshman, J., Segev, I., Burke, R., 1988. Electrotonic architecture of type identified α-motoneurons in the cat spinal cord. *J. Neurophysiol.* 60, 60-85.

Frisch, M., Trucks, G., Schlegel, H., Gill, P., Johnson, B., Robb, M., Cheeseman, J. Keith, T., Petersson, G., Montgomery, J., Raghavachari, K., Al-Laham, M., Zakrzewski, V., Ortiz, J., Foresman, J., Cioslowski, J., Stefanov, B., Nanayakkara, A., Challacombe, M., Peng, C., Ayala, P., Chen, W., Wong, M., Andres, J., Replogle, E., Gomperts, R., Martin, R., Fox, D., Brinkley, J., Defrees, D., Baker, J., Stewart, J., Head-Gordon, M., Gonzalez, C., Pople, J., 1995. Gaussian Inc., Pittsburgh.

Feringa, B., Komura, N., Van Delden, R., Ter Wiel, M., 2002. Light-driven molecular switches and rotors. *Appl. Phys.* A 75, 301-308.

Frye, L., Edidin, M., 1970. The rapid intermixing of cell surface antigens after formation of mouse-human heterokaryons. *J. Cell Sci.* 7, 319-335.

Fujiwara, T., Ritchie, K., Murakoshi, H., Jacobson, K., Kusumi, A., 2002. Phospholipids undergo hop diffusion in compartmentalized cell membrane. *J. Cell Biol.* 157, 1071-1081.

Garey, M., Johnson, D., 1979. *Computers and Intractability: A Guide to the Theory of NP-Completeness*. Freeman, San Francisco.

Geiger, B., Ayalon, O., Ginsberg, D., Volberg, T., Rodriguez Fernandez, J., Yarden, Y., Ben-Ze'ev, A., 1992. Cytoplasmic control of cell adhesion. *Cold Spring Harb. Symp. Quant. Biol.* 57, 631-642.

Gennis, R., 1989. Biomembranes: Molecular Structure and Function. *Springer*, New York.

Gokel, G., Schlesinger, P., Djedovič, N., Ferdani, R., Harder, E., Hu, J., Leevy, W., Pajewska, J., Weber, M., 2004. Functional, synthetic organic chemical models of cellular ion channels. *Bioorg. Med. Chem.* 12, 1291-1304.

Goldstein, S., Rall, W., 1974. Changes in action potential shape and velocity for changing core conductor geometry. *Biophys. J.* 14, 731-757.

Gorter, E., Grendel, F., 1968 (orig. 1925). On bimolecular layers of lipoids on the Chromocytes of the blood. . In: Branton, D., Park, R., (Eds.), 1968. *Papers on Biological Membrane Structure*. Little, Brown and Company, Boston.

Gray, J., 1982. Precis of the neuropsychology of anxiety: an enquiry into the functions of the septo-hippocampal system. *Behavioral and Brain Sciences* 5, 469-484.

Green, D. (Ed.), 1972. Membrane structure and its biological applications. *Annals of The New York Academy of Sciences*, New York.

Grossi, E., Buscema, M., Snowdon, D., Antuono, P., 2007. Neuropathological findings processed by artificial neural networks (ANNs) can perfectly distinguish Alzheimer's patients from controls in the Nun Study. *BMC Neurol.* 7:15, http://www.biomedcentral.com

Groves, J., Boxer, S., McConnell, H., 1997. Electric field-induced reorganization of two-component supported bilayer membranes. *Proc. Natl. Acad. Sci.USA* 94, 13990-13995.

Groves, J., Ulman, N., Cremer, P., Boxer, S., 1998. Supported-membrane interactions: Mechanisms for imposing patterns on a fluid lipid bilayer membrane. *Langmuir* 14, 3347-3350.

Hall, Z. (Ed.), 1992. *An introduction to molecular neurobiology*. Sinauer Associates. Sunderland.

Hao, M., Mukherjee, S., Maxfield, F., 2001. Cholesterol depletion induces large-scale domain segregation in living cell membranes. *Proc. Natl. Acad. Sci. USA* 98 (23), 13072-13077.

Harris, H., 1999. *The Birth of the Cell*. Yale University Press, New Haven.

Harris-Warwick, R., 2000. Ion channels and receptors: Molecular targets for behavioral evolution. *J. Comp Physiol*. [A];186, 605-16.

Hatt, H., Smith, D., 1975. Axon conduction block: differential channeling of nerve impulses in the crayfish. *Brain Res*. 87, 85-88.

Hering, H., Lin, C-C., Sheng, M., 2001. Lipid rafts in the maintenance of synapses, dendritic spines, and surface AMPA receptor stability. *J. Neurosci*.23, 3262-3271.

Hille, B., 2001. *Ionic Channels of Excitable Membranes*. Sinauer Associates, Sunderland.

Hodgkin, A., Huxley A., 1952a. The components of membrane conductance in the giant axon of *Loligo*. *J. Physiol*. 116, 473-496.

Hodgkin, A., Huxley A., 1952b. Currents carried by sodium and potassium ions Through the membrane of the giant axon of *Loligo*. *J. Physiol*. 116, 449-472.

Hodgkin, A., Huxley A., 1952c. The dual effect of membrane potential on sodium Conductance in the giant axon of *Loligo*. *J. Physiol*. 116, 497-506.

Hodgkin, A., Huxley A., 1952d. A quantitative description of membrane current and its application to conduction and excitation in nerve. *J. Physiol*. 117, 500-544.

Hong, K, Miller, C., 2000. The lipid-protein interface of a *Shaker* K^+ channel. *J. Gen. Physiol*. 115, 51-58.

Hughes, A., 1989. A History of Cytology. Iowa State University Press, Ames. Jain, M., 1972. *The Bimolecular Lipid Membrane: A System*. Van Nostrand Reinhold, New York.

Jefferys, J., 1993. The pathophysiology of epilepsies. In: Laidlaw, J, Richens, A., Chadwick, D., (Eds.), *A Textbook of Epilepsy*. Churchill and Livingstone, New York.

Jørgensen, K., Mouritsen, O., 1995. Phase separation dynamics and lateral organization of two-component lipid membranes. *Biophys. J*. 95, 942-954.

Kanicky, J., Shah, D. n.d. Effect of degree, type, and position of unsaturation on the pKa of long-chain fatty acids. Unpublished manuscript. *Center for Surface Science and Engineering*. University of Florida.

Killian, J., 1998. Hydrophobic mismatch between proteins and lipids in membranes. *Biochim. Biophys. Acta* 1376, 401-416.

Kinnunen, P., 1991. On the principles of functional ordering in biological membranes. *Chem. Phys. Lipids* 57, 375-399.

Kinnunen, P., Virtanen, J., 1986. A qualitative, molecular model of the nerve impulse: conductive properties of unsaturated lyotropic liquid crystals. In: Gutman, F. and Keyzer, H., (Eds.), *Modern Bioelectrochemistry*. Plenum Press, New York.

Kirkpatrick, L., Brady, S., 1999. Cytoskeleton of neurons and glia. In: Siegel, G. (Ed.), *Basic Neurochemistry*. Lippincott, Williams, and Wilkins, Philadelphia.

Koch, C., 1999. *Biophysics of computation: information processing in single neurons*. Oxford University Press, New York.

Koch, C., Segev, I., 2000. The role of single neurons in information processing. *Nat. Neurosci. Suppl.* 3, 1171-1177.

Kopysova, I., Debanne, D., 1998. Critical role of axonal A-type K^+ channels and axonal geometry in the gating of action potential propagation along CA3 pyramidal cell neurons: a simulation study. *J. Neurosci.* 18, 7436-7451.

Krnjevic, K., Miledi, R., 1959. Presynaptic failure of neuromuscular propagation in rats. *J. Physiol.* 149, 1-22.

Kusumi, A., Nakada, C., Ritchie, K., Murase, K., Suzuki, K., Murakoshi, H., Kasai, R. Kondo, J., Fujiwara, T., 2005. Paradigm shift of the plasma membrane concept from the two-dimensional continuum fluid to the partitioned fluid: high-speed single-molecule tracking of membrane molecules. *Annu. Rev. Biophys. Biomol. Struct.* 34, 351-378.

Langmuir, I., 1917. The constitution and fundamental properties of solids and liquids. II. Liquids. *J. Am. Chem. Soc.* 39, 1848-1906.

Lauritzen, I., Blondeau, N., Heurteaux, C., Widmann, C., Romney, G., Lazdunski, M., Polyunsaturated fatty acids are potent neuroprotectors. *EMBO J.* 19, 1784-1793.

Le Coutre, J., Narasimhan, L., Kumar N. Patel, C., Kaback, R., 1997. The lipid bilayer determines helical tilt angle and function in lactose permease of *Escherichia coli. Proc. Natl. Acad. Sci. USA.* 94, 10167-10171.

Lee, K., Klingler, J., McConnell, H., 1994. Electric-field-induced concentration Gradients in lipid monlayers. *Science* 263, 655-658.

Lehtonen, J., Holopainen, J., Kinnunen, P., 1996. Evidence for the formation of microdomains in liquid crystalline large unilamellar vesicles caused by hydrophobic mismatch of the constituent phospholipids. *Biophys. J.* 70, 1753-1760.

Lehtonen, J., Kinnunen, P., 1997. Evidence for phospholipid microdomain formation in liquid crystalline liposomes reconstituted with *Escherichia coli* lactose permease. *Biophys. J.* 72, 1247-1257.

Levitan, I., Kaczmarek, L., 2002. *The Neuron: Cell and Molecular Biology*. Oxford University Press, New York.

Leitner, D., Brown, F., Wilson, K., 2000. Regulation of protein mobility in cell membranes: a dynamic corral model. *Biophys. J.* 78, 125-135.

Lewis, B., Engelman, D., 1983. Bacteriorhodopsin remains dispersed in fluid phospholipid bilayers over a wide range of bilayer thicknesses. *J. Mol. Biol.* 166(2), 203-210.

Li, X-M, Momsen, M., Smaby, J., Brockman, H., Brown, R., 2001. Cholesterol decreases the interfacial elasticity and detergent solubility of sphingomyelins. *Biochemistry* 40, 5954-5963.

Liang, J., 2002. Experimental and computational studies of determinants of membrane-protein folding. *Curr. Opin. Chem. Biol.* 6, 878-884.

Llinas, R., Nicholson, C., and Precht, W., 1969. Preferred centripetal conduction of dendritic spikes in alligator Purkinje cells. *Science* 163, 184-187.

Madeja, M., 2000. Extracellular surface charges in voltage-gated ion channels. *News Physiol. Sci.* 15, 15-19.

Magee, J., Cook, E., 2000. Somatic EPSP amplitude is independent of synapse location in hippocampal pyramidal neurons. *Nature Neurosci.* 3, 895-903.

Maiti, A., Brabec, C., Roland, C., Yakobson, B., Bernhole, J., 1996. Growth and elastic properties of nanotubes. In: *Eighth Annual Workshop on Recent Developments in Electronic Structure Algorithms.* Minneapolis, MN.

Marsh, D., 1995. Lipid-protein interactions and heterogeneous lipid distribution in membranes. *Mol. Membrane Biol.* 12, 59-64.

Martens, J., Polanco-Navarro, R., Coppock, E., Nishiyama, A., Parshley, I., Grobaski, T., Tamkun, M., 2000. Differential targeting of Shaker-like potassium channels to lipid rafts. *J. Biol. Chem.* 275, 7443-7446.

Martens, J., O'Connell, K., Tamkun, M., 2004. Targeting of ion channels to membrane microdomains: localization of Kv channels in lipid rafts. *Trends Pharmacol. Sci.* 25, 16-21.

McConnell, H., Radhakrishnan, A., 2003. Condensed complexes of cholesterol and Phospholipids. *Biochim. Biophys. Acta* 1610, 159-173.

McCullough, W., Pitts, W., 1943. A logical calculus of the ideas immanent in nervous activity. *Bull. Math. Biophys.* 5, 115-133.

McNamara, J., 1999. Emerging insights into the genesis of epilepsy. Nature 24, A15-22.

Mel, B., 2002. What the synapse tells the neuron. *Science* 295, 1845-1846.

Mitchell, D., Litman, B., 1998. Effect of cholesterol on molecular order and dynamics in highly polyunsaturated phospholipid bilayers. *Biophys. J.* 75, 896-908.

Mobashery, N., Nielsen, C., Andersen, O., 1997. The conformational preference of gramicidin channels is a function of lipid bilayer thickness. *FEBS Letters* 412, 15-20.

Mouritsen, O., Bloom, M.., 1984. Mattress model of lipid-protein interaction in membranes. *Biophys. J.* 46(2), 141-153.

Mouritsen, O., Bloom, M., 1993. Models of lipid-protein interactions in membranes. In: Engleman, D., Cantor, C., Pollard, T. (Eds.), Annual Review of Biophysics and Biomolecular Structure, Vol. 22. *Annual Reviews*, Palo Alto.

Mouritsen, O., Jørgensen, K., 1992. Dynamic lipid bilayer hetereogeneity: a mesoscopic vehicle for membrane function? *BioEssays* 1, 129-136.

Mouritsen, O., Jørgensen, K., 1994. Dynamical order and disorder in lipid bilayers. *Chem. Phys. Lipids* 73, 3.

Mouritsen, O., Kinnunen, P., 1996. Role of lipid organization and dynamics for membrane functionality. In: Merz, K., Roux, B. (Eds.), *Biological membranes: A molecular perspective from computation and experiment.* Birkhäuser, Boston.

Nakada, C., Ritchie, K., Oba, Y., Nakamura, M., Hotta, Y., Iino, R., Kasai, R., Yamaguchi, K., Fujiwara, T., Kusumi, A., 2003. Accumulation of anchored proteins forms membrane diffusion barriers during neuronal polarization. *Nat. Cell Biol.* 5, 626-632.

Nelson, W., Wilson, R., Wollner, D., Mays, R., McNeill, H., Siemers, K., 1992. Regulation of epithelial cell polarity: a view from the cell surface. *Cold Spring Harb. Symp. Quant. Biol.* 57, 621-630.

Nestler, E., Hyman, S., Malenka, R., 2001. *Molecular Neuropharmacology: A Foundation for Clinical Neuroscience.* McGraw-Hill, New York.

Overton, E., 1968 (Orig., 1899). The probable origin and physiological significance of cellular osmotic properties. In: Branton, D., Park, R., (Eds.), 1968. *Papers on Biological Membrane Structure*. Little, Brown and Company, Boston.

Papazian, D., 1999. Potassium channels: some assembly required. *Neuron* 23, 7-10.

Papazian, D., Shao, X., Seoh, S.-A., Mock, A., Huang, Y., Wainstock, D., 1995. Electrostatic interactions of S4 voltage sensor in Shaker K$^+$ channel. *Neuron* 14, 1293-1301.

Parnas, I., 1972. Differential block at high frequencies of branches of a single axon innervating two muscles. *J. Neurophysiol.* 35, 903-914.

Peschke, J., Riegler, J., Möhwald, H., 1987. Quantitative analysis of membrane distortions introduced by mismatch of protein and lipid hydrophobic thickness. *Eur. Biophys. J.* 14, 385-391.

Petersen N., Hoddelius P., Wiseman P., Seger O., Magnusson K., 1993. Quantification f membrane receptor distributions by image correlation spectroscopy: concept and application. *Biophys. J.* 65, 1135-1146.

Pink, D., Chapman, D., 1979. Protein-lipid interactions in bilayer membranes: a lattice model. *Proc. Natl. Acad. Sci. USA* 76(4), 1542-1546.

Poo, M., Robinson, K., 1977. Electrophoresis of concanavalin A receptors along embryonic muscle cell membrane. *Nature* 17, 602-605.

Price, H., Wallace, R., 2001. A computational model of membrane lipid electronic properties in relation to neural signaling. *BioSystems* 59, 27-34.

Putney, J., 2003. Capacitative calcium entry in the nervous system. *Cell Calcium* 34, 339-344.

Radhakrishnan, A., McConnell, H., 2000. Electric field effect on cholesterol-phospholipid complexes. *Proc. Natl. Acad. Sci. USA* 97, 1073-1078.

Rall, W., 1977. Dendritic spines and synaptic potency. In: Porter, R., (Ed.), *Studies in neurophysiology*. Cambridge University Press, New York.

Rall, W., Burke, R., Holmes, W., Jack, J., Redman, S., Segev, I., 1992. Matching dendritic neuron models to experimental data. *Physiol. Rev.* 72, S159-S186.

Rasband, M., Schrager, P., 2000. Ion channel sequestration in central nervous system axons. *J. Physiol.* 525, 63-73.

Robertson, J., 1957. New observations on the ultrastructure of the membranes of frog peripheral nerve fibers. *J. Biophys. Biochem. Cytol.* 3, 1043-1047.

Rochefort, A., Avouris, P., Lesage, F., Salahub, D., 1999. Electrical and mechanical properties of distorted carbon nanotubes. *Phys. Rev. B*. 60, 13824-13830.

Sadava, D., 1993. *Cell Biology: Organelle Structure and Function*. Jones and Bartlett, Boston.

Salaun, C., James, D., Chamberlain, L., 2004. Lipid rafts and the regulation of exocytosis. *Traffic* 5, 255-264.

Samsonov, A., Mihalyov, I., Cohen, F., 2001. Characterization of cholesterol-sphingomyelin domains and their dynamics in bilayer membranes. *Biophys. J.* 81, 1486-1500.

Sargent, P., 1992. Electrical Signaling. In: Hall, Z. (Ed.), *An Introduction to Molecular Neurobiology*. Sinauer Associates, Sunderland.

Savtchenko, L., Gogan, P., Korogod, S., Tyč-Dumont, S., 2001a. Imaging stochastic spatial variability of active channel clusters during excitation of single neurons. *Neurosci. Res.* 39, 431-446.

Savtchenko, L., Gogan, P., Tyč-Dumont, S., 2001b. Dendritic spatial flicker of local membrane potential due to channel noise and problematic firing of hippocampal neurons in culture. *Neurosci. Res.* 41, 161-183.

Scheibel, T., Parthasarathy, R., Sawicki, G., Lin, X.-M., Jaeger, H., Lindquist, S., 2003. Conducting nanowires built by controlled self-assembly of amyloid fibers and Selective metal deposition. *Proc. Natl. Acad. Sci.* 100, 4527-4532.

Scott, A., 1995. *Stairway to the Mind: The Controversial New Science of Consciousness.* Copernicus, New York.

Shin, C., McNamara, J., 1994. Mechanisms of epilepsy. *Annu. Rev. Med.* 45, 379-389.

Simons, K., Dupree, P., Fiedler, K., Huber, L., Kabayashi, T., Kurzchalia, T., Olkkonen, V., Pimplikar, S., Parton, R., Dotti, C., 1992. Biogenesis of cell-surface polarity in epithelial cells and neurons. *Cold Spring Harb. Symp. Quant. Biol.* 57, 611-619.

Simons, K., Ikonen, E., 1997. Functional rafts in cell membranes. *Nature* 387, 569-572.

Singer, S., 1972. A fluid lipid-globular protein mosaic model of membrane structure. In Membrane structure and its biological applications, *Annals of the New York Academy of Sciences,* New York, Green, D. (Ed.) 1972.

Singer, S., Nicolson, G., 1972. The fluid mosaic model of the structure of cell Membranes. *Science* 175, 720-731.

Swadlow, H., Waxman, S., 1976. Variations in conduction velocity and excitability following single and multiple impulses of visual callosal axons in the rabbit. *Exp. Neurol.* 53, 128-150.

Tanford, C., 1989. *Ben Franklin Stilled the Waves: An Informal History of Pouring Oil on Water with Reflections of the Ups and Downs of Scientific Life in General.* Duke University Press, Durham.

Tauc, L., Hughes G., 1963. Modes of initiation and propagation of spikes in the axon of molluscan central neurons. *J. Gen. Physiol.* 46, 533-549.

Tiwari-Woodruff, S., Schulteis, C., Mock, A., Papazian, D., 1997. Electrostatic interactions between transmembrane segments mediate folding of Shaker K$^+$channel subunits. *Biophys. J.* 72, 1489-1500.

Tomishige, M., Sako, Y., Kusumi, A., 1998. Regulation mechanism of the lateral diffusion of Band 3 in erythrocyte membranes by the membrane skeleton. *J. Cell Biol.* 142, 989-1000.

Tomishige, M., Kusumi, A., 1999. Compartmentalization of the erythrocyte membrane by the membrane skeleton: intercompartmental hop diffusion of Band 3. *Mol. Biol. Cell* 10, 2475-2479.

Torshin, I., and Harrison, R., 2001. Charge centers and formation of the protein folding core. *Proteins: Structure, Function, and Genetics* 43, 353-364.

Tsui-Pierchala, B., Encinas, M., Milbrandt, J., Johnson, E., 2002. Lipid rafts in neuronal signaling and function. *Trends in Neurosciences* 25, 412-417.

Vale, R., Banker, G., Hall, Z., 1992. The neuronal cytoskeleton. In: Hall, Z. (Ed.), *An Introduction to Molecular Neurobiology.* Sinauer Associates, Sunderland.

van Essen, J., 1973. The contribution of membrane hyperpolarization to adaptation and conduction block in sensory neurones of the leech. *J. Physiol.* 230, 509-534.

Vassilev, P., Dronzin, R., Vassileva, M., Georgiev, G., 1982. Parallel arrays of microtubules formed in electric and magnetic fields. *Biosci. Rep.* 2, 1025-1029.

Vassilev, P., Dronzin, R., Valevski, G., Kanazairska, M., 1983. In vitro polymerization of tubulin modified by application of low-intensity electric and magnetic fields. *Stud. Biophys.* 94, 139-140.

Vater, W., Stracke, R., Böhm, K., Speicher, C., Weber, P., Unger, E., 1998. *Behavior of individual microtubules and microtubule bundles in electric fields.* Presented paper at 6th Foresight Conference on Molecular Nanotechnology.

Vinogradova, O., 2001. Hippocampus as comparator: role of the two input and two output systems of the hippocampus in selection and registration of information. *Hippocampus* 11, 578-598.

Wallace, R., 1995. Microscopic computation in human brain evolution. *Behav. Sci.* 40, 133-158.

Wallace, R., 1996a. Microcomputational evolution of the neural membrane. *Nanobiology* 4, 25-37.

Wallace, R., 1996b. Quantum computation in the neural membrane: Implications for the evolution of consciousness. In: Hameroff, S., Kaszniak, A., Scott, A. (Eds.), *Toward a Science of Consciousness: The First Tucson Discussions and Debates.* The MIT Press, Cambridge.

Wallace, R., 1999. Computational aspects of neural membrane biophysics. In: Leszczynski, J. (Ed.), *Computational Molecular Biology.* Elsevier, New York.

Wallace, R., Price, H., 1999. Neuromolecular computing: a new approach to human brain evolution. *Biol. Cyber.* 81, 189-197.

Wallace, R., 2004. Neural membrane field effects in a cytoskeleton corral: microdomain regulation of impulse propagation. *Int. J. Quantum Chem.* 100, 1038-1046.

Wallace, R., 2007. Neural membrane microdomains as computational systems: toward molecular modeling in the study of neural disease. *BioSystems* 87, 20-30.

Wallis, C., Wenegieme, E., Babitch, J., 1992. Characterization of calcium binding to brain spectrin. *J. Biol. Chem.* 5, 4333-4337.

Wallis, C., Babitch, J., Wenegieme, E., 1993. Divalent cation binding to erythrocyte spectrin. *Biochemistry* 32, 5045-5050.

Wang, T-Y., Leventis, R., Silvius, J., 2000. Fluorescence-based evaluation of the partitioning of lipids and lipidated peptides into liquid-ordered lipid microdomains: A model for molecular partitioning into "lipid rafts". *Biophys. J.* 79, 919-933.

Wang, T-Y., Leventis, R., Silvius, J., 2001. Partitioning of lapidated peptide sequences into liquid-ordered domains in model and biological membranes. *Biochemistry* 40, 13031-13040.

Whatley, V., Harris, R., 1996. The cytoskeleton and neurotransmitter receptors. *Int. Rev. Neurobiol.* 39, 113-143.

Williamson, I., Alvis, S., East, J., Lee, A., 2002. Interactions of phospholipids with the potassium channel KcsA. *Biophys. J.* 83(4), 2026-2038.

Winckler B., Forscher P., Mellman I., 1999. A diffusion barrier maintains distribution of membrane proteins in polarized neurons. *Nature* 397, 698-701.

Zajchowski, L., Robbins, S., 2002. Compartmentalized signaling in membrane Microdomains. *Eur. J. Biochem.* 269, 737-752.

Zuckermann, M., 1993. Self-sustained potential oscillations and the main phase transition of lipid bilayers. *Biophys. J.* 64, 1369-1370.

Chapter IX

Scaffolding Proteins that Regulate the Actin Cytoskeleton in Cell Movement

S. J. Annesley and P. R. Fisher
Microbiology Department, La Trobe University, Melbourne, Australia.

Abstract

Actin is the main component of the microfilament system in all eukaryotic cells and is essential for most intra- and inter-cellular movement including muscle contraction, cell movement, cytokinesis, cytoplasmic organisation and intracellular transport. The polymerisation and depolymerisation of actin filaments in nonmuscle cells is highly regulated and the reorganisation of the actin cytoskeleton can occur within seconds after chemotactic stimulation. There are many proteins which are involved in the regulation of the actin cytoskeleton. These include receptors which receive chemotactic stimuli, G proteins, second messengers, signalling molecules, kinases, phosphatases and transcription factors. These proteins are varied and numerous and are involved in multiple pathways. Despite the large number of proteins, there are not enough to coordinate the various responses of the cytoskeleton. An additional level of regulation is conferred by scaffolding proteins.

Due to the presence of numerous protein interaction domains, scaffolding proteins can tether various proteins to a certain location within the cell to facilitate the rapid transfer of signals from one protein to the next. This colocalisation of the components of a particular pathway also helps to prevent unwanted crosstalk with components of other pathways. Tethering receptors, kinases, phosphatases and cytoskeletal components to a particular location within a cell helps ensure efficient relaying and feedback inhibition of signals to enable rapid activation and inactivation of responses. Scaffolding proteins are also thought to stabilise the otherwise weak interactions between particular proteins in a cascade and to catalyse the activation of the pathway components. There are numerous scaffolding proteins involved in the regulation of the cytoskeleton and this chapter has focussed on examples from several groups of scaffolding proteins including the MAPK scaffolds, the AKAPs, scaffolds of the post synaptic density and actin binding scaffolding proteins.

1. Introduction

Actin is the main component of the microfilament system in all eukaryotic cells and is essential for a wide variety of functions including muscle contraction, cell movement, cytokinesis, cytoplasmic organisation to intracellular transport [Van Troys et al., 1999]. Actin is ubiquitous in eukaryotes and is one of the most highly conserved proteins in evolution. For example, actin of humans and the protist *Euplotes crassa* still share 61 % identity. Actin is even more conserved in evolution than histone H4 [Van Troys et al., 1999].

Actin is present in two forms - the 42 kDa globular monomeric actin [G-actin] which can reversibly assemble into filamentous actin [F-actin] [McGough, 1998]. In resting cells about half of the actin is present in the monomeric state and the other half is present in the filamentous state [Eichinger et al., 1998]. The polymerisation and depolymerisation of actin filaments in nonmuscle cells is highly regulated. The reorganisation of the actin cytoskeleton can occur within seconds after chemotactic stimulation and these changes correspond to morphological changes.

The signalling pathways leading to reorganisation of the cytoskeleton generally involves activation of a receptor through binding of a ligand and transmission of this signal through G proteins, signalling molecules such as GTPases, second messengers such as Ca^{2+} and its associated molecules, kinases, phosphatases and cytoskeletal components. The movement of the cell is concomitant with the formation and breakdown of cell adhesion sites at the leading edge and trailing edge respectively. These cell adhesion sites contain integrins which mediate attachment to extracellular matrix components. Clearly the rearrangement of the cytoskeleton is complex and involves numerous proteins.

The signalling pathways leading to movement of the actin cytoskeleton involve many proteins, yet the number of specific cellular behaviours that are elicited by and are reliant on these pathways is even greater. Additionally a single stimulus can elicit more than one response. Hence there are not enough proteins for each to have an individual biological role, which implies that the signalling proteins must work in conjunction with each other [Pawson & Nash, 2000]. So how do the pathways maintain specificity and prevent cross talk between alternate pathways? One way that cells do this is via scaffolding proteins.

Scaffolding proteins have many postulated roles in signalling pathways. They are thought to tether various proteins to a certain location within the cell to facilitate the rapid transfer of signals from one protein to the next [Smith & Scott, 2001]. The colocalisation of the components of a particular pathway also helps to prevent unwanted crosstalk with components of other pathways [Whitmarsh & Davis, 1998]. Tethering receptors, kinases, phosphatases and cytoskeletal components to a particular location within a cell helps ensure efficient relaying and feedback inhibition of signals to enable rapid activation and inactivation of responses. Scaffolding proteins are also thought to stabilise the otherwise weak interactions between particular proteins in a cascade and to catalyse the activation of the pathway components [Burack & Shaw, 2000].

Most scaffolding proteins are large in size presumably due to their ability to simultaneously bind various proteins. However some smaller scaffolding proteins such as MP1 (MEK partner 1) which is only 14.5 kDa in size have also been identified and MP1 has been shown to bind at least two members (MEK1 and ERK1) of a signalling cascade

[Vomastek *et al.*, 2004]. They also often contain many protein-protein interaction domains such as SH2, SH3, PH, and PDZ domains amongst many others, which aid in tethering different proteins involved in a particular cascade. The protein interaction domains have been conserved throughout evolution due to their biological significance and are represented in nearly all eukaryotes [Liu *et al.*, 2006]. In some cases the prevalence of a domain increases with multicellularity. For example the PDZ domain is found in only two proteins in yeast whereas 545 PDZ domains have been identified in humans [Zimmermann, 2006]. Additionally some domains such as the SH2 domain are not represented in fungi, mainly due to the lack of tyrosine phosphorylation pathways [*Liu et al.*, 2006]. Many protein interaction domains have been identified and some of these are listed in Table 1.

Many of the scaffolding proteins identified to date, especially the MAPK family members, dimerise to form homo- and hetero-oligomers and this dimerisation appears to be a conserved feature [Elion, 2001]. The dimerisation may allow phosphorylation in *trans* between protein kinases attached to different subunits of the dimer [Hunter, 2000].

As exemplified by overexpression experiments, the stoichiometry of the scaffolding protein to other components in the pathway is tightly regulated to ensure sufficient concentrations of all components of the pathway are present. Too much scaffold can titrate out and separate the binding partners, and consequently inhibit signalling [Symons *et al.*, 2006]. An example of this is the scaffolding protein Ksr which was identified as a positive and negative regulator of signalling. When Ksr was overexpressed it was shown to suppress signalling, however at normal levels it acts as a positive regulator, increasing signalling [Levchenko *et al.*, 2000].

There are several major families of scaffolding proteins involved in the regulation of the cytoskeleton. These include amongst others the MAPK (Mitogen Activated Protein Kinase) scaffolding proteins, the AKAPs (A-Kinase Anchoring Proteins), the post synaptic density (PSD) scaffolding proteins and actin binding scaffolding proteins including IQGAP and filamin. This article will focus on these groups.

1.1. MAPK Scaffolding Family

The mitogen activated protein kinases (MAPKs) are present in all eukaryotic organisms and are expressed in virtually all mammalian tissues [Sabbagh *et al.*, 2001]. MAPKs respond to a variety of extracellular stimuli such as growth factors, mitogens, cytokines and environmental stress [Whitmarsh & Davis, 1998] and they relay these messages mainly to transcription factors to alter gene expression. The signalling pathways these proteins are involved in are diverse, including those controlling proliferation, differentiation, apoptosis and cell movement [Pullikuth *et al.*, 2005]. MAPK cascade scaffolds are widely divergent, indicating that they have evolved independently for the individual requirements of subsets of kinases and upstream activating events [Elion, 2001].

A MAPK cascade generally consists of three protein kinases: a MAPK, a MAPK activator (MEK or MKK) and a MKK activator (MEKK or MKKK) and the particular cascade is named after the last kinase of the series [Schaeffer & Weber, 1999]. Some MAPK cascades also contain an additional kinase, a MAPKKKK which phosphorylates the MKK activator. The first kinase in the series, MKKK, is activated in response to various stimuli binding to a receptor. Ligand binding to the receptor results in the recruitment of adaptor proteins specific to the receptor type and/or activation of small GTP-binding proteins, both of which can activate MKKK proteins. For example tyrosine kinase receptors often result in recruitment of Rho GTPases which can then activate a MKKK [Davis, 2000]. Activation of MKKK leads to MKK serine/threonine phosphorylation which in turn activates the MAPK by dual phosphorylation on threonine and tyrosine residues in the activation loop [Ito et al., 1999]. Phosphorylation of both residues on the MAPK is essential for it to perform its various functions as shown by mutational analysis proving that phosphorylation of one of the residues does not activate the kinase whereas dual phosphorylation at these sites results in a >1000 fold increase in the activity of the MAPK [Widmann et al., 1999].

The MAPK's are proline-directed serine/threonine kinases. The phosphorylation of the MAPK by the upstream kinase results in a conformational change that creates a surface pocket which is specific for a proline residue. The MAPK generally recognizes a proline at the +1 position of a potential substrate [Schaeffer & Weber, 1999]. Potential substrates of MAPKs are more often than not transcription factors, however, other targets include cytoskeletal proteins, protein kinases and phosphatases [Symons et al., 2006].

In mammals MAPK cascades have been shown to be involved in diverse pathways regulating cell fate including differentiation and proliferation, response to extracellular stress and apoptosis. Many of the MAPK substrates are transcription factors, however other substrates such as cytoskeletal proteins, protein kinases and phosphatases have also been identified [Ho et al., 2006; Widmann et al., 1999]. Three major mammalian MAPK cascades have been identified, the ERK (extracellular signal-related kinase), the JNK/SAPK (c-Jun N-terminal kinase/stress-activated protein kinase]) and p38 [Fusello et al., 2006] cascades.

1.1.1. The ERK cascade

Eight ERK proteins have been identified in mammals, numbered 1 through 8, and the cascades involving these proteins are required for regulating processes as diverse as cell growth and differentiation as well as cytoskeleton-dependent focal adhesion and cell spreading. ERK1 and 2 were the first ERKs to be identified. They share 90 % sequence identity and participate with the same members of a MAPK cascade [Bogoyevitch & Court, 2004]. Both proteins have been extensively studied and hence will be the focus of this section. The members of this pathway include Raf-1 (a MKKK), MEK1/2 (a MKK) and ERK1/2 (a MAPK), and many other associated regulatory proteins. Raf-1 acts as a scaffolding molecule by binding several components of the pathway and localizing them to the plasma membrane upon stimulation. The ERK1/2 cascade is initiated through the binding of growth factors such as EGF (epidermal growth factor) and PDGF (platelet-derived growth factor) to numerous receptors. These receptors include tyrosine kinase receptors, cytokine receptors, G-protein coupled receptors and integrins [Widmann et al., 1999].

Domain	Size (amino acids)	Structure	Recognition Site	Examples	References
SH2 (Src homology 2)	~100	A spine consisting of an antiparallel β sheet dividing the domain into two distinct sides. One side binds PTyr [phosphotyrosine] the other contains residues which interact with residues C-terminal to the PTyr on the target. A conserved pocket binds the PTyr.	Short peptide motifs containing PTyr residues. Group I prefer PTyr-hydrophilic-hydrophilic-hydrophobic and Group II prefer PTyr-hydrophobic-hydrophobic recognition sequence. Residues C-terminal to PTyr determine substrate specificity. Binding to peptide with optimal sequence is relatively high.	Found in proteins involved in protein tyrosine kinase pathways such as phospholipid metabolism, tyrosine phosphorylation and dephosphorylation, gene expression, protein trafficking and cytoskeletal architecture.	Kuriyan & Cowburn, 1997 Pawson, 1995 Cohen et al., 1995 Machida & Mayer, 2005
SH3 (Src homology 3)	50-70	Consists of 2 antiparallel β sheets each comprised of 3 β strands which fold into a β sandwich. One side contains a hydrophobic pocket which binds the recognition motif.	Bind to proline-rich target sequences containing the PXXP motif. The 1st X tends to be a proline and the 2nd X tends to be an aliphatic residue. The target peptides generally adopt a polyproline type II helix which can bind the domain in either orientation. Specificity is determined by residues N- or C-terminal to the PXXP motif.	Found in proteins involved in signal transduction, cytoskeletal organisation and membrane traffic.	Morais et al., 1996 Bar-Sagi et al., 1993 Pawson, 1995 Kuriyan & Cowburn, 1997 Cesareni et al., 2002
PH (Pleckstrin homology)	100-120	PH fold contains 2 antiparallel β sheets consisting of 3 and 4 strands respectively. The structure is capped by an amphiphatic C-terminal α helix. On one side of the PH domain is a narrow cleft containing 3 variable loops and clusters of positive charges, this is the site for binding ligand.	Most bind phosphoinositides or inositol phosphates and they do this with varying affinities. PH domains with low affinities may localise to membranes through the presence of multiple PH domains on a single protein.	Found in a wide range of signalling and cytoskeletal proteins. Proteins are generally cytoplasmic but associate with the plasma membrane & are often involved in the intracellular localisation of proteins.	Ludbrook et al., 1997 Chung et al., 2001 Funamoto et al., 2001 Maffucci & Falasca, 2001 Lemmon et al., 2002

Table 1. Continued

Domain	Size (amino acids)	Structure	Recognition Site	Examples	References
PDZ (PSD-95, discs large, zona occludens 1)	80-90	Comprise 6 β strands (βA-βF) and 2 α helices (αA & αB) which fold into a 6-stranded β sandwich. Target proteins bind as an antiparallel β strand in a cavity formed by the βB strand, the αB helix and a loop connecting βA & βB strands. PDZ interactions are reversible and versatile and the binding affinities are moderate.	Recognise motifs of 3-7 residues or PDZ binding motifs (e.g. the E[S/T]DV motif of certain ion channel subunits) generally at the C-terminus of target proteins. PDZ domains can form homotypic or heterotypic interactions with other PDZ domains. Proteins with PDZ domains often contain other protein interaction domains. Specificity appears to be determined by the interaction of the first residue of the αB helix and the side chain of the -2 residue of the C-terminal ligand.	Proteins containing PDZ domains are ubiquitously expressed and have diverse roles eg. Assembly & regulation of neuronal synapses and establishment & maintenance of epithelial cell polarity & are found in a range of proteins including protein kinases, tyrosine phosphatases and a variety of proteins involved in ion-channel and receptor clustering.	Morais et al., 1996 Pawson & Scott, 1997 Kuriyan & Cowburn, 1997 Huber,2001 Hung & Sheng, 2002 Zimmermann, 2006
Immunoglobulin (Ig)-like	~100	Each domain contains 2 β sheets which are comprised of 3-5 β strands. The 2 β sheets are packed tightly together to form a β sandwich which is further stabilised by a conserved disulfide bond, however this bond is absent in some examples.	Most Ig-domains are able to interact with other Ig-like domains. The fold also facilitates interactions with other proteins and DNA molecules. The domains interact with other proteins mainly through the faces of the β sheets & therefore can interact with other proteins through any accessible part of their surface.	Cell adhesion molecules, membrane bound receptors such as tyrosine receptors, transcription factors and cytoskeletal proteins.	Williams & Barclay, 1988 Wisemann et al., 2000 Nagata et al., 1999 Noegel et al., 1989
PTB (Phosphotyrosine binding)		Contains a core fold which consists of 2 perpendicular antiparallel β sheets (β1-4 & β5-7) packed to form a β sandwich capped by a C-terminal helix (α3). Ligand binds in the groove between β5 and α3, phospholipid binds in a highly basic area composed of residues from loop regions near the N-terminus.	Recognise peptide sequences containing variations of the NPXY motif which is typically located in the juxtamembrane regions of integral membrane proteins. Also bind to the head group of phospholipids.	Occurs in proteins involved in signal transduction, membrane trafficking and cytoskeletal dynamics, such as neuronal development, immune response, tissue homeostasis and cell growth.	DiNitto & Lambright, 2006 Uhlik et al., 2005

Domain	Size	Structure	Binding	Function	Reference
homology)		calcium-binding helix-loop-helix motifs (EF hands, however not all bind calcium), which are linked by an antiparallel β sheet. Most EH domains are at the N-terminus of the protein.	NPF motif. The NPF motif enters a conserved hydrophobic pocket which binds the peptide, bringing the asparagine residue of the peptide in close proximity to the highly conserved tryptophan residue in the EH domain.	regulate endocytic membrane transport events, the regulation of actin dynamics, and various roles in signal transduction.	Caplan, 2005
WW (refers to 2 tryptophan residues [W] present in these domains)	40	Fold as a stable antiparallel 3 stranded β sheet structure which forms a shallow binding pocket for ligands.	Recognise peptides containing a proline-rich core motif (generally PPXY or PPLP) which is usually flanked by additional prolines.	Found in proteins involved in numerous cellular processes including RNA processing & transcription, receptor signalling and protein trafficking.	Kay et al., 2000; Sudol et al., 2005
LIM (lin-11, isl-1 & mec-3)	50-60	Double zinc finger motifs with the consensus sequence $(CX_2CX_{16-23}HX_2C(X_2) CX_2CX_{16-21}CX_2H/D/C)$. The conserved cysteine, histidine & aspartic acid residues form 2 tetrahedral pockets which bind zinc & stabilise the secondary & tertiary structure.	No common LIM binding motif has been identified however, LIM domains can associate with each other, with motifs found on transcription factors and other protein interaction domains.	Proteins containing LIM domains are involved in various cellular processes including cytoskeletal organisation, cell lineage specification and organ development.	Bach, 2000; Brown et al., 2001; Khurana et al., 2002
EVH1 (enabled/vasodilator-stimulated phosphoprotein homology 1)	115	The overall fold is highly conserved and consists of a compact β sandwich closed along one edge by a long α helix. There is a cluster of three aromatic sidechains which form the recognition site for the proline rich targets.	Bind to proteins containing proline rich sequences. Two classes bind different motifs: Class I recognise FPxϕP motif [where ϕ is a hydrophobic residue] and Class II recognise PPxxF motif. The binding is of low affinity but high specificity. Specificity is achieved through residues flanking the core motif.	Exist primarily in proteins which are involved in the regulation of the actin cytoskeleton and in postsynaptic proteins.	Ball et al., 2002
IQ	~20	General sequence is [I,L,V]QXXXRXXXX[R,K] which forms a basic amphipathic helix. Critical hydrophobic residues reside at positions 1, 8 and 14. Basic amino acids often flank the core motif.	Bind calmodulin.	Present in wide range of proteins including myosins, phosphatases, Ras exchange proteins, neuronal growth proteins and voltage operated channels.	Bahler & Rhoads, 2002

Table 1. Continued

Domain	Size (amino acids)	Structure	Recognition Site	Examples	References
VCA (Verprolin, cofilin homology-acidic) or VPH (Verprolin homology)		V region contains the motif KLKK which is essential for actin binding. Also contains two conserved serines which are phosphorylated, enhancing interaction with Arp2/3 complex.	The V region binds to G actin and the CA region binds to the Arp2/3 complex promoting actin nucleation.	Present in WASP family members which are involved in the regulation of actin polymerisation.	Cory et al., 2003 Kato et al., 2002 Yamaguchi et al., 2000
SAM (Sterile Alpha Motif)	~70	The core consists of a five helix bundle comprised of hydrophobic residues. Helices 3,4 and 5 are essential for the high affinity interactions.	Can self associate to form homo- or hetero-SAM domain interactions and also form heterotypic interactions with non-SAM containing proteins.	Exist in a wide number of proteins such as signalling proteins and transcription factors and also to RNA. Proteins are present in all subcellular locations, and are involved in diverse biological functions from chromatin remodelling to apoptosis.	Kim & Bowie, 2003 Kwan et al., 2006

As seen in Figure 1, ligand binding to the various receptors ultimately results in tyrosine phosphorylation of the receptor and the recruitment of various adaptor proteins to the receptor where they facilitate the activation of Ras through the exchange of GDP for GTP at its active site [Pouyssegur et al., 2002]. Raf-1 binds a group of proteins called the 14-3-3 proteins. These proteins bind to the kinase domain of Raf-1 and stabilise the inactive configuration of Raf-1 in which the regulatory domain masks the catalytic domain. Ras has a high affinity for Raf-1 and once activated it is able to bind to the NH_2-terminal regulatory domain of Raf-1 and displace the 14-3-3 protein. The displacement of the 14-3-3 protein alters the structure of Raf-1 so the catalytic domain is accessible to dephosphorylation by PP2A. Only Raf-1 which is dephosphorylated at these residues is able to initiate the MAPK cascade [Dhillon & Kolch, 2002]. The binding affinity of Ras for Raf-1 is very high, higher even than the affinity of Ras for Ras-GAP. Termination of Raf-1 activation occurs through phosphorylation of Raf-1 at another serine residue by the cAMP-dependent kinase, PKA thereby diminishing the affinity of Ras for Raf-1 [Dhillon & Kolch, 2002].

Ras activated Raf-1 binds its downstream target kinase, MEK1 through a proline-rich sequence and phosphorylates MEK1 at a serine/threonine residue. MEK1 in turn binds ERK1/2 and activates it through dual phosphorylation on a threonine and tyrosine residue in the Thr-Glu-Tyr motif. This phosphorylation causes a conformational change in the ERK2 activation lip creating a proline-specific pocket [Schaeffer & Weber, 1999]. Activated ERK1/2 can then dissociate from the scaffold and translocate to specific locations within the cell such as the nucleus where it can bind to transcription factors or to the cytoplasm where it binds cytoskeletal proteins. ERK1/2 phosphorylates a serine and threonine residue on its substrates in a proline directed manner. The most stringent recognition sequence for the ERK1/2 proteins is Pro-Leu-Ser/Thr-Pro [Widmann et al., 1999].

The ERK1/2 cascades are activated by numerous growth factors binding to many different receptors and have various substrates which they bind. They are also present in nearly all types of mammalian cells. To accommodate all these varied responses, additional levels of regulation exist to ensure flexibility yet specificity to each cascade and also insulation from regulation by other stimuli [Pullikuth et al., 2005].

In addition to the scaffolding protein Raf-1, other scaffolding proteins seem to be employed in the ERK1/2 cascades. An example of an additional scaffolding protein is Ksr (Kinase suppressor of Ras). Ksr appears to be evolutionarily conserved with homologs identified in mammals, *Drosophila, C. elegans* and *Xenopus* [Denouel-Galy et al., 1997]. Ksr shows high structural homology to Raf-1, but despite a putative kinase domain in the C-terminus it is devoid of any kinase activity [Roy & Therrien, 2002]. Figure 1 provides an illustration of this MAPK cascade and how many of the components interact due to the two scaffolding components Raf-1 and KSR.

Like Raf-1, Ksr is bound by a 14-3-3 protein which may serve to sequester Ksr to the cytoplasm. In response to stimuli such as ceramide, activated Ras induces the translocation of Ksr to the plasma membrane where it binds to the γ subunits of heterotrimeric G-proteins. Ksr has also been shown to constitutively associate with 14-3-3, MEK and a Rho family member regardless of Ras activation, whereas its interaction with Raf-1 and MAPK is Ras dependent. It appears then that Ras-dependent localisation of Ksr may bring MEK in close proximity to Raf-1 and a MAPK and aids in assembling of the cascade [Roy & Therrien, 2002].

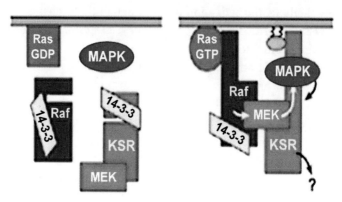

[Morrison, 2001]

Figure 1. Scaffolding proteins Raf-1 and Ksr in an ERK (MAPK) cascade. The two scaffolding proteins Raf-1 and Ksr both bind a protein, 14-3-3 which holds these proteins in the cytoplasm. Upon activation of Ras, Raf-1 is recruited to the membrane where it binds Ras with a very high affinity. The binding of Ras displaces the 14-3-3 protein, changing the structure of Raf-1 to an active configuration. The activation of Ras also recruits Ksr to the membrane where it binds to the β subunit of a heterotrimeric G protein (Gβ). Ksr brings MEK and ERK (MAPK) in close contact with the other kinase members and initiates the phosphorylation cascade from Raf-1 to MEK and finally to ERK [Morrison, 2001]. (Reproduced with permission of the Company of Biologists).

Another additional scaffolding protein of an ERK1/2 cascade is MP1 (MEK partner 1). MP1 has been shown to interact in ERK cascades in response to adhesion factors but not in response to other factors such as PDGF. MP1 tightly associates with p14, a protein that acts as an adaptor linking MP1 to late endosomes [Teis et al., 2002]. This association is very stable and the MP1/p14 complex is able to directly bind two members of the ERK1/2 cascade, these being ERK1 and MEK1 but not their closely related isoforms ERK2 and MEK2 respectively. This selectivity suggests that there may also be different but as yet unidentified components which would selectively regulate ERK2 and MEK2 [Pullikuth et al., 2005].

MP1/p14 associates with MEK1 through a proline-rich sequence which contains a site for PAK (p21-activated kinase) phosphorylation. MP1/p14 is able to bind activated PAK (p21-activate kinase) which can then phosphorylate and activate MEK1. PAK is activated in response to cell adhesion factors and by phosphorylating MEK1 it can couple the MEK1-ERK1 activation to upstream adhesion signals [Pullikuth et al., 2005]. MP1/p14 is also able to interact with Rho (a GTPase) and ROCK (a Rho kinase). ROCK is able to phosphorylate various kinases and a cytoskeletal protein, cofilin which can then counteract the membrane protrusion stimulated by the Rho proteins. This inhibition is known to be important for focal adhesion turnover and cell spreading [Pullikuth et al., 2005]. Once activated ERK1 is released from the complex with MEK1 and MP1 allowing the movement of ERK1 molecules to their sites of action [Sharma et al., 2005]. Taken together this particular ERK cascade provides an example of how different stimuli (adhesion factors), can recruit members of the ERK cascade through adaptor proteins (p14) and scaffolding proteins (MP1) to specific compartments of the cell (late endosomes) in order to elicit a particular behaviour (cell adhesion and spreading).

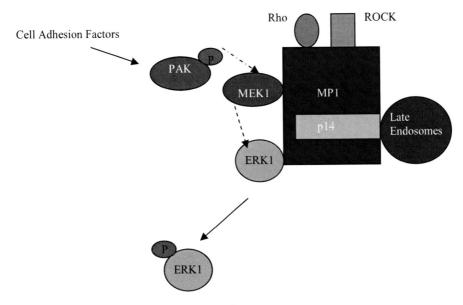

Figure 2. The MP1 Scaffold. MP1 is able to interact directly with two members of the MAPK cascade, MEK1 and ERK1. MP1 associates very strongly with the adaptor protein p14. This association links MP1 and the members of the complex to the late endosomes. This MAPK cascade is initiated by cell adhesion factors which lead to the activation and phosphorylation of PAK1. Once activated, PAK1 can phosphorylate MEK1 and MEK1 in turn phosphorylates ERK1 (as denoted by the broken arrows). Activated ERK1 is released from the complex and translocates to its sites of action. MP1 is also able to interact directly with Rho and ROCK. Rho is a GTPase and ROCK is a Rho kinase which, in addition to phosphorylating and activating Rho, can phosphorylate various kinases and the cytoskeletal protein cofilin.

The strength and duration of signals transmitted through ERK1/2 can also affect the type of response. For example in PC-12 cells stimulation of the ERK1/2 cascade through EGF stimulates proliferation yet stimulation by NGF stimulates differentiation of cells. The different responses are thought to be linked to the duration of the ERK1/2 activation. EGF stimulates ERK1/2 transiently with activity levels returning to basal standards within 1-2 hours. Conversely NGF stimulates ERK1/2 in a more sustained manner [Widmann et al., 1999]. It seems that there are many factors which aid in the regulation of MAPK cascades, including adaptor and scaffolding proteins and duration of expression.

1.1.2. JNK/SAPK Cascades

This family of MAPKs are activated by a variety of genotoxic and cytotoxic cellular stresses including heat shock, UV irradiation, hyperosmolarity, ischemia and cytokines such as interleukin-1 [Nihalani et al., 2001; Ho et al., 2006]. To date 14 associated MKKKs (including MEKK1-4, ASK1, TAK1, MST, SPRK, MLK1-3, DLK, MUK and TPL2), 2 MKKs (MKK4 and 7) and three JNK kinases (JNK1-3) and their 10 isoforms resulting from alternative splicing have been identified in mammals [Ho et al., 2006; Nihalani et al., 2001; Widmann et al., 1999]. JNK3 is expressed predominantly in the brain and testis whilst JNK1 and 2 are ubiquitously expressed [Ito *et al.*, 1999]. The JNKs, like other MAPKs are activated by dual phosphorylation on threonine and tyrosine residues of the Thr-Pro-Tyr motif and they phosphorylate substrates at a Ser/Thr-X-Pro motif [Widmann *et al.*, 1999]. The numerous members of these cascades reflect the number of distinct signalling pathways that these cascades are involved in [Ito *et al.*, 1999]. Distinct members of JNK cascades have been implicated in various responses including apoptosis, proliferation, and embryonic morphogenesis [Nihalani *et al.*, 2001].

There are a number of signalling proteins which are able to activate the JNK cascade and this activation can operate through a variety of cell surface receptors including the TNF receptor family, GPCR, tyrosine kinase receptors and cytokine receptors [Widmann *et al.*, 1999]. The type of receptor that is stimulated by a particular ligand determines which adaptor proteins are recruited. For example, GPCRs are linked to the adaptor proteins β-arrestins which control the desensitization and internalization of the receptors. They have also been shown to act as MAPK scaffolds themselves binding many members of the cascade and recruiting the signalling complexes to activated GPCRs. An example involves the AT1aR (angiotensin type 1a receptor) GPCR. β-arrestin 2 binds all three members of the MAPK cascade, JNK3, MKK4 (indirect interaction) and ASK. Upon activation of the receptor, β-arrestin 2 is recruited to the receptor along with its associated members of the MAPK cascade and aids in the activation of JNK3 [Willoughby & Collins, 2005].

Tyrosine kinase receptors activate members of the Rho family of GTPases which in turn phosphorylate and activate MLK and MEKK family members. Cytokine receptors and the IL-1 receptor appear to mediate JNK activation through a group of adaptor proteins of the TRAF group which have been shown to phosphorylate MEKK1 and ASK1. Alternatively the adaptor protein Nck may mediate JNK activation by Eph receptors [Davis, 2000].

Most JNK substrates identified are transcription factors including c-Jun, Elk-1, p53 and NFAT4. Phosphorylation of these substrates can lead to increased or decreased rates of transcriptional activity, it can also lead to structural changes which may protect the transcription factor from subsequent modifications, thereby stabilizing them [Widmann *et al.*, 1999]. However, there are some non-nuclear substrates such as the Bcl-2 family member BAD and the 14-3-3 protein [Willoughby & Collins, 2005].

The diversity and localisation of these cascades is often aided by scaffolding proteins.

Several JNK scaffolding proteins have been identified, these include JIP (JNK-interacting protein, JSAP1 (JNK stress activated protein 1) and JLP (JNK-associated leucine zipper protein) [Ito *et al.*, 1999; Nihalani *et al.*, 2001; Lee *et al.*, 2002a]. These scaffolding proteins appear to bind particular members of a JNK cascade in response to specific stress stimuli.

1.1.2.1. The JIP scaffolds

Four JIP genes and several splice isoforms have been identified in mammals. Two of the encoded proteins JIP1 and JIP2 are closely related, whereas JIP3 is structurally unrelated [Davis, 2000]. Unlike the other JIP proteins, JIP4 is involved in activating the p38 MAPK and not the JNK MAPK [Kelkar et al., 2005]. The JIP1 and 2 proteins contain an SH3 domain and a PTB domain within their carboxyl-terminal domain. The PTB domain has been shown to interact with several receptors and members of the Rho family. The function of the

SH3 domain is unclear, however, this domain has been shown in other proteins to function in protein-protein interactions [Davis, 2000]. All JIP proteins interact specifically with members of the MLK (mixed lineage kinase) family of MKKKs but not with other MKKKs such as the MEKK proteins. They also interact with MKK7 but not MKK4 [Nihalani et al., 2001] and JNK1 and 2.

As seen in Figure 3 JIP binds to a MLK protein in its monomeric inactive state through its leucine zipper domain as well as binding a receptor or adaptor protein. Upon appropriate stimulation mediated through the adaptor protein the MLK protein dissociates allowing the two leucine zipper domains to interact and form a MLK dimer. Dimerisation initiates autophosphorylation and subsequent catalytic activation. The interaction of the two leucine zipper domains in the MLK protein to form stable dimers is of high affinity and is the most favourable configuration. The JIP protein therefore provides a mechanism of regulation for this JNK cascade by tethering MLK in an inactive state prior to stimulation. The dissociation and activation of the MLK protein results in recruitment of JNK to the JIP scaffold by an unknown mechanism and also results in phosphorylation of JIP1-bound MKK7. MKK7 can then phosphorylate the bound JNK protein [Nihalani et al., 2001]. By binding and aggregating all three components of the cascade JIP may therefore act as a scaffolding protein.

Like other scaffolding proteins JIP proteins can form homo- and hetero-oligomers and belong to the group of phosphoproteins [Nihalani et al., 2001]. JIP1, 2 and 3 have been shown via a yeast two hybrid screen to interact with the tetratricopeptide repeat (TPR) domain of the light chain of the microtubule motor protein kinesin [Kelkar et al., 2005]. JIP1 and JIP2 interact with kinesin through their COOH terminus whereas JIP3 interacts via a leucine zipper domain. In immunoprecipitation experiments, kinesin, JIP1, a MKKK protein and a receptor, Reelin, coprecipitated suggesting that kinesin, a microtubule motor protein, acts to localise signalling complexes through a scaffolding protein [Verhey et al., 2001].

1.1.2.2. The JSAP Scaffold

JSAP is another scaffolding protein of the JNK cascade and is expressed as a result of alternative splicing of the JIP3 gene [Nihalani et al., 2001]. JSAP preferentially binds all three JNKs (with a higher preference for JNK3 [Ito et al., 1999]), the MKKs MKK/SEK1, 4 and 7, and the MKKK MEKK1 [Takino et al., 2005]. All three interactions occur at unique sites on JSAP1.

Figure 4 is a cartoon depicting the JNK cascade which involves JSAP as a scaffolding protein. In this figure it can be seen that MEKK1 interacts with inactive SEK1 and JSAP1, however inactive SEK1 does not interact directly with JSAP1 until it is activated. It appears that when stimulated MEKK1 phosphorylates SEK1 and facilitates its binding to the scaffold protein JSAP1. SEK1 can then activate JNK through dual phosphorylation. Once activated JNK phosphorylates JSAP1 and is subsequently dissociated from the scaffold. Phosphorylated JSAP1 has little binding affinity for JNK. Once dissociated, JNK is free to translocate to the nucleus and to phosphorylate its transcription factor substrates. JSAP1 contains a leucine zipper motif which may mediate its homo- or hetero-oligomerisation [Ito et al., 1999]. It is unknown whether this dimerisation is required for its function, however it is known to occur in many other scaffolding proteins [Elion, 2001].

1.1.2.3. The JLP scaffold

The third JNK scaffolding protein is JLP. JLP shows high sequence homology (69 % identity) to the other two scaffolding proteins discussed (JSAP1 and JIP). JLP is a 180 kDa protein that is ubiquitously expressed and is located primarily in the cytoplasm. However, JLP is translocated to the nucleus in response to stress signals [Lee et al., 2002a]. JLP associates with the MKKK MEKK3, the MKK MKK4, as well as JNK1 and a member of a different MAPK cascade p38α. MKK4 has previously been shown to activate MAPK members of both the JNK and p38 cascades. Unlike other scaffolding proteins JLP is able to directly bind target transcription factors such as Max and c-Myc which are substrates for both JNK and p38 members [Lee et al., 2002a]. JLP has also been shown to directly interact with the $G\alpha_{12}$ or $G\alpha_{13}$ subunit of the heterotrimeric G protein G12 or G13 respectively. G proteins are known to activate JNK cascades however JLP is the first mammalian scaffold identified that links $G\alpha_{12}$ or $G\alpha_{13}$ to the JNK signalling module [Kashef et al., 2005].

JLP contains two leucine zipper domains and three putative SH2 and SH3 binding sites. The leucine zipper domains have been shown to be the regions which bind the transcription factors and recently the second leucine zipper domain has been shown to bind kinesin light chain 1 (KLC1) [Nguyen et al., 2005]. The other JNK scaffold mentioned previously, the JIP family members and JSAP also interact with kinesin, albeit through a different domain. Kinesin's are a family of motor proteins that move cargo along microtubules in an ATP dependent manner. JLP therefore serves as a link between the kinesin motor proteins and the JNK signalling complex proteins [Nguyen et al., 2005].

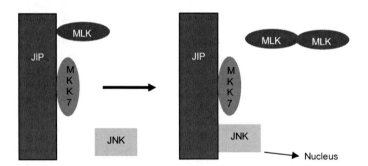

Figure 3. The JIP scaffold. JIP associates with inactivated MLK and MKK7. An adaptor protein (not shown on this diagram) facilitates the activation of MLK which stimulates the protein to dimerise, autophosphorylate and dissociate from the complex. This dissociation results in the phosphorylation of MKK7 and the recruitment of JNK to the complex which is phosphorylated by MKK7. Phosphorylated JNK can then dissociate from the complex and translocate to its substrate targets such as transcription factors in the nucleus.

The SH2 and SH3 binding sites in JLP could potentially facilitate interactions with SH2 and SH3 containing kinases which could link to other signalling pathways. JLP binds JNK1 and p38α at different sites and can therefore tether both molecules simultaneously. JLP can form oligomers and this may further facilitate the tethering of JNK and p38. Thus JLP acts as a scaffolding protein by bringing all three members of a MAPK cascade together as well as downstream targets of both the JNK and p38 MAPKs. Binding of the transcription factors to its upstream activators may accelerate transmission of signals. Interactions of JLP with other signalling molecules, possibly through the SH2 and SH3 binding sites could also facilitate subcellular trafficking of a signalling complex to different subcellular sites [Lee et al., 2002a].

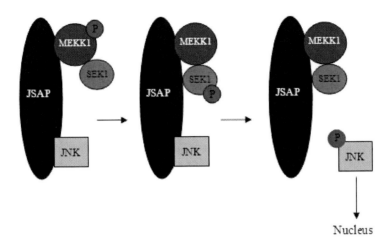

Figure 4. JSAP Scaffold. Prior to initiation of the cascade JSAP interacts directly with two members of the MAPK cascade, MEKK1 and JNK. Once MEKK1 is stimulated it phosphorylates SEK1 which, in this activated state can bind to the scaffold, JSAP. SEK1 is then able to phosphorylate JNK which subsequently phosphorylates JSAP and results in the dissociation of JNK from the scaffold. Dissociated JNK is then free to translocate to the nucleus and phosphorylate its various transcription factor substrates.

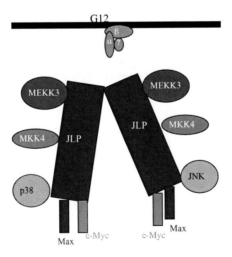

Figure 5. The JLP Scaffold. JLP is able to directly bind all three members of the MAPK cascade - the MKKK, MEKK3; the MKK, MKK4; and two different MAPKs, JNK and p38. JLP is a dimer and as such is able to bind both MAPKs simultaneously within the cell. This MAPK cascade is initiated by stress signals which activate G proteins. JLP directly binds the alpha subunit of the heterotrimeric G proteins G12 or G13 (G12 depicted in this figure). Activation of G proteins stimulates the phosphorylation cascade leading to phosphorylation-mediated activation of JNK and p38, and translocation of JLP to the nucleus where it can directly bind to transcription factors such as Max and c-Myc. JNK or p38 then phosphorylate its transcription factor targets.

1.1.3. p38 MAPK Cascade

The mammalian p38 cascade is homologous to the yeast osmosensing Hog1 pathway. These MAPK cascades are activated like JNK cascades by cellular stress such as UV irradiation, heat shock, protein synthesis inhibitors and certain cytokines. The members of these pathways include the MAPK members, p38α, β, γ and δ, the MKK members MKK4, 3 and 6 and the MKKK members which include TAK1, ASK1, MLK3 and SPRK [Widmann et al., 1999; Ito et al., 1999]. p38α and β share more than 70 % sequence identity and are ubiquitously expressed, whereas p38γ and δ share 60 % sequence identity to p38α and are only expressed in specific tissues such as the brain [Katsoulidis et al., 2005; Dean et al., 2004]. The p38 kinases are activated by dual phosphorylation at a Thr-Gly-Tyr motif.

Several potential scaffolding proteins have been identified which interact with specific members of the p38 cascade and are expressed in select tissues. These include the JIP family members JIP2, JLP and JIP4, and OSM (osmosensing scaffold for MEKK3) [Robidoux et al., 2005; Uhlik et al., 2003]. As the p38 kinases like the JNK kinase cascades are activated by cellular stresses it is not surprising that many of the proteins which act as scaffolds for JNK members also act as scaffolds for p38 members. This is the case for many of the JIP family members such as JIP2 and the JLP protein whose role as a scaffold for p38 was described in the preceding section.

Another JIP family member, JIP4 has been identified by Kelkar et al. [2005]. It is functionally distinct from other JIP members as it does not activate JNK but has been shown to activate p38 MAP kinase. The *jip4* gene encodes at least three proteins JIP4, the previously described JLP and SPAG9 (sperm-associated antigen 9 protein) of unknown function. These proteins all result from alternative splicing [Kelkar et al., 2005]. JIP4 is structurally most similar to JIP3. Like JIP3, JIP4 contains a putative transmembrane domain which indicated that this protein may span the cytoplasmic membrane. However, JIP4 was found to be widely distributed throughout the cytoplasm with no localisation to any organelles. Like other JIP members JIP4 also binds the motor protein kinesin and does this through a leucine zipper domain.

In studies conducted by Kelkar et al. [2005] JIP4 was shown to interact with the MAP3K, ASK1, and the MAPK family members, JNK and p38 as illustrated in Figure 6. Even though JIP4 can bind JNK and p38 it is only able to activate p38. Why JIP4 binds yet does not activate JNK is unclear and the authors suggested that JNK may act as a regulator of JIP4 by competing with p38 for binding. No MKK member was shown to interact directly with JIP4, so this interaction may occur indirectly via the ASK1 or p38 proteins as has been shown in other MAPK cascades such as the cascade involving β$_2$-arrestin as a scaffold. In this cascade β$_2$-arrestin interacts with MKK4 indirectly via interactions with the MKKK, ASK1, and the MAPK JNK3 [McDonald et al., 2000]. Kelkar et al. [2005] did however demonstrate that in MKK3 and MKK6 double knockout mice, JIP4 is unable to activate p38. Hence these two MKK members may be involved in the JIP4 cascade.

Another potential p38 scaffolding protein is OSM. This protein was identified by Uhlik et al. [2003] in a two hybrid screen using MEKK3, a known p38 MKKK protein as bait. As seen in Figure 7 OSM interacts directly with all three members of a MAPK cascade: p38, MKK3 and MEKK3. OSM also interacts directly with actin and a GTPase Rac1. OSM is located throughout the cytoplasm however upon exposure of cells to sorbitol, OSM and the bound members of the cascade were relocalised to ruffle-like structures rich in actin and Rac1. Once stimulated OSM binds actin and Rac1 and activates p38. Other stimulants were used such as anisomycin and no relocalisation or activation of p38 was observed [Uhlik *et al.*, 2003]. This indicates that OSM acts as a scaffolding molecule for a Rac-MEKK3-MKK3 cascade in response to hyperosmotic shock caused by treatment with sorbitol.

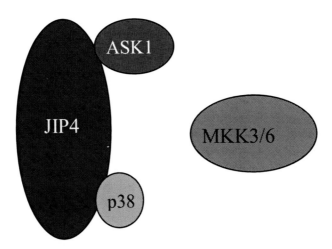

Figure 6. The JIP4 scaffold. JIP4 is able to interact with all three members of a p38 signalling module. JIP4 interacts directly with the MKKK ASK1 and the MAPK p38 and indirectly with the MKKs, MKK3 and 6.

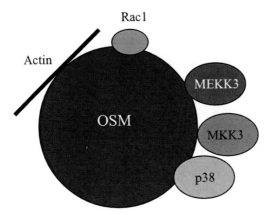

Figure 7. The OSM scaffold. OSM is located in the cytoplasm and interacts with all three members of the p38 module, MEKK3, MKK3 and p38. Upon stimulation with sorbitol OSM and its bound proteins are relocalised to ruffle like structures which are rich in actin. OSM then binds to actin and Rac1 which results in the initiation of the cascade and the activation of p38.

1.2. AKAPs (A-Kinase Anchoring Proteins)

The second messenger cyclic AMP (cAMP) is involved in a signal transduction cascade that has been extensively studied. Most of the effects that are mediated by cAMP are through its binding to PKA (cAMP-dependent protein kinase A). Mammalian PKA is a tetramer which is composed of two catalytic subunits and two regulatory subunits. The catalytic subunits are found in three isoforms encoded by three different genes (Cα, Cβ and Cγ) and all isoforms have essentially the same kinetic and physiochemical properties [Colledge & Scott, 1999]. The R subunits are expressed from four different genes RIα, RIβ, RIIα and RIIβ. The PKA tetramer assembles to form a heterotetrameric enzyme of two different forms depending on the R subunits involved. PKA type I contains RIα and RIβ dimers and is primarily cytoplasmic, whereas PKA Type II contains RIIα and RIIβ dimers and associates with specific cellular structures and organelles [McConnachie et al., 2006]. The discrete localisation of Type II PKA within the cell is due to its association with scaffolding proteins called AKAPs. AKAPs are a family of functionally related proteins which are defined based on their ability to bind the R subunits of PKA.

AKAPs have two conserved domains. The first is the PKA-binding motif which forms an amphipathic helix of 14-18 residues that interacts with a hydrophobic pocket formed on the N-terminus of the R subunit dimer [Schillace & Scott, 1999; Diviani & Scott, 2001]. Most AKAPs identified have been shown to bind to RII dimers, however some interactions have been shown between AKAPs and RI dimers such as AKAP$_{CE}$ in *C. elegans* [Angelo & Rubin, 1998]. The affinity of AKAPs for RII is about 100 fold higher than that for RI subunits [Carlisle-Michel & Scott, 2002]. The other conserved feature of AKAPs is a targeting motif which directs the PKA-AKAP complex to discrete locations within the cell such as the plasma membrane, actin cytoskeleton, mitochondria, endoplasmic reticulum, nuclear membrane, centrosomes and vesicles [Schillace & Scott, 1999].

AKAPs are defined as scaffolding proteins as they can colocalise many components of a signal transduction pathway in close proximity to specific substrates [Dell'Acqua et al., 2006]. As these complexes contain signal termination proteins such as phosphatases, and phosphodiesterases and signal transduction enzymes such as kinases, they are capable of upregulating and downregulating specific signalling pathways [McConnachie et al., 2006]. About 50 AKAPs have been identified [McConnachie et al., 2006], however this section will discuss four in detail due to their involvement in regulation of the cytoskeleton. They are gravin, ezrin, CG-NAP/AKAP450 and WAVE-1 a member of the WASP family. Like all AKAPs these proteins not only bind to PKA but also other kinases and phosphatases and they can regulate the bidirectional phosphorylation events at specific compartments in the cell.

1.2.1. Gravin

Gravin is a 250 kDa protein which acts as a scaffold by binding PKA, PKC, PP2B (protein phosphatase 2B), β$_2$-AR (β$_2$-adrenergic receptor), GRK2 (G-protein-linked receptor kinase 2) and by transiently binding to β-arrestin and clathrin [Fan et al., 2001; Diviani & Scott, 2001].

Gravin contains many domains or sites which facilitate its binding with the associated proteins. Membrane association is achieved through three domains, the first of which is a putative N-myristoylation site. N-myristoylation is a post-translational modification which provides weak and reversible interactions between gravin and the membrane. A second membrane domain was identified which shows homology to the membrane effector domain of MARCKS (myristoylated alanine-rich C-kinase substrate) proteins. This domain has been shown in MARCKS proteins to provide binding to membranes in a manner reversible by

Ca^{2+}/calmodulin binding [Malbon et al., 2004a]. Recently this has also been demonstrated for Gravin [Tao et al., 2006]. The third membrane association domain is provided by a set of sites located near the midpoint of the protein. These sequences are conserved amongst Gravin and AKAP79 and their homologs and are involved in the binding of the β$_2$-adrenergic receptor (β$_2$–AR) [Malbon et al, 2004b].

Gravin binds the protein kinases and protein phosphatase PP2B at unique conserved sites. A putative F-actin binding domain resides within the PKC binding domain and may be involved in the translocation of the complex. Also a putative SH3 binding domain was identified with which the non-tyrosine kinase Src can associate. These kinases are known regulators of GPCR-signalling complexes [Malbon et al., 2004b].

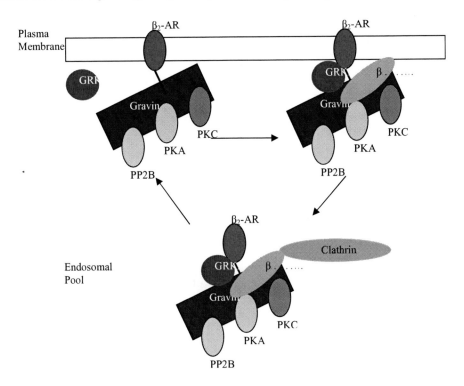

Figure 8. The Gravin Scaffold. Gravin binds several protein kinases and a phosphatase PP2B. The protein is also able to interact with the β$_2$-AR. Upon stimulation of the receptor the gravin-β$_2$-AR interaction is enhanced bringing the gravin-associated proteins in close proximity to the receptor which would allow for attenuation of the signal. GRK2 is phosphorylated at the membrane and recruits β-arrestin from the cytosol. β-arrestin associates with clathrin which translocates the complex to an endosomal pool where PP2B dephosphorylates the receptor. This disrupts the association of β-arrestin and clathrin and the complex is translocated back to the plasma membrane.

A fundamental feature of cell signalling is the attenuation of a signal following stimulation, this process is referred to as desensitization. Protein phosphorylation is often a key feature of this process. In the case of the β$_2$-AR, the desensitization involves phosphorylation of the receptor via the protein kinases PKA, PKC and GRK2 which is illustrated in Figure 8. Gravin has been shown to associate with the β$_2$-AR in unstimulated cells, however upon agonist stimulation this association is enhanced. This brings the other gravin-associated proteins such as PKA, PKC, GRK and PP2B into close proximity to the receptor, permitting an initial attenuation of the signal through phosphorylation of the receptor via the associated kinases (PKA, PKC and GRK). Phosphorylation of the C-terminal region of the membrane bound receptor by GRK allows the recruitment of β-arrestin from the cytosol which can associate with clathrin and translocate the complex to an intracellular endosomal pool via clathrin-dependent endocytosis. This process is necessary for subsequent resensitisation of the receptor. Once the complex has been sequestered to the endosome, PP2B dephosphorylates the receptor thereby disrupting its association with β-arrestin and clathrin and the complex is then translocated back to the plasma membrane [Lin et al., 2000]. Gravin is an example of a mobile scaffold which maintains the ensemble of protein kinases and phosphatases through translocation from the plasma membrane to vesicles involved in trafficking the complex during desensitization and resensitisation [Fan et al., 2001].

1.2.2. Ezrin

Ezrin belongs to a family of closely related cytoskeletal proteins termed ERM proteins, named after its three members ezrin, radixin and moesin. These AKAPs link integral membrane proteins to the actin cytoskeleton. ERM proteins are found in all multicellular organisms and share a high degree of sequence identity and structural conservation [Fievet et al., 2007]. The conserved structure consists of three major domains, an N-terminal globular FERM (four-point one ERM) domain of approximately 300 residues, followed by a 160 residue region which is an α-helical domain predicted to form coiled coils and an actin binding C-terminal domain of approximately 90 residues [Finnerty et al., 2003]. The FERM domain is composed of three subdomains, F1, F2 and F3 which are arranged in the shape of a cloverleaf. The central α-helical domain connects the FERM domain to the F-actin binding site present in the C-terminus [Fievet et al., 2007]. The three ERM members are expressed early in development in different tissues or cells within the organism. In mammals Ezrin is expressed mainly in epithelial cells and it is enriched at the apical surface [Berryman et al., 1993], while radixin is present in the liver [Tsukita et al., 1989] and also in the cochlear stereocilia [Pataky et al., 2004; Kitajiri et al., 2004] and moesin is found primarily in endothelial cells [Lankes & Furthmayr, 1991] and in some epithelial cells [Berryman et al., 1993].

ERM proteins are conformationally regulated by a head to tail interaction that masks sites for membrane associated proteins and F-actin [Gary & Bretscher, 1995; Reczek & Bretscher, 1998]. As seen in Figure 9 in the inactive configuration the ERM proteins are inactive and localise mainly to the cytoplasm. Activation of ERM proteins is achieved through disruption of the head to tail interaction by binding to PIP2 and phosphorylation of a conserved threonine in the actin binding site of the C-terminus. PIP2 binds in a cleft between subdomains F1 and F3 in the FERM domain, this binding is thought to alter the conformational change leading to disruption of the interaction between C- and N-termini [Hamada et al., 2000]. This interaction has been shown to be critical for translocation of ERM proteins to the plasma membrane. Once localised to the plasma membrane ERM proteins can integrate with additional membrane associated proteins. Plasma membrane localised ERM proteins are then phosphorylated at the conserved threonine residue which stabilises the active configuration [Yonemura et al., 2002; Fievet et al., 2004]. Several protein kinases can phosphorylate ezrin at this residue including Protein kinase C which has been shown to carry out this phosphorylation *in vitro* [Ng et al., 2001] Additionally, Akt can phosphorylate ezrin at the conserved threonine in response to Na+/glucose transport, leading to association of ezrin with the actin cytoskeleton and the translocation of the Na+/H+ exchanger NHE3 [Fievet et al., 2007]. Ezrin may be phosphorylated and its active state stabilised by different kinases depending on the type of complex ezrin is involved in and the stimuli present.

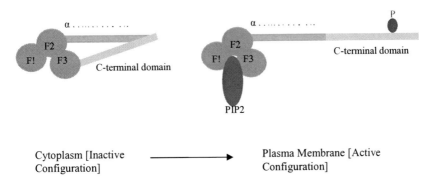

Figure 9. Activation of ERM proteins. ERM proteins contain a conserved structure consisting of an N-terminal FERM domain constructed from three subdomains F1, F2 and F3, followed by a central α-helical domain and a C-terminal domain. ERM proteins are held in the cytoplasm in an inactive configuration through the C-terminal domain binding to the FERM domain. Binding of PIP2 in a cleft between the F1 and F3 subdomains and phosphorylation of a conserved threonine residue in the C-terminus disrupts the interaction of the C-terminus with the FERM domain. This active configuration leads to translocation of ERM proteins to the plasma membrane where it can interact with additional plasma membrane associated proteins.

Of the three family members only ezrin has been shown to be essential for cell survival with ezrin-deficient mice dying shortly after birth [Saotome et al., 2004]. Further discussion will focus on the A-kinase anchoring, ERM protein ezrin. Ezrin is able to interact with many proteins and these interactions occur either through direct binding or through association of Ezrin with an adaptor protein with the best characterised adaptor being EBP50 (ERM-binding protein of 50kDa).

Ezrin interacts directly with membrane proteins in addition to PIP2 and these interactions help localise ezrin to the plasma membrane. Ezrin can directly bind the Na^+/H^+ exchanger NHE1 and this interaction is required for control of cell shape [Denker et al., 2000]. Ezrin also directly binds the hyaluronan receptor CD44 and this interaction has been shown to be important for cell motility [Legg et al., 2002]. Additional interactions with membrane proteins occur through the interaction of ezrin with EBP50. EBP50 is another scaffolding protein that contains two PDZ domains which can interact with numerous proteins, and a C-terminal region which binds to the FERM domain of Ezrin [Reczek & Bretscher, 1998]. EBP50 interacts with the cystic fibrosis transmembrane conductance regulator (CFTR) [Short et al., 1998], the β2-adrenergic receptor [Cao et al., 1999] and the Na^+/H^+ exchanger NHE3 [Yun et al., 1998] via its PDZ domains.

Ezrin is an AKAP and binds the RII subunit of PKA. Through Ezrin's interaction with numerous membrane proteins Ezrin is able to localise PKA to the membrane where it can phosphorylate its substrates including CFTR and NHE3 which it can activate or inhibit, respectively [Sun et al., 2000a; Sun et al., 2000b; Dransfield et al., 1997; Lamprecht et al., 1998; Weinman et al., 2000]. The complexes formed are important for trafficking of membrane proteins such as the recycling of β2-andrenergic receptors from the endosome to the plasma membrane after agonist stimulated endocytosis [Cao et al., 1999] and the localisation of the CFTR [Moyer et al., 1999, 2000]

Ezrin forms multiprotein complexes which are essential for the morphogenesis of the apical domain of epithelial cells, including orginisation of actin filaments and delivery of membrane proteins. Ezrin has also been shown to play an important role in Fas-mediated apoptosis. Fas is a member of the death family proteins and when activated recruits numerous proteins to form the death inducing signalling complex that initiates the apoptotic cascade. Ezrin directly binds to Fas via its FERM domain and may play a role in localising Fas and its associated molecules to the plasma membrane to receive signals from apoptotic stimuli [Fais et al., 2005]. The Fas-Ezrin interaction is essential for Fas-mediated apoptosis as mutants in which Ezrin was down regulated showed defects in apoptosis [Parlato et al., 2000].

Through its association with EBP50 ezrin is also important for linking lipid rafts in T cells to the actin cytoskeleton, and plays a negative role in immune synapse formation [Itoh et al., 2002]. These examples show how ezrin can act as a scaffold binding numerous receptors, cell adhesion molecules and scaffolding proteins to link various proteins from the plasma membrane to the underlying actin cytoskeleton.

1.2.3. CG-NAP (centrosome and golgi localised protein kinase N (PKN)-associated protein) also called AKAP450/AKPA350

CG-NAP is a giant protein predicted to form a coiled coil over most of its length except for small regions (~200 amino acids) at both the C- and N-terminal regions [Gillingham & Munro, 2000]. The protein is localised to the centrosome throughout the cell cycle, the midbody at telophase and the Golgi apparatus at interphase in cultured cell lines [Takahashi et al., 1999]. The protein interacts with many components of signal transduction cascades including three protein kinases (PKA, PKCε and PKN) and two phosphatases (PP1 and PP2A) [Takahashi et al., 2000], phosphodiesterase 4D [Tasken et al., 2001], casein kinase 1δ/ε [Sillibourne et al., 2002], cdc42 interacting protein 4 [Larocca et al., 2004] and Ran [Keryer et al., 2003]. CyclinE-cdk2 has been shown to be involved in the process of centrosome duplication [Hinchcliffe et al., 1999] and Nishimura et al. [2005] have shown that CG-NAP recruit Cyclin E-cdk2 to the centrosome and therefore may be involved in centrosome duplication.

CG-NAP contains two RII binding sites at its C-terminus and may therefore bind two PKA holoenzymes in one signalling complex. The centrosomal targeting domain resides in the C-terminus and shows high homology to another centrosomal AKAP, pericentrin. These two AKAPs may compete with each other for centrosome binding or they may work in a coordinated fashion [Carlisle-Michel & Scott, 2002]. CG-NAP also binds to the N-terminal region of PKN, a Rho-activated kinase which phosphorylates intermediate filament proteins indicating that the complex may be important for cytoskeletal reorganisation events. PKN is a substrate of PP2A which can dephosphorylate PKN and decrease its kinase activity. PP2A binds to CG-NAP through its regulatory subunit. An immature, non- or hypophosphorylated

PKCε can also associate with CG-NAP until it is sufficiently phosphorylated whereby it dissociates from the scaffold and can respond to incoming second messenger signals [Takahashi et al., 2000]. CG-NAP therefore acts as a scaffold by localising many kinases and phosphatases and it coordinates the activity of these enzymes at centrosomes and in the Golgi apparatus.

1.2.4. WAVE1

WAVE1 is a member of the WASP family of proteins. This family is named after its founding member Wiskott-Aldrich syndrome protein (WASP) which, when mutated, causes a rare X-linked immunodeficiency disease [Westphal et al., 2000]. WAVE1 functionally couples small Rho GTPases, Rac and Cdc42 (activated by ligand binding a receptor) to the Arp2/3 complex, which is a group of seven related proteins that nucleate actin polymerization, and can thereby elicit changes in the actin cytoskeleton in response to the signal [Yamazaki et al., 2005]. The C-terminus of WAVE1 contains an acidic domain which is responsible for binding and activating the Arp2/3 complex [Calle et al., 2004]. WASP proteins also contain a central proline rich sequence which facilitates binding to several SH3 containing proteins and to an actin binding protein, profilin. WASP members also contain a verprolin homology (VPH) domain that is responsible for binding monomeric actin [Westphal et al., 2000].

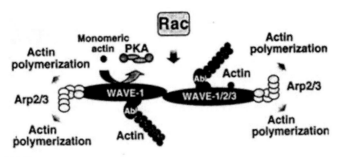

[Diviani & Scott, 2001].

Figure 10. WAVE1, an AKAP at the cytoskeleton. WAVE1 forms homo- or hetero-dimers with other WAVE isoforms, WAVE2/3. Activated Rac1 or Cdc42 binds to WAVE1 and causes the relocalisation of WAVE1 and its associated proteins, such as the kinases Abl and PKA to sites rich in actin. WAVE1 can directly bind actin, actin binding proteins and the Arp2/3 complex to promote actin polymerisation. Actin can compete with PKA for binding to WAVE1 and therefore sufficient concentrations of actin may displace PKA. (Reproduced with permission of the Company of Biologists).

WAVE1 has been shown to bind to the RII subunit of PKA and it does this through the VPH domain. It appears that actin competes for the RII binding site, the significance of this is unclear but sufficient concentrations of actin may displace the anchored PKA. Thus, PKA may be dynamically regulated at sites of actin reorginisation [Westphal et al., 2000]. WAVE1 can also form homo- or hetero-dimers with other WAVE isoforms (WAVE2 & 3). WAVE1 may therefore tether PKA to the cytoskeleton through the actin based interactions of WAVE2 or 3. WAVE1 can also bind a tyrosine kinase Abl (Abelson) at its SH3 domain. Rac-activated stimulation by Platelet-derived growth factor (PDGF) results in the rapid redistribution of WAVE1, PKA and Abl from focal adhesions to sites of actin polymerization. The assembly of the WAVE1 complex is dependent on this extracellular signal and it appears that WAVE1 not only facilitates the coupling of Rac to the Arp2/3 complex but also coordinates the location and action of PKA at sites of actin reorganisation [Diviani & Scott, 2001].

1.3. PSD (Post Synaptic Densities) Scaffolding Proteins

PSDs are disc-like structures approximately 30-40 nm thick and 400 nm wide which are observed under electron microscopy as thickenings of the postsynaptic membranes [Ziff, 1997]. These areas are specialised complexes which contain and organise many components of the postsynaptic response including receptors for the neurotransmitter glutamate, receptor associated proteins, signal transduction molecules, cytoskeletal and regulatory proteins [Irie et al., 2002]. There is an abundance of proteins in the PSD, some estimating the total number to be as many as a few hundred [Sheng, 2001].

The PSD is highly enriched in three types of glutamate receptors - the NMDA (N-methyl-D-aspartate) receptors, the AMPA (α-amino-3-hydroxy-5-methyl-4-isoxazolepropionic acid) receptors and the mGluRs (group 1 metabotropic glutamate receptors) [Sheng, 2001]. These receptors are specifically targeted to the postsynaptic membrane where they are responsible for fast signalling at these synapses. The NMDA receptors are a consistent, stable feature of excitatory synapses, they are permeable to monovalent and calcium ions both of which induce synaptic plasticity, such as long term potentiation.

AMPA receptors are glutamate-gated monovalent cation channels whose activation provides most of the postsynaptic depolarisation that drives neuronal firing [Fukata et al., 2005]. Synaptic transmission at low frequency is dependent primarily on AMPA receptors [Leonard et al., 1998]. The presence of AMPA receptors in excitatory synapses is highly variable with a significant fraction of the synapses not containing these receptors [Sheng, 2001]. The distribution of AMPA receptors in excitatory synapses is dependent on synaptic activity. AMPA receptors are dynamically regulated with receptors being delivered into and out of the synapse rapidly in response to stimulus [Sheng, 2001].

The mGluRs are linked to the activation of phospholipase C and mediate excitatory affects by eliciting a release of calcium from intracellular stores [Tappe & Kuner, 2006]. The N terminus of these receptors is extracellular followed by a transmembrane region and the C terminus is located on the intracellular side of the membrane [Leonard et al., 1998]. There is a complex network of proteins which transmit the glutamate signal received by the various receptors through signalling cascades to effector substrates such as the cytoskeleton. These proteins interact with each other via numerous scaffolding proteins. There are a large number of scaffolding proteins present in the PSD and this section will focus on those involved in the regulation of the cytoskeleton including the MAGUK (membrane-associated guanylate kinases) family, cortactin, homer, and shank scaffolding proteins.

1.3.1. MAGUK (membrane-associated guanylate kinases) family

The MAGUK family of scaffolding proteins are membrane-associated cortical cytoskeletal proteins which are involved in the trafficking of glutamate receptors. Members of this family include PSD-95/SAP90, PSD93, SAP97 and SAP102 [Schluter et al., 2006]. The most extensively studied of these are PSD-95 and SAP97 and they are the focus of this section. The MAGUKs consist of three PDZ domains at the N-terminus followed by an SH3 domain, and a C-terminal guanylate kinase (GK) domain. Both PSD-95 and SAP97 are able to bind to AMPA receptors, however they do so via different mechanisms. SAP97 is able to directly bind to the GluR1 subunit of AMPA receptors via its PDZ domain [Schluter et al., 2006], whereas PSD-95 binds to the receptor indirectly through a protein called stargazin. Stargazin is a transmembrane protein which can bind to all four subunits of AMPA receptors and traffic them to the plasma membrane. The C-terminus of stargazin binds PSD-95 and links the scaffolding protein to the receptor [Fukata et al., 2005].

PSD-95 also directly binds to the C-terminus of NR2 subunits of the NMDA receptors via the first and second PDZ domains whereas SAP97 does not coprecipitate with NMDA receptors and hence, may be involved in the regulation of AMPA but not NMDA receptors [Leonard et al., 1998]. PSD-95 and SAP97 are able to interact with protein kinases, phosphatases, cytoskeletal proteins and signal transduction molecules via their five protein-protein interaction domains. Some examples of PSD-95 and SAP-97 binding partners are given below.

PSD-95 and SAP97 associate with each other as a heteromeric complex via the N-terminal segment of SAP97 and the SH3 domain of PSD-95. This interaction may influence the interactions of each of these MAGUKs with other proteins. For example SAP97 which is normally not located in dendritic spines was strongly recruited to these spines when PSD-95 was overexpressed. Conversely, PSD-95 normally triggers the accumulation of AMPA receptors to synaptic spines however overexpression of SAP97 strongly inhibited this process [Cai et al., 2006]. It seems that each of these MAGUKs may work in synergy with each other promoting and inhibiting interactions with other proteins. The MAGUKs are important for the localisation and maturation of glutamate receptors and the coupling of these receptors to a complex of proteins involved in cytoplasmic signalling pathways.

Table 2. Interacting partners of PSD-95 and SAP97.

Scaffolding Protein	Protein Domain	Interacting Protein	Role of interacting protein	Reference
PSD-95	PDZ1, 2 and 3	SynGAP	Regulates Ras activation in response to NMDA receptor stimulation	Rockliffe & Gawler, 2006
PSD-95	GK	SPAR	A GTPase for Rap. Regulates the size and shape of dendritic spines.	Sheng, 2001
PSD-95	GK	GKAP	Couples PSD-95 to Shank	Sala et al., 2001
PSD-95	PDZ	Neuronal nitrate synthase (nNOS)	Facilitates activation of nNOS by NMDA receptor mediated Ca^{2+} influx	Ishii et al., 2006
PSD-95	PDZ3	Neuroligins	Synaptic surface proteins	Levinson et al., 2005
SAP97	PDZ	NrCAM	A cell adhesion molecule	Dirks et al., 2006
SAP97	N-terminal domain	CASK	Another MAGUK	Lee et al., 2002b

1.3.2. Cortactin

There are several isoforms of cortactin, a ubiquitous protein present in the majority of cell types, including neurons where it is present in the PSDs [Weed et al., 1998]. Overexpression of cortactin has been linked to several human diseases including breast and bladder cancer [Lua & Low, 2005]. Cortactin consists of numerous protein interaction domains including an N-terminal acidic region which has been shown to bind to the Arp2/3 complex and activate it. This is followed by a region containing six complete copies and one incomplete copy of a 37 amino acid tandem repeat responsible for binding F-actin. The next domain is an alpha helical region which is rich in proline, threonine, serine and tyrosine residues that harbour sites of phosphorylation [Lua & Low, 2005]. The kinase Fyn, a protein involved in postsynaptic signalling pathways phosphorylates cortactin in this region [Iki et al., 2005].

The C-terminal region contains an SH3 domain that interacts with numerous proteins including cortactin-binding protein 1 and CBP90, two brain-specific proteins and ZO1, a cell-cell adhesion complex protein [Webb et al., 2006; Campbell et al., 1999]. The SH3 domain of cortactin also interacts with regulators of the actin cytoskeleton including dynamin2 [Mizutani et al., 2002], GTPase regulators including BPGAP1 which is a Rho GTPase activating protein [Lua & Low, 2005], N-WASP [Kinley et al., 2003], and WASP interacting protein (WIP) [McNiven et al., 2000] as well as an additional PSD scaffolding protein, Shank [Naisbitt et al., 1999].

Cortactin does not bind any glutamate receptors directly but does so indirectly through binding additional scaffolding proteins such as Shank. The PDZ domain of Shank binds to GKAPs (guanylate kinase associated proteins) which in turn bind to the GK domain of PSD-95. As mentioned earlier PSD-95 interacts directly with transmembrane receptors in the PSD such as the NMDA and AMPA receptors [Daly, 2004]. Cortactin is able to promote the nucleation of actin in response to glutamate binding to various receptors in the PSD. Thereby cortactin acts as a scaffold linking postsynaptic signalling in the PSD to the actin cytoskeleton.

1.3.3. Homer

Homer proteins are scaffolding molecules that regulate the localisation of group 1 metabotropic glutamate receptors (mGluR) [Irie et al., 2002]. Three Homer genes have been identified, *Homer* 1, 2 and 3 and these genes are alternatively spliced to form 15 long and short isoforms [Duncan et al., 2005]. The long forms are tetramers which oligomerise due to their C-terminal coiled coil domains. This oligomerisation allows Homer to interact with four ligand proteins at the same time [Hayashi et al., 2006]. This coiled coil domain is absent in the short forms of Homer. The other domain present in all Homer isoforms is the N-terminal EVH1 domain. The EVH1 domains are highly conserved and bind to a proline rich motif present in mGluRs [Xiao et al., 2000]. The long forms are constitutively expressed, whereas the short forms are expressed in an activity dependent manner. The long forms due to their ability to oligomerise are able to couple postsynaptic proteins to the receptor, whereas the short forms which are unable to oligomerise, act to compete with the long form of Homer and block its function [Hayashi et al., 2006].

Homer is able to bind many proteins apart from the mGluR through its EVH1 domain. These proteins include amongst others the receptors for ryanodine [Hwang et al., 2003] and IP$_3$ (inositol [1,4,5]-triphosphate) [Yuan et al., 2003], members of the Rho family of small GTPases [Shiraishi et al., 1999], Shank [Tu et al., 1999] an additional PSD scaffolding protein (discussed in section 1.2.4.4), TRPC [transient receptor potential canonical] channels [Yuan et al., 2003], dynamin III [Gray et al., 2003], syntakin 13 [Minakami et al., 2000] and actin [Shiraishi et al., 1999]. Homer is able to regulate the trafficking and clustering of mGluRs through these various interactions. For example dynamin III, a protein involved in endocytosis enables Homer to mediate the trafficking of mGluRs. Additionally, the Homer complex can promote the accumulation of F-actin in synapses and as it binds actin directly may link the mGluRs to the actin cytoskeleton. Homer aids in the targeting and clustering of mGluRs, and signalling proteins to the plasma membrane.

1.3.4. Shank

Shank proteins are relatively large scaffolding proteins (>200 kDa in molecular mass) and three isoforms have been identified named Shank 1 to Shank 3 [Sheng & Kim, 2000]. These isoforms are generated by alternative splicing events and their presence and level of expression varies amongst different tissues. All three isoforms however are found in the PSD [Lim et al., 1999]. The Shank members share a similar domain structure consisting of several protein interaction domains. The structure begins with 5-6 N-terminal ankyrin repeats, followed by an SH3 domain, a PDZ domain, a long proline rich region and a sterile alpha motif (SAM) domain [Gundelfinger et al., 2006]. Numerous Shank binding partners have been identified these include α-fodrin which binds to the ankyrin repeats. α-fodrin interacts with actin and calmodulin and thereby links Shank to the actin cytoskeleton [Boeckers et al., 2001]. The ankyrin repeats are also responsible for Shank binding to sharpin, a PSD protein which contains a region homologous to a protein kinase C binding protein [Lim et al., 2001]. The SH3 domain of Shank binds Densin 180, a membrane targeted PSD protein [Quitsch et al., 2005].

The PDZ domain is able to facilitate the interactions with numerous proteins including GKAP (guanylate kinase-associated protein) via its C-terminus which aids in recruitment of Shank to postsynapses [Naisbitt et al., 1999]. GKAP interacts with the PSD scaffolding protein PSD-95 and thereby this interaction links Shank to NMDA and AMPA receptors [Boeckers et al., 2002]. The PDZ domain is also responsible for the interaction of Shank with numerous transmembrane receptors such as the somatostatin receptor, the α-latrotoxin receptor, the cystic fibrosis transmembrane conductance regulator and the Ca$_v$1.3 L-type Ca^{2+} channel [Gundelfinger et al., 2006].

The proline rich region contains proline rich motifs which are binding sites for many interaction domains such as SH3, EVH1 and WW domains. Homer, a scaffolding protein discussed earlier, is able to interact with the proline rich region of Shank via its EVH1 domain. This interaction links Shank proteins to the mGluRs through their interaction with Homer [Du et al., 1998]. Shank is able to interact with an additional scaffolding protein cortactin (discussed in Section 1.2.4.2) [Naisbitt et al., 1999]. This interaction links Shank to the regulation of the actin cytoskeleton.

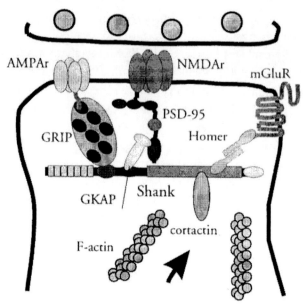

[Sheng & Kim, 2000].

Figure 11. Scaffolding proteins in the PSD. The three transmembrane glutamate receptors of the PSD are bound to different PSD scaffolding proteins. The AMPA receptors (AMPAr) are bound directly by GRIP (Not discussed in the text, also bound by MAGUK family members either directly or indirectly and not shown on this figure) The NMDA receptors [NMDAr] interact with the MAGUK family of scaffolding proteins represented by PSD-95 in this figure, and the mGluR interact with Homer. Cortactin is a scaffolding protein which interacts with F-actin. Shank is able to interact with all of the scaffolding proteins depicted in this figure and as such acts as a master scaffold linking all the glutamate receptors to the actin cytoskeleton. (Reproduced with permission of the Company of Biologists).

Shank is found in a deeper part of the PSD than other scaffolding proteins such as the MAGUK family members which are located close to the membrane [Sheng & Kim, 2000]. Shank is able to interact with numerous additional PSD scaffolding proteins and indirectly to all three glutamate receptors and as such may act as a master scaffold linking all receptor complexes in the PSD as illustrated in Figure 11 [Sheng & Kim, 2000].

1.4. Actin Binding Protein Scaffolds

The dynamic reorganisation of the cytoskeleton which occurs within seconds after chemotactic stimulation is facilitated by a large family of proteins called actin binding proteins (ABP). ABP's have been identified as the major regulators of these dynamic rearrangements that occur when a cell moves, divides or takes up particles and liquid. They control the polymerisation of the G-actin monomers into filaments, the steady state equilibrium between F and G-actin and the 3D organisation of the filamentous network. Many of these actin binding proteins act as scaffolds in signalling pathways interacting with many proteins in addition to actin. Two such actin binding scaffolds will be described here, IQGAP and filamin.

1.4.1. Filamin (ABP280)

Filamin belongs to a large family of actin binding proteins which are responsible for forming and stabilizing 3D cortical actin networks. Homologs of filamin are present in all eukaryotes and in mammals three filamin isoforms have been identified, FLNA, B and C. The three isoforms share strong sequence homology over the entire sequence with the exception of the two hinge regions which show greater divergence [Feng & Walsh, 2004]. FLNA and B are ubiquitously expressed in all tissues whereas FLNC is largely restricted to skeletal and cardiac muscle. Filamins have been shown to be essential for normal development, with mutations leading to developmental defects of many organs including the brain, bone and cardiovascular system [Feng & Walsh, 2004]. Filamin A is a 280 kDa protein and as it is the most abundant of the three isoforms will be the focus of this discussion.

Filamin is comprised of two major domains and forms a homodimer. At the N-terminus resides an F-actin binding domain consisting of two calponin homology (CH) domains of approximately 110 residues named after the first protein in which they were identified, calponin. This actin binding domain is shared amongst many actin binding proteins including α-actinin, β-spectrin and dystrophin. Following the actin binding domain is the rod domain which is comprised of a series of 24 repeat elements that form sandwiches of β-sheets resembling the structure of immunoglobulin domains. Sequence insertions immediately before repeats 16 and 24 predict two hinges which are susceptible to cleavage by the protease calpain. The last repeat (24th) is responsible for the dimerisation of the protein which enables filamin to crosslink two F-actin filaments. As with other immunoglobulin-like domains these domains are responsible for protein-protein interactions. Filamin has been reported to interact directly with more than 50 proteins [Nakamura et al., 2006], and further research will no doubt identify more interacting partners.

Figure 12 provides an illustration of some of the filamin interacting proteins and the locations of their binding sites. These binding partners include several receptors including members of the GPCR (G-protein coupled receptors) such as dopamine D2/D3 and the calcium sensing receptor, the Fcg receptor and the insulin receptor, platelet glycoproteins Ibα, β1 and β2 integrins, many signalling proteins including Ras-related small GTPases such as Rac, Rho, Cdc42, RalA and FilGAP, GEFs including Trio, Lbc, Pak1 and ROCK, kinases such as PKC, PKA and members of the MAPK family and other structural proteins such as caveolin-1 [Scott et al., 2006; Ohta et al., 2006; Awata et al., 2001; Hjalm et al., 2001]. Most of these binding partners interact with the C-terminal region of filamin from repeats 14-24. Only three proteins have been shown to interact with filamin between repeats 1-14. These include PKC illustrated in Figure 12 which has been shown to bind filamin between repeats 1-4 and repeats 22-24, however the significance of binding between repeats 1-4 has not been established [Tigges et al., 2003]. The other two proteins are furin which binds filamin between repeats 13 and 14 [Liu et al., 1997] and Cyclin B1 which binds filamin repeat 9 [Cukier et al., 2007].

Filamin contains many phosphorylation consensus sequences most of which are located in or near the hinge regions. Protein kinases which phosphorylate filamin include PKA [Jay et al., 2000], PKC [Tigges et al., 2003], p21-activated kinase [Vadlamudi et al., 2002], Cdk1 [Cukier et al., 2007] and CaM kinase II (Ca^{2+}/calmodulin-dependent protein kinase II) [Ohta & Hartwig, 1995]. Phosphorylation by these kinases provides a mechanism of regulation of filamin. PKA-mediated phosphorylation provides increased resistance to the calcium activated protease calpain and can alter filamin's interaction with Rho GTPases. Phosphorylation by CaM kinase II or Cdk1 decreases filamin's actin crosslinking activity [Cukier *et al.*, 2007; Ohta & Hartwig, 1996].

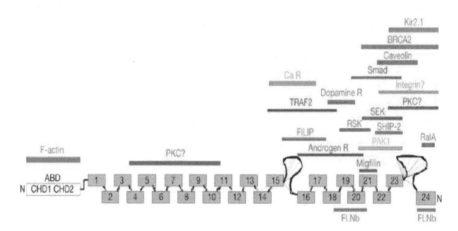

Figure 12. Filamin interacting proteins. This figure is a schematic representation of some of the known filamin interacting proteins and the region of filamin to which they bind. As evident in this figure most proteins tend to interact with the C-terminal repeats in the rod domain except for actin which is bound by the N-terminal actin binding domain. (Reprinted by permission from Macmillan Publishers Ltd. (Nature Cell Biology), Feng & Walsh, 2004, copyright 2004).

Filamin acts as a scaffold in diverse signal transduction cascades by binding various receptors and intracellular signalling molecules such as protein kinases and G proteins and physically linking these signalling complexes to the actin cytoskeleton. Several examples of signalling pathways in which filamin acts as a scaffold are described below.

Filamin is involved in a MAPK cascade involving MEKK1, SEK-1 and SAPK (a member of the ERK family). Filamin binds constitutively to SEK-1 (a MKK) between repeats 21 to 23. Bound SEK1 is then able to be phosphorylated by the upstream kinase MEKK1. Phosphorylated SEK1 is then able to phosphorylate and activate SAPK which phosphorylates c-Jun and initiates programmed cell death. Although filamin does not interact directly with the other two members of the cascade, mutational analysis has revealed that filamin is required for efficient signalling between the three components [Marti *et al.*, 1997]. Filamin has been shown to directly bind other MKK's including MEK1 and MKK4 which activate ERK and JNK respectively. Filamin does not bind the other members of the MAPK cascade in these signalling pathways either, but again is essential for efficient signalling [Scott *et al.*, 2006].

Activation of SAPK was shown to be dependent on the expression of filamin, with filamin-deficient cell lines unable to activate SAPK in response to the cellular stress TNF-α (Tumour Necrosis Factor). These cells also exhibited an 80 % reduction in stimulation via LPA (Lysophosphophatidic acid) [Marti *et al.*, 1997]. Direct regulation of filamin may occur through its association with receptors and GTPase's, however the specific components were not identified for this pathway. Likewise filamin may be regulated via phosphorylation by the protein kinases listed earlier-filamin has been shown to be phosphorylated in response to

LPA and other stimuli by kinases such as Ribosomal S6 kinase (RSK) [Woo et al., 2004; Marti et al., 1997]. The exact mechanisms of this pathway are still to be elucidated, however it is clear that filamin plays a direct and essential role in the MAPK cascade leading to activation of SAPK in response to both LPA and TNF-α.

Filamin is able to interact with other scaffolding proteins such as β-arrestin to form an additional level of complexity through a double scaffold. Filamin binds β-arrestin via its 22nd repeat which is in close proximity to the binding sites for the MAP2K members MEK1 and MKK4 [Scott et al., 2006]. β-arrestin has been shown in other MAPK signalling pathways to bind MAP3K members including ASK1 and also to the MAPK JNK, but it does not bind directly to the MAP2K [Mc Donald et al., 2000]. Likewise in the ERK signalling pathway β-arrestin may bind the MAP3K members and ERK and interact indirectly through filamin with the MAP2K. As filamin is concentrated to the cell periphery where it binds the cytoskeleton, filamin may localise β-arrestin and the other MAPK members to this cell compartment [Scott et al., 2006].

Filamin is able to bind furin, a protein responsible for the proteolytic maturation of proproteins within the trans-Golgi and endosomal network. This interaction occurs between repeats 13 and 14 of filamin and the cytosolic domain of furin. Furin is primarily located in the trans-Golgi network but cycles to the cell surface where it is bound by filamin. Filamin can tether furin to the surface and regulate the rate of furin internalization. Filamin deficient cell lines internalized furin at a 2.3 fold higher rate, than the wild type. The efficient sorting of furin from the early endosomes to the Golgi network was also altered in filamin deficient cell lines suggesting that filamin not only controls the rate of furin internalization but also aids in the efficient trafficking of furin from the early endosome stage onwards [Liu et al., 1997].

Filamin can concentrate furin to regions of the cell surface that contain potential substrates including MT-MMP1 (membrane type 1 matrix metalloprotease) which localises to the cell surface due to its cytosolic domain. MMP are proteins which are involved in the degradation of extracellular matrix proteins [Zhu et al., 2007]. Colocalised furin may cleave this substrate at the cell surface. The internalization motif of furin is masked when bound to filamin and hence the rate of internalization is reduced. However disruption of this interaction through unknown regulatory mechanisms would enable the motifs to interact with the internalization machinery and relocate furin to intracellular compartments. Filamin is also important for appropriate localisation of late endosomes and lysosomes in the cell as demonstrated by fluorescence microscopy with filamin-deficient cell lines showing incorrect localisation of vesicles [Liu et al., 1997].

Other mutational experiments have demonstrated the essential role of filamin in many signalling processes. Glogauer et al. [1998] have shown that filamin binds to β1-integrin and this interaction localised filamin to focal adhesions in response to shear stress. This resulted in modulation of the cytoskeleton to stiffen the cells which made them more resistant to physical strain. Cells lacking filamin were unable to produce a stiffening response to shear stress.

Filamin has also been shown to be involved in the regulation of cell polarity with filamin null cells exhibiting impaired locomotion which is partially caused by their reduced ability to polarise [Ohta et al., 2006]. Filamin can crosslink actin filaments and also interacts with many other proteins involved in the regulation of the actin cytoskeleton. These proteins include Rho GTPases, GEFs (guanine nucleotide exchange factors), Pak1 which promotes actin assembly and many transmembrane proteins involved in locomotion and adhesion. Filamin is able to localise these proteins to promote retraction and suppress leading lamellae formation which aids in the regulation of cell polarity [Ohta et al., 2006].

1.4.2. IQGAP

IQGAP proteins belong to a family of conserved actin binding proteins which have been identified in many eukaryotic organisms from yeasts to mammals [Briggs & Sacks, 2003]. They can form dimers with each monomer binding F-actin and crosslinking these filaments [Bashour et al., 1997; Fukata et al., 1997]. In mammals three isoforms have been identified IQGAP1, 2 and 3. All three isoforms share a high degree of sequence similarity and domain structure yet differ in tissue distribution. IQGAP1 is expressed in all tissues, IQGAP3 is enriched in the brain and the lung and IQGAP2 is predominantly expressed in the liver and stomach but has been identified in other tissues including platelets [Brandt & Grosse, 2007]. IQGAP1 has been the most extensively studied and will be the focus of this section.

IQGAP1 is a 189 kDa protein that contains a conserved domain structure consisting of an N terminal CH (Calponin homology) domain, a WW domain, an IQ domain, a GAP-related domain and a RasGAP domain, shown schematically in Figure 12. The CH domain binds to F-actin (as described for filamin, Section 1.4.1) [Mateer et al., 2004], the WW domain is a known protein interaction domain (refer to Table 1) however no binding partners for this domain in IQGAPs have been identified to date. The next two domains, the IQ and GAP-related domains lend the protein its name.

The IQ domain in IQGAP1 is constructed from four tandem IQ motifs which are involved in binding numerous proteins including calmodulin [Hart et al., 1996; Ho et al., 1999; Joyal et al., 1997], myosin essential light chain [Weissbach et al., 1998], and a Zn^{2+} and Ca^{2+} binding protein, S100B [Mbele et al., 2002]. The GAP-related domain shares high sequence similarity to Ras GTPase activating proteins yet does not contain any GAP activity [Briggs & Sacks, 2003]. This domain mediates the binding of Rho GTPases, Cdc42 and Rac1 but not RhoA or Ras [Hart et al., 1996; Ho et al., 1999; Kuroda et al., 1996]. Finally, the C-terminal RasGAP domain interacts with the microtubule binding protein CLIP70 (cytoplasmic linker protein 70) [Fukata et al., 2002], E-cadherin [Kuroda et al., 1998] and β-catenin [Briggs et al., 2002].

The multiple partners of IQGAP indicate that it is an important protein involved in cell movement. In support of this IQGAP has been shown to be necessary for cell-cell adhesion [Noritake et al., 2005] and cytokinesis [Machesky, 1998], is overexpressed in cancer cells [Clark et al., 2000; Nabeshima et al., 2002] and is localised to lamellipodia of motile cells [Kuroda et al., 1996]. IQGAP binds Cdc42 and inhibits its GTPase activity, which stabilises the active GTP form of Cdc42. In turn, active Cdc42 enhances the ability of IQGAP to crosslink F-actin filaments. Active Cdc42 also stimulates N-WASp, a nucleation promoting factor which stimulates the Arp2/3 complex to generate branched actin meshworks from pre-existing filaments [LeClainche et al., 2007]. N-WASp contains several domains, two of which are the CRIB (Cdc42-Rac interactive binding domain) and the VCA or C-terminal catalytic domain. These two domains interact with each other and hold the N-WASp protein in an inactive state. Binding of Cdc42 to the CRIB domain abolishes its interaction with the VCA domain which is then free to interact with Arp2/3, G-actin and an actin filament barbed end [Kim et al, 2000]. The C-terminal region of IQGAP can also interact with the CRIB domain of N-WASp and appears to act in synergy with Cdc42 to activate N-WASp [LeClainche et al., 2007].

IQGAP also stimulates actin polymerisation through formins. Formins are actin nucleating proteins which initiate the formation of linear actin filaments through processive elongation at the growing (barbed) end. IQGAP1 binds to the Rho-activated form of Dia1 (a formin protein) and recruits it to sites of actin assembly such as the leading edge of migrating cells. It is thought that IQGAP1 binding to Dia1 stabilises its active conformation [Brandt et al., 2007].

IQGAP1 is involved in cell-cell adhesion. Cell to cell adhesion is achieved through the interaction of cadherins present on adjacent cells. Cadherins are a family of cell surface adhesion molecules which are regulated by Ca^{2+}. The cytoplasmic domain of E-cadherin binds to β-catenin or γ-catenin and this complex is coupled to the actin cytoskeleton through α-catenin [Bracke et al., 1996]. IQGAP1 binds directly to E-cadherin and β-catenin and reduces the ability of E-cadherin to interact with the cytoskeleton. This weakens the cell-cell attachment which is necessary for cells to detach from each other and move [Kuroda et al., 1998; Li et al., 1999].

In addition to interaction with the actin cytoskeleton IQGAP1 also interacts with the microtubule cytoskeleton. Microtubules are a main element of the cytoskeleton and are essential for cell division, migration and vesicle transport. IQGAP1 interacts with a microtubule tip protein CLIP70 at the leading edge of migrating cells. This interaction localises IQGAP and its binding partners to microtubules linking the plus ends of microtubules to the actin meshwork and promotes cell polarisation during migration [Fukata et al., 2002].

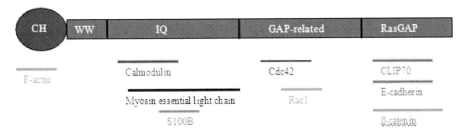

Figure 13. IQGAP interacting proteins. This figure provides a schematic representation of the known binding partners of IQGAP and the protein interaction domain to which each binds. No binding partners have been identified as yet for the WW domain, but in other proteins this domain has been shown to mediate protein-protein interactions.

Because it interacts with both the actin cytoskeleton and the microtubular cytoskeleton, IQGAP provides a mechanism for crosstalk between them and the pathways described above. IQGAP's role in the processes is regulated by its interactions with Cdc42 and Ca^{2+}/calmodulin and through phosphorylation. Activated Cdc42 enhances both the actin crosslinking activity of IQGAP [Fukata et al., 1997] and its interaction with the microtubule cytoskeleton through stimulation of binding to CLIP70 [Fukata et al., 2002]. Active Cdc42 and Rac1 additionally inhibit the interaction of IQGAP with E-cadherin and β-catenin. This prevents IQGAP from inhibiting cell-cell adhesions [Kuroda et al., 1998].

Like many actin binding proteins IQGAP is regulated by Ca^{2+}/calmodulin. Calmodulin interacts with IQGAP1 through the four tandem IQ motifs and this interaction is mediated by Ca^{2+}. Calmodulin can interact with IQ1 and IQ2 only when Ca^{2+} is present whereas calmodulin interacts with IQ3 and 4 regardless of the presence or absence of Ca^{2+}. The binding of Ca^{2+}/calmodulin prevents IQGAP from stabilising active Cdc42 and inhibits actin polymerisation. Conversely, the displacement of active Cdc42 enables the interaction of IQGAP with E-cadherin and β-catenin and cell adhesion is inhibited [Li & Sacks, 2003].

Phosphorylation of IQGAP provides an additional level of regulation. IQGAP is held in an inactive configuration through interaction of its C-terminal and N-terminal domains. Phosphorylation of Serine1443 relieves this inhibition allowing IQGAP to interact with its binding partners such as Cdc42 and N-WASp to promote actin polymerisation [LeClainche et al., 2007]. IQGAP has been shown to be phosphorylated by PKC, and this phosphorylation event was shown to alter the conformation of IQGAP so that the C-terminus is free to interact with Cdc42 [Brandt & Grosse, 2007].

Most of the proteins with which IQGAP interacts are involved in regulation of the actin or microtubule cytoskeleton. These interactions enable IQGAP to act as a scaffold in many processes which involve the regulation of the cytoskeleton such as in cytokinesis, cell invasion and metastasis, cell migration and cell polarity.

1.5. Conclusion

The cytoskeleton is a highly dynamic structure which can rapidly reorganise in response to various stimuli. This reorganisation is important for a cell to respond to various stimuli, for intracellular and intercellular transport, for maintenance of cell shape, cell division, growth and development. In order for a cell to reorganise its cytoskeleton so rapidly and in response to various stimulation cues, numerous proteins are employed in signal transduction pathways to aid in the cytoskeletal rearrangement. These proteins range from receptors, G proteins, signalling molecules and second messengers to kinases, phosphatases and cytoskeletal components. These proteins are often involved in many pathways and located in different compartments of the cell.

Scaffolding proteins are important proteins in the regulation of the cytoskeleton as they are able to localise many of the components of a particular pathway to a particular location within the cell and assist in the efficient relaying of the response. Scaffolding proteins can tether members of a complex through protein interaction domains which abound on these proteins. They can also sequester binding partners to a particular pathway, thereby avoiding crosstalk between components involved in multiple pathways. Scaffolding proteins can also stabilise weak interactions between particular proteins in a cascade and catalyse activation of the pathway components. Due to these roles scaffolding proteins are essential members of signalling pathways that regulate the cytoskeleton and without them the efficiency, selectivity and rapidity of responses would not be possible. Many scaffolding proteins have been identified to date, however growing interest will no doubt lead to the identification of many more.

References

[1] Van Troys, M., Vandekerckhove, J. & Ampe, C. (1999). Structural modules in actin-binding proteins: towards a new classification. *Biochim Biophys Acta, 1448*, 323-348.
[2] Mc Gough. A. (1998). F-actin binding proteins. *Curr Biol, 8*, 166-176.
[3] Eichinger, L., Bahler, M., Dietz, M., Eckerskorn, C. & Schleicher, M. (1998). Characterization and cloning of a *Dictyostelium* Ste20-like protein kinase that phosphorylates the actin-binding protein severin. *J Biol Chem, 273*, 12952-12959.
[4] Pawson, T. & Nash, P. (2000). Protein-protein interactions define specificity in signal transduction. *Genes & Dev, 14*, 1027-1047.
[5] Smith, F. D. & Scott, J. D. (2001). Signaling complexes: Junctions on the intracellular information super highway. *Curr Biol, 12*, R32-R40.
[6] Whitmarsh, A. J. & Davis, R. J. (1998). Structural organization of MAP-kinase signaling modules by scaffold proteins in yeast and mammals. *Trends Biochem Sci, 23*, 481-485.
[7] Burack, W. R. & Shaw, A. S. (2000). Signal transduction: hanging on a scaffold. *Curr Opin Cell Biol, 12*, 211-216.
[8] Vomastek, T., Schaeffer, H. J., Tarcsafalvi, A., Smolkin, M. E., Bissonette, E. A. & Weber, M. J. (2004). Modular construction of a signaling scaffold: MORG1 interacts with components of the ERK cascade and links ERK signaling to specific agonists. *PNAS, 101*, 6981-6986.
[9] Liu, B. A., Jablonowski, K., Raina, M., Arce, M., Pawson, T. & Nash, P. D. (2006). The human and mouse complement of SH2 domain proteins – establishing the boundaries of phosphotyrosine signaling. *Mol Cell, 22*, 851-868.
[10] Zimmermann, P. (2006). The prevalence and significance of PDZ domain-phosphoinositide interactions. *Biochim Biophys Acta, 1761*, 947-956.
[11] Kuriyan, J. & Cowburn, D. (1997). Modular peptide recognition domains in eukaryotic signaling. *Annu Rev Biophys Biomol Struct, 26*, 259-288.
[12] Pawson, T. (1995). Protein modules and signaling networks. *Nature, 373*, 573-580.
[13] Cohen, G. B., Ren, R. & Baltimore, D. (1995). Modular binding domains in signal transduction proteins. *Cell, 80*, 237-248.
[14] Machida, K. & Mayer, B. J. (2005). The SH2 domain: versatile signalling module and pharmaceutical target. *Biochim Biophys Acta, 1747*, 1-25.
[15] Morais Cabral, J. H., Petosa, C., Sutcliffe, M. J., Raza, S., Byron, O., Poy, F., Marfatia, S. M., Chishti, A. H., & Liddington, R. C. (1996). Crystal structure of a PDZ domain. *Nature, 382*, 649-652.
[16] Bar-Sagi, D., Rotin, D., Batzer, A., Mandiyan, V. & Schlessinger, J. (1993). SH3 domains direct cellular localization of signalling molecules. *Cell, 74*, 83-91.
[17] Cesareni, G., Panni, S., Nardelli, G. & Castagnoli, L. (2002). Can we infer peptide recognition specificity mediated by SH3 domains? *FEBS Letters, 513*, 38-44.

[18] Ludbrook, S. B., Eccleston, J. F. & Strom, M. (1997). Cloning and characterisation of a rhoGAP homolog from *Dictyostelium discoideum*. *J Biol Chem, 272*, 15682-15686.
[19] Chung, C. Y., Potikyan, G. & Firtel, R. A. (2001). Control of cell polarity and chemotaxis by Akt/PKB and PI3 kinases through the regulation of PAKa. *Mol Cell, 7*, 937-947.
[20] Funamoto, S., Milan, K., Meili, R. & Firtel, R. A. (2001). Role of phosphatidylinositol 3' kinase and a downstream pleckstrin homology domain-containing protein in controlling chemotaxis in *Dictyostelium. J. Cell Biol., 153*, 795-809.
[21] Maffucci, T. & Falasca, M. (2001). Specificity in pleckstrin homology (PH) domain membrane targeting: a role for a phosphoinositide-protein co-operative mechanism. *FEBS Letters, 506*, 173-179.
[22] Lemmon, M. A., Ferguson, K. M. & Abrams, C. S. (2002). Pleckstrin homology domains and the cytoskeleton. *FEBS Letters, 513*, 71-76.
[23] Pawson, T. & Scott, J. D. (1997). Signaling through scaffold, anchoring and adaptor proteins. *Science, 278*, 2075-2080.
[24] Huber, A. (2001). Scaffolding proteins organize multimolecular protein complexes for sensory signal transduction. *Eur J Neurosci, 14*, 769-776.
[25] Hung, A. Y. & Sheng, M. (2002). PDZ domains: Structural modules for protein complex assembly. *J Biol Chem, 277*, 5699-5702.
[26] Williams, A. F. & Barclay, A. N. (1988). The immunoglobulin superfamily-domains for cell surface recognition. *Ann Rev Immunol, 6*, 381-405.
[27] Wisemann, C., Muller, Y. A. & de Vos, A. M. (2000). Ligand-binding sites in Ig-like domains of receptor tyrosine kinases. *J Mol Med, 78*, 247-260.
[28] Nagata, T., Gupta, V., Sorce, D., Kim, W-Y., Sali, A., Chait, B. T., Shigesada, K., Ito, Y. & Werner, M. (1999). Immunoglobulin motif DNA recognition and heterodimerization of the PEBP2/CBF Runt domain. *Nature Struct Biol, 6*, 615-619.
[29] Noegel, A. A., Rapp, S., Lottspeich, F., Schleicher, M. & Stewart, M. (1989). The *Dictyostelium* gelation factor shares a putative actin binding site with α–actinins and dystrophin and also has a rod domain containing six 100-residue motifs that appear to have a cross-beta conformation. *J Cell Biol, 109*, 607-618.
[30] DiNitto, J. P. & Lambright, D. G. (2006). Membrane and juxtamembrane targeting by PH and PTB domains. *Biochim Biophys Acta, 1761*, 850-867.
[31] Uhlik, M. T., Temple, B., Bencharit, S., Kimple, A. J., Siderovski, D. P. & Johnson, G. L. (2005). Structural and evolutionary division of phosphotyrosine binding (PTB) domains. *JMB, 345*, 1-20.
[32] Naslavsky, N. & Caplan, S. (2005), C-terminal EH-domain-containing proteins: consensus for a role in endocytic trafficking, EH? *J Cell Sci, 118*, 4093-4101.
[33] Kay, B. K., Williamson, M. P. & Sudol, M. (2000). The importance of being proline: the interaction of proline-rich motifs in signalling proteins with their cognate domains. *FASEB J, 14*, 231-241.
[34] Sudol, M., Recinos, C. C., Abraczinskas, J., Humbert, J. & Farooq, A. (2005). WW or WoW: The WW domains in a union of bliss. *IUBMB Life, 57*, 773-778.
[35] Bach, I. (2000). The LIM domain: regulation by association. *Mech Develop, 91*, 5-17.

[36] Brown, S., Coghill, I. D., McGrath, M. J. & Robinson, P. A. (2001). Role of LIM domains in mediating signalling protein interactions. *IUBMB Life, 51*, 359-364.

[37] Khurana, T., Khurana, B. & Noegel, A. A. (2002). LIM proteins: association with the actin cytoskeleton. *Protoplasma, 219*, 1-12.

[38] Ball, L. J., Jarchau, T., Oschkinat, H. & Walter, U. (2002). EVHI domains: structure, function and interactions. *FEBS Letters, 513*, 45-52.

[39] Bahler, M. & Rhoads, A. (2002). Calmodulin signalling via the IQ motif. *FEBS Letters, 513*, 107-113.

[40] Cory, G. O. C., Cramer, R., Blanchoin, L. & Ridley, A. J. (2003). Phosphoryaltion of the WASP-VCA domain increases its affinity for the Arp2/3 complex and enhances actin polymerisation by WASP. *Mol Cell, 11*, 1229-1239.

[41] Kato, M., Miki, H., Kurita, S., Endo, T., Nakagawa, H., Miyamoto, S. & Takenawa, T. (2002) WICH, a novel Verprolin homology domain-containing protein that functions cooperatively with N-WASP in actin-microspike formation. *Biochem Biophys Res Commun, 291*, 41-47.

[42] Yamaguchi, H., Miki, H., Suetsugu, S., Ma, L., Kirschner, M. W. & Takenawa, T. (2000). Two tandem verprolin homology domains are necessary for a strong activation of Arp2/3 complex-induced actin polymerisation and induction of microspike formation by N-WASP. *PNAS, 97*, 12631-12636.

[43] Kim, C. A. & Bowie, J. U. (2003). SAM domains: uniform structure, diversity of function. *Trends Biochem Sci, 28*, 625-628.

[44] Kwan, J. J., Warner, N., Maini, J., Chan Tung, K. W., Zakaria, H., Pawson, T. & Donaldson, L.W. (2006). *Saccharomyces cerevisiae* Ste50 binds the MAPKKK Ste11 through a head-to-tail SAM domain interaction. *JMB, 356*, 142-154.

[45] Elion, E. A. (2001). The Ste5p scaffold. *J Cell Sci, 114*, 3967-3978.

[46] Hunter, T. (2000). Signaling-2000 and Beyond. *Cell, 100*, 113-127.

[47] Symons, A., Beinke, S. & Ley, S. C. (2006). MAP kinase kinase kinases and innate immunity. *Trends Immunol, 27*, 40-48.

[48] Levchenko, A., Bruck, J. & Sternberg, P. W. (2000). Scaffold proteins may biphasically affect the levels of mitogen-activated protein kinase signaling and reduce its threshold properties. *PNAS, 97*, 5818-5823.

[49] Sabbagh, Jr. W., Flatauer, L. J., Bardwell, A. J. & Bardwell, L. (2001). Specificity of MAP kinase signaling in Yeast differentiation involves transient versus sustained MAPK activation. *Mol Cell, 8*, 683-691.

[50] Pullikuth, A., McKinnon, E., Schaeffer, H-J. & Catling, A. D. (2005). The MEK1 scaffolding protein MP1 regulates cell spreading by integrating PAK1 and Rho signals. *Mol Cell Biol, 25*, 5119-5133.

[51] Schaeffer, H. J. & Weber, M. J. (1999). Mitogen-activated protein kinases: specific messages from ubiquitous messengers. *Mol Cell Biol, 19*, 2435-2444.

[52] Davis, R. J. (2000). Signal transduction by the JNK group of MAP Kinases. *Cell, 103*, 239-252.

[53] Ito, M., Yoshioka, K., Akechi, M., Yamashita, S., Takamatsu, N., Sugiyama, K., Hibi, M., Nakabeppu, Y., Shiba, T. & Yamamoto, K-I. (1999). JSAP-1 a novel Jun N-

terminal protein kinase (JNK)-binding protein that functions as a scaffold factor in the JNK signaling pathway. *Mol Cell Biol, 19,* 7539-7548.

[54] Widmann, C., Gibson, S., Jarpe, M. B. & Johnson, G. L. (1999). Mitogen-activated protein kinase: Conservation of a three-kinase module from yeast to human. *Physiolog Rev, 79,* 143-180.

[55] Ho, D. T., Bardwell, A. J., Grewal, S., Iverson, C. & Bardwell, L. (2006), Interacting JNK-docking sites in MKK7 promote binding and activation of JNK mitogen-activated protein kinases. *J Biol Chem, 281,* 13169-13179.

[56] Fusello, A. M., Mandik-Nayak, L., Shih, F., Lewis, R. E., Allen, P. M. & Shaw, A.S. (2006). The MAPK scaffold kinase suppressor of Ras is involved in ERK activation by stress and proinflammatory cytokines and induction of arthritis. *J Immun, 177,* 6152-6258.

[57] Bogoyevitch, M. A. & Court, N. W. (2004). Counting on mitogen-activated protein kinases-ERKs 3, 4, 5, 6, 7 and 8. *Cellular Signalling, 16,* 1345-1354.

[58] Pouyssegur, J., Volmat, V. & Lenormand, P. (2002). Fidelity and spatio-temporal control in MAP kinase (ERKs) signalling. *Biochem Pharmacol, 64,* 755-763.

[59] Dhillon, A. S. & Kolch, W. (2002). Untying the regulation of the Raf-1 kinase. *Archives of Biochem Biophy, 404,* 3-9.

[60] Denouel-Galy, A., Douville, E. M., Warne, P. H., Papin, C., Laugier, D., Calothy, G., Downward, J. & Eychene, A. (1997). Murine Ksr interacts with MEK and inhibits Ras-induced transformation. *Curr Biol, 8,* 46-55.

[61] Roy, F. & Therrien, M. (2002). MAP kinase module: The Ksr connection. *Curr Biol, 12,* R325-R327.

[62] Morrison, D. K. (2001). KSR: a MAPK scaffold of the Ras pathway? *J Cell Sci, 114,* 1609-1612.

[63] Teis, D., Wunderlich, W. & Huber, L. A. (2002). Localisation of the MP1-MAPK scaffold complex to endosomes is mediated by p14 and required for signal transduction. *Develop Cell, 3,* 803-814.

[64] Sharma, C., Vomastek, T., Tarcsafalvi, A., Catling, A. D., Schaeffer, H-J., Eblen, S. T. & Weber, M. J. (2005). MEK partner 1 (MP1): Regulation of oligomerization in MAP kinase signaling. *J Cell Biochem, 94,* 708-719.

[65] Nihalani, D., Meyer, D., Pajni, S. & Holzman, L. B. (2001). Mixed lineage kinase-dependent JNK activation is governed by interactions of scaffold protein JIP with MAPK module components. *EMBO J, 20,* 3447-3458.

[66] Willoughby, E. A. & Collins, M. K. (2005). Dynamic interaction between the dual specificity phosphatase MKP7 and the JNK3 scaffold protein β–arrestin 2. *J Biol Chem, 280,* 25651-25658.

[67] Lee, C. M., Onesime, D., Reddy, C. D., Dhanasekaran, N. & Reddy, E. P. (2002a). JLP: A scaffolding protein that tethers JNK/p38MAPK signaling modules and transcription factors. *PNAS, 99,* 114189-14194.

[68] Kelkar, N., Standen, C. L. & Davis, R. J. (2005). Role of the JIP4 scaffold protein in the regulation of mitogen-activated protein kinase signaling pathways. *Mol Cell Biol, 25,* 2733-2743.

[69] Verhey, K. J., Meyer, D., Deehan, R., Blenis, J., Schnapp, B. J., Rapoport, T. A. & Margolis, B. (2001). Cargo of Kinesin identified as JIP scaffolding proteins and associated signaling molecules. *J Cell Biol, 152*, 959-970.

[70] Takino, T., Nakada, M., Miyamori, H., Watanabe, Y., Sato, T., Gantulga, D., Yoshioka, K., Yamada, K. M. & Sato, H. (2005). JSAP1/JIP3 cooperates with focal adhesion kinase to regulate c-Jun N-terminal kinase and cell migration. *J Biol Chem, 280*, 37772-37781.

[71] Kashef, K., Lee, C. M., Ha, J. H., Reddy, E. P. & Dhanasekaran, D. N. (2005). JNK-interacting leucine zipper protein is a novel scaffolding protein in the Gα13 signalling pathway. *Biochem, 44*, 14090-14096.

[72] Nguyen, Q., Lee, C. M., Lee, A. & Reddy, E. P. (2005). JLP associates with kinesin light chain 1 through a novel leucine zipper-like domain. *J Biol Chem, 280*, 30185-30191.

[73] Katsoulidis, E., Li, Y., Mears, H. & Platanias, L. C. (2005). The p38 Mitogen-activated protein kinase pathway in Interferon signal transduction. *J Interferon Cytokine Res, 25*, 749-756.

[74] Dean, J. L. E., Sully, G., Clark, A. R. & Saklatvala, J. (2004). The involvement of AU-rich element-binding proteins in p38 mitogen-activated protein kinase pathway-mediated mRNA stabilization. *Cellular Signalling, 16*, 1113-1121.

[75] Robidoux, J., Cao, W., Quan, H., Daniel, K. W., Moukdar, F., Bai, X., Floering, L. M. & Collins, S. (2005). Selective activation of mitogen-activated protein (MAP) kinase kinase 3 and p38 alpha MAP kinase is essential for cyclic AMP-dependent UCP1 expression in adipocytes. *Mol Cell Biol, 25*, 5466-5479.

[76] Uhlik, M. T., Abell, A. N., Johnson, N. L., Sun, W., Cuevas, B. D., Lobel-Rice, K. E., Horne, E. A., Dell'Acqua, M. L. & Johnson, G. L. (2003). Rac-MEKK3-MKK3 scaffolding for p38 MAPK activation during hyperosmotic shock. *Nature Cell Biol, 5*, 1104-1110.

[77] McDonald, P. H., Chow, C. W., Miller, W. E., Laporte, S. A., Field, M. E., Lin, F. T., Davis, R. J. & Leftkowitz, R. J. (2000). Beta-arrestin 2: a receptor regulated MAPK scaffold for the activation of JNK3. *Science, 290*, 1574-1577.

[78] Colledge, M. & Scott, J. D. (1999). AKAPs: from structure to function. *Trends Cell Biol, 9*, 216-221.

[79] McConnachie, G., Langeberg, L. K. & Scott, J. D. (2006). AKAP signalling complexes: getting to the heart of the matter. *Trends Mol Med, 12*, 317-323.

[80] Schillace, R. V. & Scott, J. D. (1999). Organization of kinases, phosphatases, and receptor signaling complexes. *J Clin Investig, 103*, 761-765.

[81] Diviani, D, & Scott, J. D. (2001). AKAP signalling complexes at the cytoskeleton. *J. Cell Sci, 114*, 1431-1437.

[82] Angelo, R. & Rubin, C. S. (1998). Molecular characterization of an anchor protein (AKAP$_{CE}$) that binds the RI subunit (R$_{CE}$) of type I protein kinase A from *Caenhorhabditis elegans*. *J Biol Chem, 273*, 14633-14643.

[83] Carlisle-Michel, J. J. & Scott, J. D. (2002). AKAP mediated signal transduction. *Annu Rev Pharmacol Toxicol, 42*, 235-257.

[84] Dell'Acqua, M. L., Smith, K. E., Gorski, J. A., Horne, E. A., Gibson, E. S. & Gomez, L. L. (2006). Regulation of neuronal PKA signalling through AKAP targeting dynamics. *J. Cell Biol*, *85*, 627-633.

[85] Fan, G-F., Shumay, E., Wang, H-Y. & Malbon, C. C. (2001). The scaffold protein Gravin (cAMP-dependent protein kinase-anchoring protein 250) binds the β_2-adrenergic receptor via the receptor cytoplasmic Arg-329 to Leu-413 domain and provides a mobile scaffold during desensitization. *J Biol Chem*, *276*, 24005-24014.

[86] Malbon, C. C., Tao, J. & Wang, H. Y. (2004a). AKAPs (A-kinase anchoring proteins) and molecules that compose their G-protein-coupled receptor signalling complexes. *Biochem J*, *379*, 1-9.

[87] Tao, J., Shumay, E., McLaughlin, S., Wang, H-Y. & Malbon, C. C. (2006). Regulation of AKAP-membrane interactions by calcium. *J Biol Chem*, *281*, 23932-23944.

[88] Malbon, C. C., Tao, J., Shumay, E. & Wang, H-Y. (2004b). AKAP (A-kinase anchoring protein) domains: beads of structure-function on the necklace of G-protein signalling. *Biochem Soc Trans*, *32*, 861-864.

[89] Lin, F., Wang, H-Y. & Malbon, C. C. (2000). Gravin-mediated formation of signaling complexes in β_2-adrenergic receptor desensitization and resensitization. *J Biol Chem*, *275*, 19025-19034.

[90] Fievet, B., Louvard, D. & Arpin, M. (2007). ERM functions in epithelial cell orginisation and functions. *Biochim Biophys Acta*, *1773*, 653-660.

[91] Finnerty, C. M., Chambers, D., Ingraffea, J., Faber, H. R., Karplus, A. P. & Bretscher, A. (2003). The EBP50-moesin interaction involves a binding site regulated by direct masking on the FERM domain. *J Cell Sci*, *117*, 1547-1552.

[92] Berryman, M., Franck, A. & Bretscher, A. (1993). Ezrin is concentrated in the apical microvilli of a wide variety of epithelial cells whereas moesin is found primarily in endothelial cells. *J Cell Sci*, *105*, 1025-1043.

[93] Tsukita, S., Hieda, Y. & Tsukita, S. (1989). A new 82-kDa barbed end-capping protein (radixin) localised in the cell-to-cell adherens junction: purification and characterisation. *J Cell Biol*, *108*, 2369-2382.

[94] Pataky, F., Pironkova, R. & Hudspeth, A. J. (2004). Radixin is a constituent of stereocilia in hair cells. *PNAS*, *101*, 2601-2606.

[95] Kitajiri, S., Fukumoto, K., Hata, M., Sasaki, H., Katsuno, T., Nakagawa, M., Ito, J., Tsukita, S. & Tsukita, S. (2004). Radixin deficiency causes deafness associated with progressive degeneration of cochlear stereocilia. *J Cell Biol*, *166*, 559-570.

[96] Lankes., W. T. & Furthmayr, H. (1991). Moesin: a member of the protein 4.1-talin-ezrin family of proteins. *PNAS*, *88*, 8297-8301.

[97] Gary, R. & Bretscher, A. (1995). Ezrin self-association involves binding of an N-terminal domain to a normally masked C-terminal domain that includes the F-actin binding site. *Mol Biol Cell*, *6*, 1061-1075.

[98] Reczek, D. & Bretscher, A. (1998). The carboxy-terminal region of EBP50 binds to a site in the amino-terminal domain of ezrin that is masked in the dormant molecule. *J Biol Chem*, *273*, 18452-18458.

[99] Hamada, K., Shimizu, T., Matsui, T., Tsukita, S., Tsukita, S. & Hakoshima, T. (2000). Structural basis of the membrane-targeting and unmasking mechanisms of the radixin FERM domain. *EMBO J, 19*, 4449-4462.

[100] Yonemura, S., Matsui, T., Tsukita, S. & Tsukita, S. (2002). Rho-dependent and – independent activation mechanisms of ezrin/radixin/moesin proteins: an essential role for poly-phosphoinositides in vivo. *J Cell Sci, 115*, 2569-2580.

[101] Fievet, B. T., Gautreau, A., Roy, C., DelMaestro, L., Mangreat, P., Louvard, D. & Arpin, M. (2004). Phosphoinositide binding and phosphorylation act seqeuentially in the activation mechanism of ezrin. *J Cell Biol, 164*, 653-659.

[102] Ng, T., Parsons, M., Hughes, W. E., Monypenny, J., Zicha, D., Gautreau, A., Arpin, M., Gschmeissner, S., Verveer, P. J., Bastiaens, P. I. H. & Parker, P. J. (2001). Ezrin is a downstream effector of trafficking PKC-integrin complexes involved in the control of cell motility. *EMBO J, 20*, 2723-2741.

[103] Saotome, I., Curto, M. & McClatchey, A. I. (2004). Ezrin is essential for epithelial organisation and villus morphogenesis in the developing intestine. *Dev Cell, 6*, 855-864.

[104] Denker, S. P., Huang, D. C., Orlowski, J., Furthmayr, H. & Barber, D. L. (2000). Direct binding of the Na^+-H^+ exchanger NHE1 to ERM proteins regulates the cortical cytoskeleton and cell shape independently of H(+) translocation. *Mol Cell, 6*, 1425-1436.

[105] Legg, J. W., Lewis, C. A., Parsons, M., Ng, T. & Isacke, C. M. (2002). A novel PKC-regulated mechanism controls CD44 ezrin association and directional cell motility. *Nat Cell Biol, 4*, 399-407.

[106] Short, D. B., Trotter, K. W., Reczek, D., Kreda, S. M., Bretscher, A., Boucher, R. C., Stutts, M. J. & Milgram, S. L. (1998). An apical PDZ protein anchors the cystic fibrosis transmembrane conductance regulator to the cytoskeleton. *J Biol Chem, 273*, 19797-19801.

[107] Cao, T. T., Deacon, H. W., Reczek, D., Bretscher, A. & von Zastrow, M. (1999). A kinase-regulated PDZ-domain interaction controls endocytotic sorting of the beta2-adrenergic receptor. *Nature, 401*, 286-290.

[108] Yun, C. H., Lamprecht, G., Forster, D. V. & Sidor, A. (1998). NHE3 kinase A regulatory protein E3KARP binds the epithelial brush border Na+/H+ exchanger NHE3 and the cytoskeletal protein ezrin. *J Biol Chem, 273*, 25856-25863.

[109] Sun, F., Hug, M. J., Bradbury, R. A. & Frizzell, R. A. (2000a). Protein kinase A associates with cystic fibrosis transmembrane conductance regulator via an interaction with ezrin. *J Biol Chem, 275*, 14360-14366.

[110] Sun, F., Hug, M. J., Lewarchik, C. M., Yun, C. H., Bradbury, N. A. & Frizzell, R.A. (2000b). E3KARP mediates the association of ezrin and protein kinase A with the cystic fibrosis transmembrane conductance regulator in airway cells. *J Biol Chem, 275*, 29539-29546.

[111] Dransfield, D. T., Bradford, A. J., Smith, J., Martin, M., Roy, C., Mangeat, P. H. & Goldenring, J. R. (1997). Ezrin is a cyclic AMP-dependent protein kinase anchoring protein. *EMBO J, 16*, 35-43.

[112] Lamprecht, G., Weinman, E. J. & Yun, C-H. C. (1998). E3KARP in the cAMP-mediated inhibition of NHE3. *J Biol Chem*, 273, 29972-29978.
[113] Weinman, E. J., Steplock, D., Donowitz, M. & Shenolikar, S. (2000). NHERF associations with sodium-hydrogen exchanger isoforms 3 (NHE3) and ezrin are essential for cAMP-mediated phosphorylation and inhibition of NHE3. *Biochem*, 39, 6123-6129.
[114] Moyer, B. D., Denton, J., Karlson, K. H., Reynolds, D., Wang, S., Mickle, J. E., Milewski, M., Cutting, G. R., Guggino, W. B., Li, M. & Stanton, B. A. (1999). A PDZ-interacting domain in CFTR is an apical membrane polarisation signal. *J Clin Invest*, 104, 1353-1361.
[115] Moyer, B. D., Duhaime, M., Shaw, C., Denton, J., Reynolds, D., Karlson, K. H., Pfeiffer, J., Wang, S., Mickle, J. E., Milewski, M., Cutting, G. R., Guggino, W. B., Li, M. & Stanton, B. A. (2000). The PDZ-interacting domain of cystic fibrosis transmembrane conductance regulator is required for functional expression in the apical plasma membrane. *J Biol Chem*, 275, 27069-27074.
[116] Fais, S., De Milito, A. & Lozupone, F. (2005). The role of FAS to ezrin association in FAS-mediated apoptosis. *Apoptosis*, 10, 941-947.
[117] Parlato, S., Giammariolo, A. M., Logozzi, M., Lozupone, F., Matarrese, P., Luciani, F., Falchi, M., Malorni, W. & Fais, S. (2000). CD95 (APO1/Fas) linkage to the actin cytoskeleton through ezrin in human T lymphocytes: A novel regulatory mechanism of the CD95 apoptotic pathway. *EMBO J*, 19, 5123-5134.
[118] Itoh, K., Sakakibara, M., Yamasaki, S., Takeuchi, A., Arase, H., Miyazaki, M., Nakajima, N., Okada, M. & Saito, T. (2002). Negative regulation of immune synapse formation by anchoring lipid raft to cytoskeleton through Cbp-EBP50-ERM assembly. *J Immunol*, 168, 541-544.
[119] Gillingham, A. K. & Munro, S. (2000). The PACT domain, a conserved centrosomal targeting motif in the coiled-coil proteins AKAP450 and pericentrin. *EMBO Reports*, 11, 524-529.
[120] Takahashi, M., Shibata, H., Shimakawa, M. Miyamoto, M., Mukai, H. & Ono, Y. (1999). Characterization of a novel giant scaffolding protein, CG-NAP, that anchors multiple signaling enzymes to centrosome and the Golgi apparatus. *J Biol Chem*, 274, 17267-17274.
[121] Takahashi, M., Mukai, H., Oishi, K., Isagawa, T. & Ono, Y. (2000). Association of immature hypophosphorylated protein kinase Cε with an anchoring protein CG-NAP. *J Biol Chem*, 275, 34592-24596.
[122] Tasken, K. A., Collas, P., Kemmner, W. A., Witczak, O., Conti, M. & Tasken, K. (2001). Phosphodiesterase 4D and protein kinase a type II constitute a signalling unit in the centrosomal area. *J Biol Chem*, 276, 21999-22002.
[123] Sillibourne, J. E., Milne, D. M., Takahashi, M., Ono, Y. & Meek, D. W. (2002). Centrosomal anchoring of the protein kinase CK1delta mediated by attachment to the large, coiled-coil scaffolding protein CG-NAP/AKAP450. *J Mol Biol*, 322, 785-797.
[124] Larocca, M. C., Shanks, R. A., Tian, L., Nelson, D. L., Stewart, D. M. & Goldenring, J. R. (2004). AKAP350 interaction with cdc42 interacting protein 4 at the Golgi apparatus. *Mol Biol Cell*, 15, 2771-2781.

[125] Keryer, G., Di Fiore, B., Celati, C., Lechtreck, K. F., Mogensen, M., Delouvee, A., Lavia, P., Bornens, M. & Tassin, A. M. (2003). Part of Ran is associated with AKAP450 at the centrosome: involvement in microtubule-organising activity. *Mol Biol Cell, 14*, 4260-4271.

[126] Hinchcliffe, E. H., Li, C., Thompson, E. A., Maller, J. L. & Sluder, G. (1999). Requirement of Cdk2-cyclin E activity for repeated centrosome reproduction in *Xenopus* egg extracts. *Science, 283*, 851-854.

[127] Nishimura, T., Takahashi, M., Kim, H. S., Mukai, H. & Ono, Y. (2005). Centrosome-targeting region of CG-NAP causes centrosome amplification by recruiting cyclin E-cdk2 complex. *Genes to Cells, 10*, 75-86.

[128] Westphal, R. S., Soderling, S. H., Alto, N. M., Langeberg, L. K. & Scott, J. D. (2000). Scar/WAVE-1, a Wiskott-Aldrich syndrome protein, assembles an actin-associated multi-kinase scaffold. *EMBO J, 19*, 4589-4600.

[129] Yamazaki, D., Fujiwara, T., Suetsugu, S. & Takenawa, T. (2005). A novel function of WAVE in lamellipodia: WAVE1 is required for stabilisation of lammellipodial protrusions during cell spreading. *Genes to Cells, 10*, 381-392.

[130] Calle, Y., Chou, H. C., Thrasher, A. J. & Jones, G. E. (2004). Wiskott-Aldrich syndrome protein and the cytoskeletal dynamics of dendritic cells. *J Path, 204*, 460-469.

[131] Ziff, E. B. (1997). Enlightening the postsynaptic density. *Neuron, 19*, 1163-1174.

[132] Irie, K., Nakatsu, T., Mitsuoka, K., Miyazawa, A., Sobue, K., Hiroaki, Y., Doi, T., Fujiyoshi, Y. & Kato, H. (2002). Crystal structure of the Homer 1 family conserved region reveals the interaction between the EVH1 domain and own proline-rich motif. *J Mol Biol, 318*, 1117-1126.

[133] Sheng, M. (2001). Molecular orginisation of the postsynaptic specialisation. *PNAS, 98*, 7058-7061.

[134] Fukata, Y., Tzingounis, A. V., Trinidad, J. C., Fukata, M., Burlingame, A. L., Nicoll, R. A. & Bredt, D. S. (2005). Molecular constituents of neuronal AMPA receptors. *J Cell Biol, 169*, 399-404.

[135] Leonard, A. S., Davare, M. A., Horne, M. C., Garner, C. C. & Hell, J. W. (1998). SAP97 is associated with the α-amino-3-hydroxy-5-methylisoxazole-4-propionic acid receptor GluR1 subunit. *J Biol Chem, 273*, 19518-19524.

[136] Tappe, A. & Kuner, R. (2006). Regulation of motor performance and striatal function by synaptic scaffolding proteins of the Homer1 family. *PNAS, 103*, 774-779.

[137] Schluter, O. M., Xu, W. & Malenka, R. C. (2006). Alternative N-terminal domains of PSD-95 and SAP97 govern activity-dependent regulation of synaptic AMPA receptor function. *Neuron, 51*, 99-111.

[138] Rockliffe, N. & Gawler, D. (2006). Differential mechanisms of glutamate receptor regulation of SynGAP in cortical neurones. *FEBS Letters, 580*, 831-838.

[139] Sala, C., Piech, V., Wilson, N. R., Passafaro, M., Liu, G. & Sheng, M. (2001). Regulation of dendritic spine morphology and synaptic function by Shank and Homer. *Neuron, 31*, 115-130.

[140] Ishii, H., Shibuya, K., Ohta, Y., Mukai, H., Uchino, S., Takata, N., Rose, J. A. & Kawato, S. (2006). Enhancement of nitric oxide production by association of nitric

oxide synthase with N-methyl-D-aspartate receptors via postsynaptic density 95 in genetically engineered Chinese hamster ovary cells: real-time fluorescence imaging using nitric oxide sensitive dye. *J Neurochem, 96,* 1531-1539.

[141] Levinson, J. N., Chery, N., Huang, K., Wong, T. P., Gerrow, K., Kang, R., Prange, O., Wang, Y. T. & El-Husseini, A. (2005). Neuroligins mediate excitatory and inhibitory synapse formation: Involvement of PSD-95 and neurexin-1b in neuroligin-induced synaptic specificity. *J Biol Chem, 280,* 17312-17319.

[142] Dirks, P., Thomas, U. & Montag, D. (2006). The cytoplasmic domain of NrCAM binds to PDZ domains of synapse-associated proteins SAP90/PSD95 and SAP97. *Euro J Neurosci, 24,* 25-31.

[143] Lee, S., Fan, S., Makarova, O., Straight, S. & Margolis, B. (2002b). A novel and conserved protein-protein interaction domain of mammalian Lin-2/CASK binds and recruits SAP97 to the lateral surface of epithelia. *Mol Cell Biol, 22,* 1778-1791.

[144] Cai, C., Li, H., Rivera, C. & Keinanen, K. (2006). Interaction between SAP97 and PSD-95, two MAGUK proteins involved in synaptic trafficking of AMPA receptors. *J Biol Chem, 281,* 4267-4273.

[145] Weed, S. A., Du, Y. & Parsons, J. T. (1998). Translocation of cortactin to the cell periphery is mediated by the small GTPase Rac1. *J Cell Sci, 111,* 2433-2443.

[146] Lua, B. L. & Low, B. C. (2005). Cortactin phosphorylation as a switch for actin cytoskeletal network and cell dynamics control. *FEBS Letters, 579,* 577-585.

[147] Iki, J., Inoue, A., Bito, H. & Okabe, S. (2005). Bi-directional regulation of postsynaptic cortactin distribution by BDNF and NMDA receptor activity. *Eur J Neurosci, 22,* 2985-2994.

[148] Webb, B. A., Eves, R. & Mak, A. S. (2006). Cortactin regulates podosome formation: Roles of the protein interaction domains. *Exp Cell Res, 312,* 760-769.

[149] Campbell, D. H., Sutherland, R. L. & Daly, R. J. (1999). Signalling pathways and structural domains required for phosphorylation of EMS1/Cortactin. *Cancer Res, 59,* 5376-5385.

[150] Mizutani, K., Miki, H., He, H., Maruta, H. & Takenawa, T. (2002). Wiskott-Aldrich syndrome protein in podosome formation and degradation of extracellular matrix in src-transformed fibroblasts. *Cancer Res, 62,* 669-674.

[151] Kinley, A. W., Weed, S. A, Weaver, A. M., Karginov, A. V., Bissonette, E., Cooper, J. A. & Parsons, J. T. (2003). Cortactin interacts with WIP in regulating Arp2/3 activation and membrane protrusion. *Curr Biol, 13,* 384-393.

[152] McNiven, M. A., Kim, L., Krueger, E. W., Orth, J. D., Cao, H. & Wong, T. W. (2000). Regulated interactions between dynamin and the actin-binding protein cortactin modulate cell shape. *J Cell Biol, 151,* 187-198.

[153] Naisbitt, S., Kim, E., Tu, J. C., Xiao, B., Sala, C., Valtschanoff, J., Weinberg, R. J., Worley, P. F. & Sheng, M. (1999). Shank, a novel family of postsynaptic density proteins that binds to the NMDA receptor/PSD-95/GKAP complex and cortactin. *Neuron, 23,* 569-582.

[154] Daly, R. J. (2004). Cortactin signalling and dynamic actin networks. *Biochem J, 382,* 13-25.

[155] Duncan, R. S., Hwang, S-Y. & Koulen, P. (2005). Effects of Vesl/Homer proteins on intracellular signalling. *Exp Biol Med, 230,* 527-535.

[156] Hayashi, M. K., Ames, H. M. & Hayashi, Y. (2006). Tetrameric hub structure of postsynaptic scaffolding protein homer. *J Neurosci, 26,* 8492-8501.

[157] Xiao, B., Tu, J. C. & Worley, P. F. (2000). Homer: a link between neural activity and glutamate receptor function. *Curr Opin Neurobiol, 10,* 370-374.

[158] Hwang, S. Y., Wei, J., Westhoff, J. H., Duncan, R. S., Ozawa, F., Volpe, P., Inokuchi, K. & Koulen, P. (2003). Differential functional interaction of two Vesl/Homer protein isoforms with ryanodine receptor type 1: a novel mechanism for control of intracellular calcium signalling. *Cell Calcium, 34,* 177-184.

[159] Yuan, J. P., Kiselyov, K., Shin, D. M., Chen, J., Shcheynikov, N., Kang, S. H., Dehoff, M. H., Schwarz, M. K., Seeburg, P. H., Muallem, S. & Worley, P. F. (2003). Homer binds TRPC family channels and is required for gating of TRPC1 by IP3 receptors. *Cell, 114,* 777-789.

[160] Shiraishi, Y., Mizutani, A., Bito, H., Fujisawa, K., Narumiya, S., Mikoshiba, K. & Furuichi, T. (1999). Cupidin, an isoform of Homer/Vesl, interacts with the actin cytoskeleton and activated rho family small GTPases and is expressed in developing mouse cerebellar granule cells. *J Neurosci, 19,* 8389-8400.

[161] Tu, J. C., Xiao, B., Naisbitt, S., Yuan, J. P., Petralia, R. S., Brakeman, P., Doan, A., Aakalu, V. K., Lanahan, A. A., Sheng, M. & Worley, P. F. (1999). Coupling of mGluR/Homer and PSD-95 complexes by the Shank family of postsynaptic density proteins. *Neuron, 23,* 583-592.

[162] Gray, N. W., Fourgeaud, L., Huang, B., Chen, J., Cao, H., Oswald, B. J., Hemar, A. & McNiven, M. A. (2003). Dynamin 3 is a component of the postsynapse, where it interacts with mGluR5 and Homer. *Curr Biol, 13,* 510-515.

[163] Minakami, R., Kato, A. & Sugiyama, H. (2000). Interaction of Vesl-1L/Homer 1c with Syntaxin 13. *Biochem. Biophys Res Commun., 272,* 466-471.

[164] Sheng, M. & Kim, E. (2000). The Shank family of scaffold proteins. *J Cell Sci, 113,* 1851-1856.

[165] Lim, S., Naisbitt, S., Yoon, J., Hwang, J. I., Suh, P. G., Sheng, M. & Kim, E. (1999). Characterisation of the shank family of synaptic proteins. Multiple genes, alternative splicing and differential expression in brain and development. *J Biol Chem, 274,* 29510-29518.

[166] Gundelfinger, E. D., Boeckers, T. M., Baron, M. K. & Bowie, J. U. (2006). A role for zinc in postsynaptic density assembly and plasticity. *Trends Biochem Sci, 31,* 366-373.

[167] Boeckers, T. M., Mameza, M. G., Kreutz, M. R., Bockmann, J., Weise, C., Buck, F., Richter, D., Gundelfinger, E. D. & Kreienkamp, H. J. (2001). Synaptic scaffolding proteins in rat brain. Ankyrin repeats of the multidomain Shank protein family interact with the cytoskeletal protein alpha-fodrin. *J Biol Chem, 276,* 40104-40112.

[168] Lim, S., Sala, C., Yoon, J., Park, S., Kuroda, S., Sheng, M. & Kim, E. (2001). Sharpin, a novel postsynaptic density protein that directly interacts with the shank family of proteins. *Mol Cell Neurosci, 17,* 385-397.

[169] Quitsch, A., Berhorster, K., Liew, C. W., Richter, D. & Kreienkamp, H. J. (2005). Postsynaptic Shank antagonises dendrite branching induced by leucine-rich repeat protein Densin 180. *J Neurosci*, *25*, 479-487.

[170] Boeckers, T. M., Bockmann, J., Kreutz, M. R. & Gundelfinger, E. D. (2002). ProSAP/Shank proteins-a family of higher order organising molecules of the postsynaptic density with an emerging role in human neurological disease. *J Neurochem*, *81*, 903-910.

[171] Du, Y., Weed, S. A., Xiong, W. C., Marshall, T. D. & Parsons, J. T. (1998). Identification of a novel cortactin SH3 domain-binding protein and its localisation to growth cones of cultured neurons. *Mol Cell Biol*, *18*, 5838-5851.

[172] Feng, Y. & Walsh, C. A. (2004). The many faces of filamin: A versatile molecular scaffold for cell motility and signalling. *Nature Cell Biol*, *6*, 1034-1038.

[173] Nakamura, F., Pudas, R., Heikkinen, O., Permi, P., Kilpelainen, I., Munday, A. D., Hartwig, J. H., Stossel, T. P. & Ylanne, J. (2006). The structure of the GpIb-filamin A complex. *Blood*, *107*, 1925-1932.

[174] Scott, M. G. H., Pierotti, V., Storez, H., Lindberg, E., Thuret, A., Muntaner, O., Labbe-Jullie, C., Pitcher, J. A. & Marullo, S. (2006). Cooperative regulation of extracellular signal-regulated kinase activation and cell shape change by filamin A and β-arrestins. *Mol Cell Biol*, *26*, 3432-3445.

[175] Ohta, Y., Hartwig, J. H. & Stossel, T. P. (2006). FilGAP, a Rho- and ROCK-regulated GAP for Rac binds filamin A to control actin remodelling. *Nature Cell Biol*, *8*, 803-814.

[176] Awata, H, Huang, C, Handlogten, M. E. & Miller, R. T. (2001). Interaction of the calcium-sensing receptor and filamin, a potential scaffolding protein. *J Biol Chem*, *276*, 34871-34879.

[177] Hjalm, G., MacLeod, R. J., Kifor, O., Chattopadhyay, N. & Brown, E. M. (2001). Filamin-A binds to the carboxyl-terminal tail of the calcium-sensing receptor, an interaction that participates in CaR-mediated activation of mitogen-activated protein kinase. *Am Soc Biochem Mol Biol*, *276*, 34880-34887.

[178] Tigges, U., Koch, B., Wissing, J., Jockusch, B. M. & Ziegler, W. H. (2003). The F-actin cross-linking and focal adhesion protein filamin A is a ligand and *in vivo* substrate for protein kinase Cα. *J Biol Chem*, *278*, 23561-23569.

[179] Liu, G., Thomas, L., Warren, R. A., Enns, C. A., Cunningham, C. C., Hartwig, J. H. & Thomas, G. (1997). Cytoskeletal protein ABP-280 directs the intracellular trafficking of furin and modulates proproteins processing in the endocytic pathway. *J Cell Biol*, *139*, 1719-1733.

[180] Cukier, I. H., Li, Y. & Lee, J. M. (2007). Cyclin B1/Cdk1 binds and phosphorylates Filamin A and regulates its ability to cross-link actin. *FEBS Letters*, *581*, 1661-1672.

[181] Jay, D., Garcia, E. J., Lara, J. E., Medina, M. A. & de la Luz Ibarra, M. (2000). Determination of a cAMP-dependent protein kinase phosphorylation site in the C-terminal region of human endothelial actin-binding protein. *Arch Biochem Biophys*, *377*, 80-84.

[182] Vadlamudi, R. K., Li, F., Adam, L., Nguyen, D., Ohta, Y., Stossel, T. P. & Kumar, R. (2002). Filamin is essential in actin cytoskeletal assembly mediated by p21-activated kinase. *Nature Cell Biol*, *4*, 681-690.

[183] Ohta, Y. & Hartwig, J. H. (1995). Actin filament cross-linking by chicken gizzard filamin is regulated by phosphorylation in vitro. *Biochem*, *34*, 6745-6754.

[184] Marti, A., Luo, Z., Cunningham, C., Ohta, Y., Hartwig, J., Stossel, T. P., Kyriakis, J. M. & Avruch, J. (1997). Actin-binding protein-280 binds the stress-activated protein kinase (SAPK) activator SEK-1 and is required for tumor necrosis factor-α activation of SAPK in melanoma cells. *J Biol Chem*, *272*, 2620-2628.

[185] Woo, M. S., Ohta, Y., Rabinovitz, I., Stossel, T. P. & Blenis, J. (2004). Ribosomal S6 kinase (RSK) regulates phosphorylation of Filamin A on an important regulatory site. *Mol Cell Biol*, *24*, 3025-3035.

[186] Zhu, T. N., He, H. J., Kole, S., D'Souza, T., Agarwal, R., Morin, P. J. & Bernier, M. (2007). Filamin A-mediated down-regulation of the exchange factor Ras-GRF1 correlates with decreased matrix metalloproteinase-9 expression in human melanoma cells. *J Biol Chem*, *282*, 14816-14826.

[187] Glougauer, M., Arora, P., Chou, D., Janmey, P. A., Downey, G. P. & McCulloch, C. A. G. (1998). The role of actin-binding protein 280 in integrin-dependent mechanoprotection. *J Biol Chem*, *273*, 1689-1698.

[188] Briggs, M. W. & Sacks, D. B. (2003). IQGAP proteins are integral components of cytoskeletal regulation. *EMBO Reports*, *4*, 571-574.

[189] Bashour, A. M., Fullerton, A. T., Hart, M. J., Bloom, G. S. (1997). IQGAP1, a Rac- and Cdc42-binding protein, directly binds and cross-links microfilaments. *J Cell Biol*, *137*, 1555-1566.

[190] Fukata, M., Kuroda, S., Fujii, K., Nakamura, T., Shoji, I., Matsuura, Y., Okawa, K., Iwamatsu, A., Kikuchi, A. & Kaibuchi, K. (1997). Regulation of cross-linking of actin filament by IQGAP1, a target for Cdc42. *J Biol Chem*, *272*, 29579-29583.

[191] Brandt, D. T. & Grosse, R. (2007). Get to grips: steering local actin dynamics with IQGAPs. *EMBO Reports*, *8*, 1019-1023.

[192] Mateer, S. C., Morris, L. E., Cromer, D. A., Bensenor, L. B. & Bloom, G. S. (2004). Actin filament binding by a monomeric IQGAP1 fragment with a single calponin homology domain. *Cell Motil Cytoskel*, *58*, 231-241.

[193] Hart, M. J., Callow, M. G., Souza, B. & Polakis, P. (1996). IQGAP1, a calmodulin-binding protein with a rasGAP-related domain, is a potential effector for cdc42Hs. *EMBO J*, *15*, 2997-3005.

[194] Ho, Y. D., Joyal, J. L., Li, Z. & Sacks, D. B. (1999). IQGAP1 integrates Ca^{2+}/calmodulin and CDC42 signalling. *J Biol Chem*, *274*, 464-470.

[195] Joyal, J. L., Annan, R. S., Ho, Y. D., Huddleston, M. E., Carr, S. A., Hart, M. J. & Sacks, D. B. (1997). Calmodulin modulates the interaction between IQGAP1 and CDC42. Identification of IQGAP1 by nanoelectrospray tandem mass spectrometry. *J Biol Chem*, *272*, 15419-15425.

[196] Weissbach, L., Bernards, A. & Herion, D. W. (1998). Binding of myosin essential light chain to the cytoskeleton-associated protein IQGAP1. *Biochem Biophys Res Commun*, *251*, 269-276.

[197] Mbele, G. O., Deloulme, J. C., Gentil, B. J., Delphin, C., Ferro, M., Garin, J., Takahashi, M. & Baudier, J. (2002). The zinc- and calcium-binding S100B interacts and co-localises with IQGAP1 during dynamic rearrangement of cell membranes. *J Biol Chem, 277*, 49998-50007.

[198] Kuroda, S., Fukata, M., Kobayashi, M., Nomura, N., Iwamatsu, A. & Kaibuchi, K. (1996). Identification of IQGAP as a putative target for the small GTPases, CDC42 and Rac1. *J Biol Chem, 271*, 23363-23367.

[199] Fukata, M., Watanabe, T., Noritake, J., Nakagawa, M., Yamaga, M., Kuroda, S., Matsuura, Y., Iwamatsu, A., Perez, F. & Kaibuchi, K. (2002). Rac1 and Cdc42 capture microtubules through IQGAP1 and CLIP-170. *Cell, 109*, 873-885.

[200] Kuroda, S., Fukata, M., Nakagawa, M., Fujii, K., Nakamura, T., Ookubo, T., Izawa, I., Nagase, T., Nomura, N., Tani, H., Shoji, I., Matsuura, Y., Yonehara, S. & Kaibuchi, K. (1998). Role of IQGAP1, a target of the small GTPases CDC42 and Rac1, in regulation of E-cadherin-mediated cell-cell adhesion. *Science, 281*, 832-835.

[201] Briggs, M. W., Li, Z. & Sacks, D. B. (2002). IQGAP1-mediated stimulation of transcriptional co-activation by beta-catenin is modulated by calmodulin. *J Biol Chem, 277*, 7453-7465.

[202] Noritake, J., Watanabe, T., Sato, K., Wang, S. & Kaibuchi, K. (2005). IQGAP1: a key regulator of adhesion and migration. *J Cell Sci, 118*, 2085-2092.

[203] 196. Machesky, L. M. (1998). Cytokinesis: IQGAPs find a function. *Curr Biol, 8*, R202-R205.

[204] Clark, E. A., Golub, T. R., Lander, E. S. & Hynes, R. O. (2000). Genomic analysis of metastasis reveals an essential role for RhoC. *Nature, 406*, 532-535.

[205] Nabeshima, K., Shimao, Y., Inoue, T. & Koono, M. (2002). Immunohistochemical analysis of IQGAP1 expression in human colorectal carcinomas: its overexpression in carcinomas and association with invasion fronts. *Cancer Lett, 176*, 101-109.

[206] Le Clainche, C., Schlaepfer, D., Ferrari, A., Klingauf, M., Grohmanova, K., Veligoskiy, A., Didry, D., Le, D., Egile, C., Carlier, M-F. & Kroschewski, R. (2007). IQGAP1 stimulates actin assembly through the N-Wasp-Arp2/3 pathway. *J Biol Chem, 282*, 426-435.

[207] Kim, A. S., Kakalis, L. T., Abdul-Manan, N., Liu, G. A. & Rosen, M. K. (2000). Autoinhibition and activation mechanisms of the Wiskott-Aldrich syndrome protein. *Nature, 404*, 151-158.

[208] Brandt, D. T., Marion, S., Griffiths, G., Watanabe, T., Kaibuchi, K. & Grosse, R. (2007). Dia1 and IQGAP1 interact in cell migration and phagocytic cup formation. *J Cell Biol, 178*, 193-200.

[209] Bracke, M. E., Van Roy, F. M. & Mareel, M. M. (1996). The E-cadherin/catenin complex in invasion and metastasis. *Curr Top Microbiol Immunol, 213*, 123-161.

[210] Li, Z., Kim, S. H., Higgins, J. M., Brenner, M. B. & Sacks, D. B. (1999). IQGAP1 and calmodulin modulate E-cadherin function. *J Biol Chem, 274*, 37885-37892.

[211] Li, Z. & Sacks, D. B. (2003). Elucidation of the interaction of calmodulin with the IQ motifs of IQGAP1. *J Biol Chem, 278*, 4347-4352.

Chapter Sources

Chapter VIII was also published in "Membrane Microdomain Regulation of Neuron Signaling", authored by Ron Wallace, Nova Science Publishers. It was submitted for appropriate modifications in an effort to encourage wider dissemination of research.

Chapter IX was also published in "Cell Movement: New Research Trends", edited by T. Abreu and G. Silva, Nova Science Publishers. It was submitted for appropriate modifications in an effort to encourage wider dissemination of research.

Index

A

acetate, 131
acetone, 130
acetylation, 49, 57
acetylcholine, 167
acid, 123, 125, 154, 158, 185, 202, 204, 208, 221
actin-depolymerizing factor, 41
action potential (AP), x, xi, 25, 29, 35, 66, 81, 87, 91, 98, 120, 124, 129, 161, 162, 163, 165, 166, 167, 169, 170, 172, 194, 217
activation, xi, 1, 2, 6, 7, 8, 9, 13, 19, 20, 24, 27, 29, 30, 31, 35, 36, 40, 58, 59, 81, 87, 94, 133, 144, 153, 155, 156, 179, 180, 182, 187, 188, 189, 190, 191, 192, 193, 195, 202, 203, 209, 212, 215, 216, 217, 219, 222, 224, 225, 226
activation state, 13
activators, 192
active site, 187
activity level, 189
acute, 31
acute leukemia, 31
Adams, 53, 60
adaptation, 176
adenocarcinoma, 105
adenovirus, 23, 79
adenoviruses, 106
adherens junction, 218
adhesive interaction, 84
adhesive properties, 4
adipocytes, 217
administration, 58
ADP, 49
adult, 10, 38, 43, 46, 57, 58, 59, 63, 77, 93, 97, 98, 106

adulthood, 20
adults, 58
Ag, 113, 124
age, 70, 128, 130, 131
agents, 106, 113, 122
aggregates, 14, 58, 63, 114, 126
aggregation, 114
aggressiveness, 123
agonist, 33, 197, 200
aid, 107, 181, 189, 212
AKT, 98
alanine, 196
aldolase, 71, 90
Aldrich syndrome, 201, 221, 222, 226
algae, 155, 157, 158, 159
alpha, 23, 25, 27, 28, 30, 32, 33, 36, 73, 74, 78, 98, 169, 193, 204, 205, 217, 223
alternative, xi, 21, 55, 77, 79, 85, 94, 141, 161, 189, 191, 194, 205, 223
alternative hypothesis, 85
alters, 19, 22, 71, 95, 123, 187
Alzheimer, 170
Alzheimer disease, 58, 64
amino, 3, 20, 29, 33, 72, 77, 78, 183, 184, 185, 186, 200, 202, 204, 218, 221
amino acid, 3, 72, 77, 78, 183, 184, 185, 186, 200, 204
amino acids, 3, 72, 77, 78, 183, 184, 185, 186, 200
amoeboid, 150
AMPA, 40, 167, 171, 202, 203, 204, 205, 206, 221, 222
amphibia, 140
amplitude, 164, 167, 173
amyloid, 46, 58, 62, 175
analog, 154
angiogenesis, 10, 101, 120

Index

animals, 51, 84, 105, 129, 136, 150
antagonist, 31, 106, 154
antecedents, 81
antibiotics, 130
antibodies, 136
antibody, 22, 72, 86, 87, 123
anticancer, 106, 122
antigen, 35, 123, 194
antisense, 15, 23, 50, 79, 80, 84, 85, 86, 87, 88
antisense RNA, 79, 80
anti-tumor, 106, 122
antrum, 133
anxiety, 170
aortic stenosis, 45
APC, 79, 95, 140, 145
apoptosis, 10, 28, 106, 114, 168, 181, 182, 186, 190, 200, 220
apoptotic pathway, 220
application, 171, 174, 176
aqueous solution, 131
Arabidopsis thaliana, 154
argument, 163, 166
arthritis, 216
aspartate, 202, 222
assessment, 90, 131
astrocytoma, 125
asymmetry, 149, 155, 156, 157
ATF, 20
atmosphere, 130
ATP, 41, 61, 62, 71, 90, 192
ATPase, 159, 169
attachment, 3, 10, 14, 28, 39, 57, 180, 211, 220
autism, 45
autocrine, 109, 110, 112
autoradiography, 128, 130, 131, 132, 133, 135
autosomal recessive, 73, 92
availability, 16
awareness, 42, 52
axon, x, 40, 43, 59, 60, 161, 162, 163, 165, 171, 174, 175
axons, 10, 38, 39, 41, 42, 43, 59, 62, 63, 67, 162, 163, 174, 175

B

β2-adrenergic receptor, 196, 197, 199, 218
back, 8, 16, 25, 33, 75, 88, 197, 198
bacteria, 87
barrier, 107, 177
barriers, 164, 173
base pair, 76, 78
basement membrane, 6, 13, 24, 84, 104
basic fibroblast growth factor, 6, 32
Bcl-2, 190
BD, 107, 108, 120
BDNF, 43, 44, 67, 222
behavior, 40, 48, 52, 81, 108, 110, 111, 114, 119, 123, 124, 163, 166
behaviours, 180
binding energy, 44
biogenesis, 39, 53, 133, 137
bioinformatics, 44
biological processes, 10, 11, 102
biological systems, 37, 38
biology, 167
biophysics, 176
biosynthesis, 4
birth, 67, 158, 199
bladder, 118, 125, 204
bladder cancer, 204
blastoderm, 50, 51
blocks, 9, 38, 52, 108, 120, 130
blood, 71, 75, 78, 82, 90, 94, 106, 124, 170
blood group, 71, 90
blood vessels, 78
blot, 85
body shape, 150
bonds, 3, 166
bone marrow, 104, 106, 120, 121, 122, 123
Bose, 125
Boston, 168, 170, 173, 174
bovine, 32, 108, 109
boys, 70, 72, 75
brain, 6, 38, 42, 44, 46, 57, 58, 59, 61, 62, 67, 75, 76, 77, 78, 79, 80, 93, 95, 96, 97, 98, 103, 118, 125, 126, 176, 189, 194, 204, 207, 210, 223
brain development, 42, 76
brain structure, 46, 57
brain tumor, 125
branching, xi, 161, 162, 163, 165, 166, 224
breakdown, 180
breast cancer, 24, 36, 102, 103, 104, 105, 106, 107, 109, 110, 111, 119, 120, 121, 122, 123, 125
breast carcinoma, 105, 106, 119, 126
budding, 139, 140, 142, 143, 146, 147, 157
buffer, 130
bundling, 140

C

Ca^{2+}, 40, 88, 98, 99, 144, 153, 154, 155, 156, 158, 159, 165, 180, 197, 203, 205, 207, 210, 211, 212, 225
cadherin, 145, 210, 211, 212, 226
cadherins, 13, 211
Caenorhabditis elegans, 137
calcium, 20, 72, 75, 99, 139, 140, 145, 165, 174, 176, 185, 202, 207, 208, 218, 223, 224, 226
calculus, 173
calf, 113, 130
calmodulin, 74, 92, 98, 139, 140, 143, 144, 145, 185, 197, 205, 207, 210, 211, 212, 225, 226
cAMP, 46, 66, 150, 153, 187, 195, 218, 220, 224
cancer, 27, 33, 34, 35, 101, 102, 103, 104, 106, 110, 114, 115, 120, 121, 122, 123, 124, 125, 145, 146, 204, 210
cancer cells, 24, 27, 28, 104, 109, 110, 111, 115, 122, 123, 210
Candida, 140, 143
candidates, 125
carbon, 168, 169, 174
carbon nanotubes, 168, 174
carboxyl, 72, 73, 77, 78, 80, 81, 85, 86, 87, 99, 190, 224
carcinogenesis, 103
carcinoma, 10, 23, 31, 34, 105, 106, 119, 125, 126
carcinomas, 146, 226
cardiac muscle, 207
cardiovascular system, 70, 83, 207
cargo, 192
carrier, 90
casein, 87, 200
catabolism, 36
catalytic activity, 20, 41
cation, 176, 202
C-C, 171
CD95, 220
CDK, 133, 143
cDNA, 72, 76, 79, 84, 91
cell adhesion, 1, 2, 6, 10, 11, 12, 13, 14, 15, 16, 24, 31, 88, 97, 98, 99, 109, 140, 144, 145, 170, 180, 188, 189, 200, 203, 204, 210, 211, 212, 226
cell body, 108, 163, 167
cell culture, 107, 108, 109, 112, 113, 115, 116, 119, 125, 130
cell cycle, 10, 20, 41, 64, 83, 127, 128, 129, 130, 131, 132, 133, 134, 200
cell death, 119, 208

cell differentiation, 10, 97
cell division, 20, 21, 23, 117, 119, 127, 128, 150, 152, 211, 212
cell fate, 121, 182
cell growth, 7, 20, 33, 116, 133, 157, 182, 184
cell invasion, 9, 34, 119, 125, 212
cell line, 29, 30, 32, 33, 81, 84, 94, 98, 103, 104, 106, 107, 108, 110, 114, 115, 117, 119, 120, 123, 125, 128, 133, 168, 185, 200, 208, 209
cell lines, 30, 32, 94, 103, 104, 108, 110, 115, 117, 119, 120, 123, 125, 200, 208, 209
cell membranes, 24, 73, 145, 171, 172, 175, 226
cell signaling, 117
cell surface, 5, 6, 7, 8, 9, 12, 22, 24, 26, 29, 32, 34, 35, 82, 170, 173, 190, 209, 211, 214
cellular adhesion, 13, 35, 80, 84
cellular processes, 123
cellular regulation, 130
cellular signaling pathway, 81
central nervous system, 10, 70, 77, 80, 88, 99, 174
centriole, 127, 128, 129, 130, 131, 132, 133, 135, 137
centromere, 45
centrosome, 19, 21, 127, 128, 129, 131, 132, 133, 134, 135, 137, 200, 220, 221
cerebellar granule cells, 223
cerebellum, 76
cerebral cortex, 77, 83
cerebral function, 80
channels, x, 40, 53, 59, 78, 95, 117, 152, 159, 161, 163, 165, 166, 167, 168, 169, 171, 172, 173, 174, 185, 202, 205, 223
chemical, 165, 170
chemical energy, 34
chemicals, 154
chemoattractant, 105, 110, 150, 153
chemokine, 7, 24, 105, 109, 121
chemokine receptor, 105, 121
chemotaxis, 8, 18, 21, 26, 35, 102, 107, 108, 109, 124, 150, 153, 157, 158, 214
chemotherapy, 114
chicken, 225
childhood, 20, 73, 92
children, 72, 92
chloroplasts, 154
cholesterol, 78, 94, 167, 173, 174
chondrocytes, 34
choroid, 96
chromatin, 28, 38, 39, 41, 44, 46, 49, 50, 52, 57, 59, 61, 62, 63, 64, 65, 66, 67, 68, 81, 186

chromosome, 3, 37, 38, 39, 42, 44, 45, 46, 47, 48, 50, 51, 52, 53, 54, 55, 56, 59, 61, 62, 63, 66, 67, 72, 89, 90, 91, 92
chromosome map, 61
chromosomes, 44, 45, 47, 48, 52, 54, 55, 56, 59, 60, 61, 63, 64, 66, 68, 127, 135, 146
cilia, 127
cilium, 129
c-Jun kinase, 82
classes, 39, 81, 185
classification, 31, 103, 213
cleavage, 3, 4, 27, 28, 31, 33, 49, 88, 207
clone, 85
cloning, 1, 91, 213
closure, 42
clustering, 8, 10, 12, 23, 30, 82, 83, 110, 167, 168, 184, 205
clusters, x, 13, 14, 19, 20, 48, 60, 84, 108, 110, 114, 161, 163, 166, 167, 175, 183
c-Myc, 192, 193
CNS, 81, 83, 93, 98
Co, 87, 92, 96, 104, 136
CO_2, 130
coatings, 107, 112
coding, 37, 39, 57, 59, 66, 159, 167
codon, 76, 77
codons, 79
cofilin, 38, 40, 43, 46, 50, 58, 59, 68, 186, 188, 189
cognition, 40
cognitive function, 163
cognitive impairment, 70, 94, 97
cognitive level, 58
cognitive process, 59
cognitive profile, 45
coil, 166, 200, 204, 220
collagen, 24, 81, 82, 84, 94, 98, 115, 116, 117, 118, 125
colon, 36, 125
colorectal cancer, 35
communication, 53, 109, 146
compaction, 48
competition, 86
competitor, 95
complement, 30, 213
complexity, 50, 65, 75, 166, 209
complications, 70
components, xi, 2, 10, 13, 23, 30, 35, 37, 38, 46, 49, 53, 57, 59, 75, 79, 80, 85, 88, 113, 128, 140, 144, 150, 163, 165, 171, 179, 180, 181, 182, 187, 188, 191, 196, 200, 202, 208, 212, 213, 216, 225

composition, 34, 41, 63, 96, 164, 168
compounds, 102, 107, 108, 113
computation, 172, 173, 176
computer, 163
computer simulations, 163
computers, 170
computing, 176
concentration, 140, 150, 153, 164, 165, 166, 172
conditioning, 38, 109
conductance, 169, 171, 199, 205, 219, 220
conduction, x, xi, 161, 162, 163, 166, 167, 168, 171, 172, 175, 176
conduction block, x, 161, 171, 176
conductive, 171
conductor, 170
configuration, 45, 187, 188, 191, 198, 199, 212
confrontation, 115, 118, 125
connective tissue, 73
consciousness, 176
consensus, 87, 103, 140, 162, 185, 207, 214
conservation, 198
consolidation, 61
constraints, 163
construction, 117, 213
continuing, x, 161
control, x, 2, 6, 7, 9, 10, 21, 35, 41, 50, 51, 63, 64, 65, 84, 100, 109, 110, 112, 120, 127, 128, 130, 131, 144, 153, 159, 161, 165, 170, 190, 199, 206, 216, 219, 222, 223, 224
controlled, 175
conversion, 32, 152
correlation, 5, 31, 80, 131, 134, 174
cortex, 34, 77, 84, 98
cotton, 108
couples, 201
coupling, 35, 100, 146, 202, 203
creatine, 71, 75, 90
creatine kinase, 71, 75, 90
creatine phosphokinase, 75
CREB, 57, 58
critical period, 51
crossing over, 48, 54
crosslinking, 27, 208, 210, 211, 224, 225
crosstalk, xi, 27, 28, 33, 59, 102, 109, 179, 180, 211, 212
crust, 80
crystal structure, 4
crystalline, 172
C-terminal, 3, 54, 87, 183, 184, 198, 199, 203, 204, 207, 208, 210, 212, 214, 218, 224

C-terminus, 3, 4, 184, 187, 198, 199, 200, 201, 203, 205, 212
cues, 43, 150, 212
cultivation, 105
culture, 107, 108, 109, 110, 112, 113, 114, 115, 116, 117, 118, 119, 121, 123, 125, 130, 132, 170, 175
culture media, 108, 109
curcumin, 111, 122, 123
curing, 79
cycles, 50, 51, 130, 133, 134, 135, 209
cyclic AMP, 195, 217, 219
cyclins, 133
cysteine, 3, 72, 78, 80, 85, 185
cystic fibrosis, 199, 205, 219, 220
cytokeratins, 103, 104
cytokine, 2, 10, 16, 33, 109, 182, 190
cytokine receptor, 2, 10, 16, 182, 190
cytokines, 10, 105, 106, 150, 181, 189, 194, 216
cytokinesis, xi, 1, 20, 21, 33, 139, 141, 142, 143, 146, 147, 179, 180, 210, 212
cytometry, 111
cytoplasm, 80, 108, 134, 187, 188, 192, 194, 195, 198, 199
cytoplasmic membrane, 194
cytosol, x, 161, 164, 197, 198

D

D. melanogaster, 39, 44, 48, 53, 66
data set, 113, 119
database, 44
daughter cells, 20, 117
de novo, 128, 134, 137
deafness, 218
death, 42, 67, 70, 75, 81, 119, 200, 208
decay, 167
defects, 38, 40, 42, 45, 50, 74, 141, 155, 200, 207
defence, 65
deficiency, 4, 42, 80, 85, 88, 218
degradation, 4, 5, 6, 32, 46, 50, 51, 73, 126, 209, 222
degree, 162, 171
dehydrogenase, 71, 90
delivery, 79, 106, 120, 122, 123, 200
dendrites, 38, 39, 40, 42, 43, 44, 57, 59, 62, 163, 167
dendritic cell, 221
dendritic spines, 38, 40, 44, 171, 203
density, xi, 2, 9, 26, 28, 32, 34, 35, 36, 43, 92, 110, 111, 112, 179, 181, 221, 222, 223, 224
dentate gyrus, 78
dephosphorylating, 40

dephosphorylation, 183
depolarization, x, 113, 114, 161, 162, 163
deposition, 175
depression, 38, 43, 59
derivatives, 95, 152, 158
desensitization, 190, 197, 218
destruction, 75
detachment, 9, 13, 104, 110
detection, 66, 72, 90
developing brain, 96
developmental disorder, 34
developmental process, 104
diacylglycerol, 153, 154
dialysis, 165
differentiation, 10, 15, 40, 41, 76, 80, 81, 96, 97, 116, 120, 122, 149, 181, 182, 189, 215
diffusion, 8, 19, 42, 164, 165, 166, 168, 170, 173, 175, 177
dimer, 8, 181, 191, 193, 196
dimerization, 8
diploid, 127, 128, 150
dipole, 165
directionality, 111
discriminatory, 123
discs, 44, 184
disease gene, 47
disease progression, 104
disease-free survival, 103
diseases, 16, 38, 45, 204
disorder, 38, 40, 71, 75, 173
dispersion, 123
displacement, 187, 212
dissociation, 31, 164, 166, 191, 192, 193
distal, 167
distilled water, 115
distortions, 174
distribution, 2, 8, 17, 18, 19, 22, 36, 48, 52, 54, 56, 63, 78, 79, 84, 86, 95, 96, 97, 118, 149, 150, 152, 153, 154, 156, 173, 177, 202, 210, 222
disulfide, 184
divergence, 207
diversity, 2, 155, 190, 215
division, 20, 21, 23, 61, 117, 118, 119, 127, 128, 134, 150, 152, 211, 212, 214
DNA, 38, 41, 47, 48, 49, 53, 54, 57, 59, 60, 63, 64, 72, 80, 88, 91, 127, 128, 130, 131, 134, 135, 136, 184, 214
domain structure, 99, 205, 210
donkey, 46
dopamine, 207

dosage, 45
downregulating, 196
down-regulation, 19, 225
Drosophila, 38, 40, 41, 42, 43, 44, 45, 46, 47, 49, 50, 53, 55, 56, 59, 60, 61, 62, 63, 64, 65, 66, 67, 68, 142, 143, 147, 187
drug discovery, 123
drug interaction, 170
drug resistance, 10
drug-induced, 22
drugs, 22, 71
duplication, 45, 48, 61, 127, 128, 129, 130, 131, 132, 133, 135, 137, 200
duration, x, 128, 131, 161, 163, 167, 189
dyes, 108
dynamin, 205, 222
dystrophin, 70, 72, 73, 74, 75, 76, 77, 78, 79, 80, 81, 84, 86, 87, 88, 91, 92, 93, 94, 95, 96, 97, 98, 99, 207, 214

E

E-cadherin, 104, 126, 140, 145, 210, 211, 212, 226
ECM, 6, 13, 19, 22, 28, 81, 82, 83, 84, 87, 88
Eden, 3, 7, 21, 26
egg, 50, 143, 221
elaboration, 16
elasticity, 172
elastin, 45
electric field, 165, 166, 176
electrical, 162, 163, 165, 167
electron, 71, 89, 98, 128, 129, 130, 133, 202
electron microscopy, 71, 128, 129, 130, 202
electronic, 174
electrophysiological, 163
electrophysiology, 93
electrostatic, 166
electrostatic interactions, 166
elongation, 43, 80, 132, 135, 152, 211
embryo, 50, 61, 137
embryogenesis, 50, 51, 61, 62, 67, 70, 94, 101, 110, 134
embryonic development, 4, 10, 16, 49, 51, 78, 80, 81, 87
embryonic stem, 78, 95, 125
embryonic stem cells, 78, 95, 125
embryos, 144, 147
emission, 168
encoding, 24, 42, 43, 67, 153
endocrine, 105

endocytosis, 9, 25, 26, 74, 198, 200, 205
endometrial cancer, 123, 145
endoplasmic reticulum, 4, 43, 159, 165, 196
endothelial cell, 25, 27, 29, 31, 32, 33, 35, 36, 81, 113, 116, 122, 124, 125, 198, 218
endothelial cells, 25, 27, 29, 31, 35, 36, 81, 113, 116, 122, 124, 198, 218
endothelial progenitor cells, 104
energy, 16, 34, 41, 73, 75, 166
engraftment, 105
environment, 38, 53, 105, 118, 163
environmental factors, 103
environmental stimuli, 37, 38
enzymatic activity, 169
enzymes, 2, 46, 49, 71, 75, 87, 196, 201, 220
epidemiology, 72
epidermal growth factor, 29, 36, 182
epidermal growth factor receptor, 36
epigenetic, 38, 39, 42, 48, 49, 54, 57, 59, 63, 64
epigenetic mechanism, 42
epilepsy, 166, 169, 170, 173, 175
epithelia, 222
epithelial cell, 77, 87, 104, 110, 123, 133, 173, 175, 184, 198, 200, 218
epithelial cells, 77, 87, 104, 110, 133, 175, 198, 200, 218
epitope, 3, 5, 8, 12, 20, 26
epitopes, 24
equilibrium, 206
ERK proteins, 182
ERK1, 140, 180, 182, 187, 188, 189
erythrocyte, 71, 90, 164, 175, 176
erythrocyte membranes, 90, 175
erythropoietin, 10
Escherichia coli, 135, 172
ester, 113
estimating, 202
estrogen, 103, 104, 120
ethanol, 130
ethers, 93
etiology, 38
euchromatin, 47, 48
eukaryotes, 140, 156, 157, 180, 181, 207
eukaryotic cell, xi, 39, 123, 149, 155, 157, 164, 179, 180
Euro, 222
evaporation, 115
evidence, xi, 161, 162, 164, 165
evolution, 37, 48, 65, 137, 158, 168, 171, 176, 180, 181

excitability, 175
excitation, 168, 171, 175
excitatory postsynaptic potentials, 167
excitatory synapses, 202
exclusion, 13
execution, 139
exocytosis, 19, 23, 167, 174
exons, 72, 76, 77, 79
exposure, 12, 46, 48, 80, 194
external growth, 133
extracellular matrix, 1, 6, 13, 27, 34, 35, 73, 74, 78, 81, 82, 84, 92, 98, 107, 114, 180, 209, 222
extrapolation, 59
extravasation, 6
eye, 77

F

fabrication, 107
failure, x, xi, 31, 85, 141, 161, 162, 163, 166, 172
FAK, 8, 10, 12, 13, 14, 16, 22, 82, 85, 86, 88
family, 2, 8, 10, 13, 15, 16, 33, 36, 49, 54, 59, 81, 82, 96, 139, 140, 141, 142, 143, 168, 181, 186, 187, 189, 190, 192, 194, 196, 198, 199, 200, 201, 202, 205, 206, 207, 208, 210, 211, 218, 221, 222, 223, 224
family members, 82, 181, 186, 190, 192, 194, 199, 206
Fas, 200, 220
fatty acid, 171, 172
fatty acids, 171, 172
FEC, 50, 51, 52, 57
feedback, xi, 59, 179, 180
feedback inhibition, xi, 179, 180
feeding, 117
fertilization, 50
fetal, 4, 20, 108, 109, 113, 126
fetus, 77
fiber, 14, 17, 73, 88, 89, 168
fiber content, 14
fibers, 14, 15, 17, 18, 19, 22, 27, 29, 36, 71, 73, 75, 79, 82, 83, 87, 174, 175
fibrinolysis, 30
fibroblast, 33, 88, 105, 122, 124
fibroblast growth factor, 6, 32
fibroblasts, 14, 35, 77, 82, 98, 106, 113, 116, 122, 222
fibronectin, 23, 81, 84, 109
fibrosarcoma, 36
fibrosis, 75, 199, 205, 219, 220

filament, 43, 66, 74, 93, 103, 140, 145, 200, 211, 225
filopodia, 19, 60
filters, 108
fish, 113, 124
fission, 49, 140, 143, 147, 158
FITC, 46
fixation, 108
flagellum, 150
flank, 45, 185
flexibility, 43, 59, 107, 119, 187
floating, 14, 88
flow, 111, 163, 165
fluid, 70, 124, 164, 171, 172, 175
fluorescence, 24, 107, 108, 111, 118, 146, 154, 165, 209, 222
fluorophores, 117
focal adhesion kinase, 31, 33, 105, 217
folding, 123, 166, 168, 175
follicle, 13
Fox, 99, 121, 170
fragility, 48
fragmentation, 88
France, 26, 127
Fullerenes, 169
functional analysis, 93, 147
fungi, 4, 139, 140, 181
fungus, 140, 143
fusion, 87, 167

G

G protein, xi, 33, 179, 180, 188, 192, 193, 208, 212
GABAergic, 39, 61
gametophyte, 150, 151
Gamma, 136
ganglion, 41, 43, 62
gastrulation, 83
Gaussian, 170
GDP, 142, 187
gel, 117, 118, 141
gelation, 214
gels, 116, 117, 125
gene, 2, 3, 17, 21, 22, 24, 29, 38, 39, 40, 41, 44, 45, 46, 47, 48, 50, 51, 52, 53, 54, 57, 58, 59, 62, 63, 65, 66, 67, 68, 70, 72, 75, 76, 77, 78, 79, 80, 91, 93, 94, 95, 97, 98, 103, 114, 119, 120, 122, 123, 125, 137, 143, 146, 147, 153, 181, 183, 191, 194
gene expression, 2, 21, 22, 38, 41, 48, 50, 53, 57, 59, 63, 67, 98, 103, 114, 119, 125, 181, 183

gene promoter, 39, 93
gene silencing, 52
gene therapy, 79, 80, 122
gene transfer, 97, 123
generation, 26, 42, 115, 120, 125
genes, 4, 23, 39, 44, 45, 47, 48, 49, 53, 57, 59, 61, 62, 65, 67, 71, 73, 75, 87, 90, 99, 103, 154, 190, 196, 204, 223
genetic alteration, 72, 79
genetic disease, 45, 70
genetic disorders, 72
genetic linkage, 72
genetics, 38, 47, 58, 59, 93, 95
genome, 28, 37, 38, 40, 45, 47, 49, 53, 59, 63, 67, 128, 158
genomes, 153, 154
genotype, 61
germ cells, 67
germ line, 64
Germany, 1, 130
gestation, 42
GFP, 108, 115, 117, 121
Gibbs, 91
gizzard, 225
glass, 82, 86, 112, 113, 154
glia, 84, 171
glial cells, 76, 81, 95, 96
glioblastoma, 30
glioma, 15, 23, 25, 106, 118, 122, 125
gliomas, 106, 122
glucose, 199
glutamate, 38, 167, 202, 203, 204, 206, 221, 223
glutamic acid, 3
glutaraldehyde, 130
glycine, 167
glycogen, 87, 98, 99
glycogen synthase kinase, 98
glycoprotein, 3, 73, 91, 92, 93, 94, 95, 96, 98
glycoproteins, 73, 78, 81, 92, 207
glycosylated, 3, 78
glycosylation, 3
glycosylphosphatidylinositol (GPI), 1, 31, 33
goals, 2, 103
gold, 111, 165
gonads, 81, 87
GPCR, 190, 197, 207
GPI, 2, 3, 4, 5, 7, 10, 15, 27, 32, 33, 35
G-protein, 182, 187, 196, 207, 218
grading, 103
grants, 135

granule cells, 223
granules, 42, 43, 68
green fluorescent protein, 159
grids, 131
groups, xi, 75, 80, 81, 140, 166, 179, 181
growth factor, 6, 9, 10, 12, 27, 29, 30, 31, 32, 33, 36, 80, 87, 97, 98, 104, 106, 109, 123, 124, 133, 139, 140, 144, 181, 182, 187, 201
growth factors, 6, 10, 106, 109, 133, 181, 182, 187
GST, 87
guanine, 210
guidance, 43

H

hair cells, 218
hands, 185
hanging, 115, 116, 118, 125, 213
haploid, 150
haptotaxis, 102
harbour, 204
head, 164, 166
head and neck cancer, 23
healing, 105, 106, 111
health, 38, 70, 101, 119
heart, 24, 70, 75, 77, 79, 93, 118, 217
heart attack, 70
heart failure, 70
heat, 43, 57, 58, 189, 194
heat shock protein, 43
helical conformation, 140
helix, 166, 183, 184, 185, 186, 196
hematopoietic stem cell, 34
hepatocellular carcinoma, 10
hepatocyte, 6, 31, 106
hepatocyte growth factor, 6, 31, 106
hepatotoxicity, 125
HER2, 103
heterochromatin, 42, 48, 49, 51, 54, 57, 59, 60, 61, 62, 65, 66, 67, 68
heterodimer, 81, 164
heterogeneity, 78, 79, 96
high temperature, 51
high-speed, 172
hippocampus, 78, 169, 176
histidine, 185
histochemical, 71, 89, 96
histogram, 31
histone, 48, 49, 57, 62, 180
histopathology, 103

Hoechst, 108, 113, 114
homeostasis, 27, 184
homolog, 50, 51, 53, 153, 214
homologous chromosomes, 53
homology, 47, 48, 72, 88, 140, 145, 153, 154, 156, 183, 185, 186, 187, 192, 196, 200, 201, 207, 210, 214, 215, 225
hormones, 13
horse, 109
host, 6, 29
hot spots, 66
HSP27, 43
HSP60, 43
HSP90, 43
hub, 132, 223
human brain, 97, 176
human genome, 45
human mesenchymal stem cells, 121, 122
human neutrophils, 34
humans, 3, 47, 72, 91, 180, 181
hybrid, 50, 191, 194
hybridization, 49
hydro, 183
hydrogen, 220
hydrolysis, 41, 139
hydrolyzed, 88, 99
hydroxide, 117
hypercalcemia, 45
hypermethylation, 39, 61
hyperplasia, 104
hypothesis, 85, 86, 87, 131
hypoxia, 205, 121, 125

I

ICAM, 81
identification, 20, 41, 71, 72, 73, 90, 103, 108, 124, 164, 213
identity, 41, 45, 180, 182, 192, 194, 198
IFN, 106
IGF, 2, 7
IGF-1, 2, 7
IGF-I, 2
IgG, 30, 46
IL-1, 122, 190
IL-2, 5
image analysis, 117
images, 112, 118, 129, 151, 152, 154
imaging, 123, 124, 222
immune response, 16, 184

immune system, 101
immunity, 215
immunocompromised, 104
immunodeficiency, 201
immunofluorescence, 46, 50, 84, 86, 128
immunoglobulin, 81, 207, 214
immunoglobulin superfamily, 81, 214
immunoprecipitation, 39, 85, 141, 191
impairments, 59
implementation, 169
impulse conduction, 162
in situ, 29, 114
in utero, 97
in vitro, 16, 25, 26, 32, 34, 36, 86, 87, 102, 104, 105, 106, 113, 114, 116, 118, 121, 123, 124, 125, 126, 139, 141, 163, 199, 225
in vivo, 3, 16, 23, 26, 27, 31, 36, 40, 54, 74, 102, 103, 104, 106, 114, 119, 121, 124, 126, 139, 141, 165, 169, 219, 224
inactivation, xi, 8, 54, 179, 180
inactive, 43, 154, 187, 191, 198, 199, 211, 212
incidence, 77, 103, 104, 120
inclusion, 128
incubation, 110, 111, 131, 154
indication, 97, 116
indices, 58
indirect effect, 73
inducer, 22
induction, 24, 57, 66, 215, 216
inert, 48
infancy, 106
inflammation, 10, 26, 105
inflammatory response, 103
information processing, 172
inheritance, 62, 71
inherited, 70
inherited disorder, 70
inhibition, xi, 23, 32, 36, 57, 80, 87, 98, 122, 123, 125, 155, 179, 180, 188, 212, 220
inhibitor, 5, 6, 9, 26, 31, 32, 34, 104, 153, 154, 159
inhibitors, 3, 57, 87, 109, 154, 155, 194
inhibitory, 111, 156, 222
inhibitory effect, 111, 156
inhomogeneities, 168
initiation, 43, 53, 76, 175, 193, 195
injection, 79, 105, 128
injury, 10, 32, 43, 105, 109, 124
innate immunity, 215
inoculation, 106
inositol, 153, 158, 183, 205

insects, 4, 41, 53
insertion, 46, 52
inspection, 112
instability, 73, 88
insulation, 187
insulators, 50
insulin, 9, 30, 32, 207
insulin-like growth factor, 9, 30, 32
integration, 169
integrin, 3, 6, 7, 8, 9, 10, 12, 13, 14, 15, 19, 21, 22, 23, 24, 25, 26, 27, 28, 29, 31, 33, 34, 35, 36, 70, 80, 81, 82, 83, 84, 85, 86, 87, 88, 97, 98, 99, 122, 209, 219, 225
integrins, 1, 2, 3, 7, 8, 9, 10, 11, 12, 13, 14, 15, 16, 17, 19, 20, 21, 22, 23, 24, 25, 26, 27, 33, 35, 58, 81, 82, 83, 88, 98, 99, 100, 180, 182, 207
integrity, 70
intercellular adhesion molecule, 81
interface, 139, 140, 171
interference, 48, 50, 63, 98
interferon, 106, 120
interleukin, 106, 123, 189
interleukin-1, 106, 189
interleukin-2, 106
interleukin-8, 123
internalization, 5, 6, 7, 8, 9, 16, 17, 25, 32, 190, 209
internalizing, 26
interphase, 20, 50, 53, 67, 127, 128, 200
interrelations, 51
interstitial, 56
intervention, 169
intestine, 219
intravenously, 80
intrinsic, 3, 26
intron, 77
invasive, 102, 110, 124, 125
inversions, 45
invertebrates, 57
inverted repeats, 50
iodine, 13
ion channels, 40, 59, 95, 152, 167, 170, 172, 173
ionotropic glutamate receptor, 38
ions, x, 140, 161, 163, 171, 202
irradiation, 123, 189, 194
ischemia, 189
isoenzymes, 90
isoforms, 75, 76, 77, 80, 93, 96, 97, 140, 188, 189, 190, 196, 201, 204, 205, 207, 210, 220, 223
isolation, 106
isomerization, 49

J

Japan, 131, 149
JNK, 182, 189, 190, 191, 192, 193, 194, 208, 209, 215, 216, 217
joints, 75
Jun, 23, 28, 29, 31, 33, 34, 97, 98, 119, 120, 121, 122, 123, 124, 125, 182, 190, 208, 215, 217
Jung, 93, 95

K

K^+, x, 40, 161, 163, 167, 171, 172, 174, 175
keratin, 15
keratinocytes, 26, 28, 30
KH, 49
kidney, 30, 77, 79, 93, 96, 130, 165
kinase activity, 65, 158, 187, 200
kinetics, 5
King, 145, 158
knockout, 64, 77, 194
kringle domain, 12

L

labeling, 108, 113, 115, 117, 118, 170
lactose, 172
lamellae, 210
lamina, 84
laminar, 84
laminin, 15, 26, 73, 78, 81, 84, 86, 87, 94, 98
laminin-5, 26
land, 150, 154
Langmuir, 171, 172
language, 45, 61
language delay, 45, 61
laptop, 114
large-scale, 171
larva, 51
larvae, 48, 58
laser, 86, 110, 113, 134
latency, 103, 104
lattice, 174
LDH, 71
LDL, 26, 29, 32
lead, 189, 190, 213
learning, 38, 40, 46, 57, 71
learning difficulties, 71
lentiviral, 123

leucine, 190, 191, 192, 194, 217, 224
leukemia, 31
leukocyte, 35, 113
leukocytes, 29, 81, 124, 149, 150, 153
lice, 163
life cycle, 150, 157
lifetime, 127
ligand, 2, 4, 9, 12, 13, 14, 23, 26, 29, 33, 34, 35, 40, 81, 106, 167, 180, 183, 184, 187, 190, 201, 204, 224
ligands, 4, 6, 7, 8, 10, 13, 23, 50, 81, 185
limitations, 106, 165
linear, 38, 47, 59, 67, 84, 109, 111, 114, 124, 211
linkage, 90, 220
links, 6, 13, 145, 146, 189, 192, 203, 205, 213, 225
lipid, 4, 5, 8, 9, 10, 12, 26, 32, 34, 163, 164, 165, 166, 168, 169, 171, 172, 173, 174, 175, 176, 177, 200, 220
lipid rafts, 5, 8, 9, 10, 12, 26, 34, 173, 176, 200
lipids, x, 150, 161, 164, 165, 166, 167, 169, 171, 176
lipoprotein, 2, 9, 26, 28, 32, 34, 35, 36
liposomes, 172
liquid crystals, 171
liquid nitrogen, 130
liquids, 172
liver, 79, 103, 125, 198, 210
localised, 198, 200, 209, 210, 218
localization, 5, 6, 9, 14, 19, 20, 22, 25, 28, 33, 34, 39, 43, 46, 54, 59, 65, 79, 80, 95, 96, 98, 147, 150, 152, 153, 154, 155, 156, 159, 168, 173, 213
location, xi, 9, 22, 40, 46, 48, 75, 173, 179, 180, 202, 212
locomotion, 124, 209
locus, 45, 46, 48, 50, 58, 59, 72, 90, 91, 93, 94
long distance, 135
long-term memory, 58
Long-term potentiation (LTP), 43, 57, 59, 63, 66
low-density, 110
low-intensity, 176
LPA, 208
LTD, 38, 43, 59, 130
LTP, 38, 43, 57, 59, 61, 64, 66
lung, 79, 103, 106, 119, 123, 126, 146, 210
lung cancer, 146
lungs, 70, 75, 81, 87, 104, 135
lying, 116, 117, 118
lymph, 103
lymph node, 103
lymphocytes, 220
lymphoma, 106, 123

lysine, 49
lysosomes, 32, 209

M

machinery, 42, 43, 49, 59, 102, 144, 156, 209
machines, 39, 41
macromolecules, 42
magnetic field, 176
maintenance, 13, 49, 57, 59, 80, 109, 149, 151, 152, 155, 156, 158, 167, 171, 184, 212
maize, 159
males, 57, 72
malignant, 24, 30, 36, 102, 118, 121, 126
malignant cells, 36, 102, 118
malignant melanoma, 24
mammalian cell, 32, 134, 142, 152, 153, 168, 187
mammalian cells, 32, 142, 152, 153, 168, 187
mammalian tissues, 181
mammals, 4, 41, 72, 81, 141, 142, 182, 187, 189, 190, 198, 207, 210, 213
management, 170
manipulation, 41, 119
MAPK, xi, 23, 35, 82, 179, 181, 182, 187, 188, 189, 190, 192, 193, 194, 195, 207, 208, 209, 215, 216, 217
MAPKs, 105, 181, 182, 189, 192, 193
mapping, 46, 59
marrow, 104, 106, 120, 121, 122, 123
Mars, 29
Marx, 28
mask, 110
masking, 218
mass spectrometry, 144, 225
maternal, 51, 53, 90, 129, 137
matrix, 1, 6, 13, 15, 19, 21, 22, 27, 29, 34, 35, 53, 57, 73, 74, 78, 81, 82, 84, 92, 95, 98, 107, 115, 116, 117, 129, 164, 180, 209, 222, 225
matrix metalloproteinase, 225
matrix protein, 73, 78, 107, 209
maturation, 19, 34, 38, 93, 123, 129, 203, 209
MDA, 24, 110, 111, 119
measurement, 8, 124
measures, 109
mechanical energy, 34, 73
mechanical properties, 174
mechanical stress, 88
media, 105, 107, 108, 109, 110, 112, 119
mediators, 22
medulla, 46

meiosis, 45
MEK, 180, 181, 187, 188, 216
melanoma, 14, 27, 29, 32, 106, 122, 125, 168, 225
melatonin, 40
membranes, 73, 75, 78, 90, 107, 108, 110, 154, 156, 168, 169, 170, 171, 173, 174, 176, 183, 196, 202, 226
memory, 38, 40, 42, 46, 49, 57, 59, 63, 66
memory formation, 40, 57, 59, 63
mental impairment, 80
mental retardation, 45, 61, 77, 78, 80, 81, 88
mesenchymal stem cells, 101, 102, 115, 120, 121, 122, 123, 126
messages, 181, 215
messenger RNA, 35, 39
messengers, xi, 153, 179, 180, 212, 215
MET, 124
metabolism, 109, 158, 183
metabotropic glutamate receptor, 202, 204
metabotropic glutamate receptors, 202, 204
metalloproteinase, 225
metastases, 106
metastasis, 10, 36, 102, 103, 104, 106, 114, 120, 124, 140, 212, 226
metastasize, 104
metastatic cancer, 104, 120
metastatic disease, 103
metazoan, 143
methane, 46
methionine, 77
methylation, 49, 52, 54, 57, 62, 64
mGluR, 204, 205, 206, 223
mGluRs, 202, 204, 205
mice, 40, 42, 54, 64, 72, 77, 78, 79, 84, 91, 92, 93, 95, 103, 104, 106, 107, 120, 194, 199
microarray, 119
microdomains, xi, 161, 165, 166, 167, 172, 173, 176
microenvironment, 104, 105, 120, 121
microfilaments, 145, 225
microglia, 81
micrometer, 109
microRNAs (miRNAs), 42
microscope, 98, 107, 108, 110, 112, 113, 118, 119, 124, 130
microscopy, 24, 71, 84, 86, 98, 112, 113, 114, 117, 128, 129, 130, 165, 170, 202, 209
microsomes, 78
microspheres, 112
microtubule, 19, 21, 22, 33, 43, 127, 128, 129, 155, 158, 165, 176, 191, 210, 211, 212, 221

microtubules, 2, 19, 20, 21, 22, 23, 129, 133, 137, 140, 145, 150, 159, 164, 165, 176, 192, 211, 226
microvasculature, 96
migratory properties, 7
mimicking, 4
miRNAs, 38, 44, 51
mirror, 17, 18, 19
MIT, 168, 176
mitochondria, 113, 114, 196
mitogen, 20, 34, 35, 105, 144, 181, 215, 216, 217, 224
mitogen-activated protein kinase, 34, 35, 105, 144, 181, 215, 216, 217, 224
mitosis, 20, 21, 35, 127, 128, 130, 131, 132, 133, 134
MMP, 19, 209
mobility, 8, 70, 172
model system, 82, 102, 104, 114, 118, 124
modeling, 81, 103, 176
models, xi, 10, 12, 13, 53, 104, 105, 106, 120, 123, 125, 157, 161, 162, 163, 164, 170, 174
modulation, 28, 36, 73, 88, 98, 140, 144, 166, 209
modules, 164, 167, 213, 214, 216
molecular dynamics, 169
molecular mass, 205
molecular mechanisms, 71, 80, 125, 155, 156
molecular weight, 3, 4, 6, 25, 77, 78
molecules, xi, 2, 8, 10, 13, 16, 17, 19, 20, 39, 41, 54, 59, 81, 82, 86, 133, 139, 140, 145, 172, 179, 180, 184, 188, 192, 200, 202, 203, 204, 208, 211, 212, 213, 217, 218, 224
Møller, 32
monocyte, 35
monocytes, 25, 27, 120, 124
monolayer, 107, 109, 114, 118, 125
monolayers, 125
monomer, 210
monomers, 8, 206
Monte Carlo, 164
morning, 115
morphogenesis, 13, 28, 61, 83, 149, 190, 200, 219
morphology, 5, 14, 15, 17, 18, 19, 20, 23, 28, 41, 62, 63, 64, 78, 95, 103, 133, 164, 221
mortality, 103
mosaic, 164, 175
Moscow, 66, 127, 136
mother cell, 20, 141
motile cells, 17, 210
motion, 2, 64, 67

mouse, 26, 44, 50, 67, 68, 72, 73, 77, 79, 92, 94, 95, 96, 97, 104, 105, 106, 122, 125, 134, 142, 147, 170, 213, 223
mouse model, 73, 104, 106
movement, xi, 6, 16, 53, 75, 102, 104, 124, 140, 151, 153, 158, 164, 165, 179, 180, 181, 188, 210
mRNA, 3, 39, 42, 43, 44, 49, 51, 65, 66, 67, 68, 72, 76, 77, 78, 79, 121, 217
MSC, 121, 122
MSCs, 122
MTs, 150
mucosa, 119, 126
multicellular organisms, 149, 198
multicellular resistance, 125
multinucleated cells, 108
murine model, 123
muscle, xi, 17, 20, 70, 71, 72, 73, 74, 75, 76, 78, 79, 80, 87, 90, 91, 93, 95, 140, 146, 174, 179, 180, 207
muscle cells, 17, 20, 74
muscle contraction, xi, 75, 179, 180
muscle strength, 70
muscle tissue, 71, 72
muscles, 70, 75, 174
muscular contraction, 73
muscular dystrophy, 73, 77, 78, 89, 90, 91, 92, 93, 94, 95, 97
muscular tissue, 73, 75, 76, 78
mutagen, 48
mutagenesis, 40
mutant, 28, 34, 46, 51, 53, 58, 64
mutants, 3, 46, 50, 51, 52, 54, 58, 200
mutation, 3, 46, 54, 91, 97
mutations, 45, 46, 47, 70, 72, 73, 75, 78, 79, 80, 99, 207
myelin, 94
myeloid, 14
myocardium, 70
myocytes, 76
myofibroblasts, 122
myogenesis, 95
myosin, 62, 63, 73, 139, 140, 141, 142, 146, 147, 150, 157, 159, 210, 225

N

Na^+, x, 40, 161, 167, 199, 219
nanomachines, 169
nanostructures, 168
nanotubes, 169, 173
nanowires, 175
Nash, 180, 213
natural killer, 106
neck, 23, 141
necrosis, 73, 106, 225
necrotic core, 115
negative consequences, 13
negative reinforcement, 46
neovascularization, 105, 106
nephron, 96
nerve, 38, 41, 57, 59, 68, 77, 80, 94, 97, 171
nerve cells, 41
nerve growth factor, 80, 97
nervous system, 38, 41, 59, 70, 77, 81, 87, 94, 99, 167, 174
network, 10, 13, 17, 18, 19, 21, 22, 38, 74, 122, 128, 146, 163, 164, 166, 167, 202, 206, 209, 222
neural development, 41, 62, 63, 84, 96
neural network, 163, 170
neural networks, 163, 170
neural stem cell, 41
neural stem cells, 41
neurobiology, 38, 59, 171
neurochemistry, 61, 98
neurodegeneration, 66
neurodegenerative disease, 58
neurodegenerative diseases, 58
neurodegenerative disorders, 38, 43
neurogenesis, 67
neurological disease, 224
neuronal cells, 88
neuronal circuits, 57
neuronal migration, 80, 88, 99
neuronal precursor cells, 80
neurons, 38, 39, 40, 41, 43, 61, 65, 70, 76, 80, 81, 83, 123, 162, 163, 165, 166, 167, 168, 169, 171, 172, 173, 175, 177, 204, 224
neuropeptide, 41
neurophysiology, 174
neuroprotective, 42
neuropsychology, 170
neurotoxins, 33
neurotransmitter, 44, 59, 176, 202
neurotransmitters, 40, 59, 77
neutralization, 36
neutrophil, 30, 124
neutrophils, 30, 34, 35, 153
new, 164, 167, 169, 170, 176
New Science, 175

New York, 103, 169, 170, 171, 172, 173, 174, 175, 176
Nielsen, 3, 24, 27, 32, 35, 125, 173
NIH, 113
nitrate, 203
nitric oxide, 74, 92, 221
nitric oxide synthase, 74, 92, 222
nitrogen, 130
NK, 106, 193
NK-cell, 106
NMDA, 40, 43, 202, 203, 204, 205, 206, 222
NMDA receptors, 202, 203, 206
N-methyl-D-aspartate, 202, 222
NMR, 165
nodes, 147, 167
noise, 165, 175
normal, 33, 37, 38, 40, 42, 46, 58, 59, 75, 77, 84, 88, 91, 93, 103, 113, 115, 118, 125, 135, 165, 166, 181, 207
normal development, 37, 38, 59, 207
Northern Ireland, 142
novelty, 164
N-terminal, 3, 54, 65, 72, 77, 85, 86, 182, 198, 199, 200, 203, 204, 205, 208, 212, 216, 217, 218, 221
nuclear, 38, 39, 40, 41, 49, 54, 55, 56, 58, 60, 61, 65, 66, 76, 79, 80, 95, 96, 98, 108, 129, 130, 133, 134, 135, 156, 159, 190, 196
nucleation, 128, 186, 204, 210
nuclei, 40, 50, 108, 113, 114, 132, 134
nucleosomes, 41
nucleotides, 76
nucleus, 17, 18, 19, 35, 37, 38, 39, 40, 45, 48, 52, 54, 56, 59, 67, 81, 95, 131, 187, 191, 192, 193

O

observations, 57, 105, 130, 174
olfactory, 46, 78
olfactory bulb, 78
oligomerization, 34, 216
oligomers, 181, 191, 192
oncogene, 21, 26, 29, 120, 123
oocyte, 39
oocytes, 50, 67, 68, 142, 147
oogenesis, 39, 64, 134
optics, 118
organ, 78, 80, 101, 115, 125, 185
organelle, 127, 128
organelles, 194, 196
organism, 16, 37, 39, 59, 82, 139, 141, 142, 198

organization, 167, 168, 169, 171, 173, 213
orientation, 21, 35, 45, 84, 123, 129, 133, 169, 183
oscillations, 30, 177
OSM, 194, 195
osteoblasts, 113
osteoclasts, 19
ovarian cancer, 27, 28, 106, 123
ovarian cancers, 106
ovary, 222
overlay, 118
overload, 116
oxide, 221
oxygen, 144

P

p38, 23, 27, 29, 82, 182, 190, 192, 193, 194, 195, 217
p53, 190
packaging, 38, 41, 46
PAI-1, 5, 6, 9, 15, 19, 24, 26
pairing, 38, 45, 46, 50, 51, 53, 54, 57, 60, 61
pancreatic islet, 121
paracrine, 105
paradigm shift, 167
parameter, 75
Paris, 169
particles, 108, 111, 165, 206
paternal, 53, 137
pathology, 58, 59, 70
pathophysiology, 171
pathways, xi, 7, 16, 22, 23, 25, 26, 28, 29, 49, 50, 57, 98, 105, 139, 140, 179, 180, 181, 182, 183, 190, 192, 194, 196, 203, 204, 206, 208, 209, 211, 212, 216, 222
patients, 31, 34, 35, 58, 70, 71, 72, 73, 77, 78, 79, 80, 88, 90, 91, 103, 170
patterning, 45, 65
PC12 cells, 80, 84, 85, 86, 87, 88, 96, 97, 98, 99
PCM, 129
PCR, 43, 46, 72, 91, 121
PCS, 129
PD, 34, 90
PDGF, 2, 182, 188, 201
PDZ domains, 40, 53, 92, 181, 184, 199, 203, 214, 222
pemphigus, 30
peptide, 3, 15, 26, 28, 31, 168, 176, 183, 184, 185, 213
peptides, 3, 124, 141, 169, 176, 183, 185

Index

performance, 221
peripheral nerve, 77, 94, 174
peripheral nervous system, 94
permeability, 71, 169
peroxisomes, 157
pertussis, 18, 26
pH, 130
phagocytosis, 112, 142
phenotype, 61, 78, 79, 84, 103, 104, 105, 121
phenotypes, 45
phenotypic, 106, 126
pheochromocytoma, 97
phosphatases, xi, 40, 179, 180, 182, 184, 185, 196, 198, 200, 201, 203, 212, 217
phosphatases, 60
phosphate, 2, 7, 9, 30, 32, 130
phosphates, 183
phosphatidic acid, 154
phosphatidylcholine, 155
phosphodiesterase, 46, 200
phosphoinositides, 157, 158, 183
phospholipase C, 149, 158, 202
phospholipids, 165, 172, 176, 184
phosphoprotein, 185
phosphorylates, 40, 133, 181, 187, 189, 191, 193, 200, 204, 208, 213, 224
phosphorylation, 31, 33, 35, 40, 49, 58, 62, 81, 82, 87, 90, 98, 99, 123, 141, 181, 182, 183, 187, 188, 189, 190, 191, 192, 193, 194, 196, 197, 198, 199, 204, 207, 208, 211, 212, 219, 220, 222, 224, 225
photon, 31
physical interaction, 54
physiological regulation, 152
PI3K, 87, 153, 154, 155, 156
PKC, 197, 207
plants, 4, 41, 54, 150, 153, 154, 157, 159
plasma, 2, 4, 5, 6, 8, 9, 15, 28, 30, 31, 82, 156, 167, 172, 182, 183, 187, 196, 197, 198, 199, 200, 203, 205, 220
plasma membrane, 2, 4, 5, 8, 9, 15, 28, 30, 82, 156, 167, 172, 182, 183, 187, 196, 197, 198, 199, 200, 203, 205, 220
plasmid, 79
plasmids, 84
plasminogen, 1, 6, 9, 23, 24, 25, 26, 27, 28, 29, 30, 31, 32, 33, 34, 35, 36
plastic, 82, 111, 115, 116
plasticity, 37, 38, 42, 43, 57, 59, 62, 202, 223
platelet, 87, 99, 182, 201, 207
platelet aggregation, 88, 99

platelets, 94, 210
platforms, 8, 119
play, 5, 10, 13, 40, 57, 59, 102, 128, 139, 150, 151, 200
PLC, 153, 154, 155, 156
PLD, 154, 155, 156
plexus, 96
point mutation, 3, 54, 97
polarity, 16, 19, 103, 104, 146, 149, 150, 151, 152, 153, 154, 155, 156, 158, 173, 175, 184, 209, 212, 214
polarization, 17, 18, 30, 145, 146, 154, 167, 173
polarized, 166, 177
pollen, 150, 155, 157, 158
pollen tube, 150, 155, 157, 158
polycarbonate, 107
polyglutamine, 63
polymerase, 39, 72
polymerase chain reaction, 72
polymerization, 130, 154, 176, 201
polymers, 40
polymorphism, 46, 62
polymorphisms, 72
polymorphonuclear, 35, 123, 124
polypeptide, 3
polyploid, 128
polyproline, 183
poor, 4, 58
poor performance, 58
population, 20, 64, 84, 105, 118, 120, 124
pore, 107, 109
pores, 39, 107
Portugal, 101
position effect, 48, 68
positive correlation, 53
postmortem, 58
potassium, x, xi, 53, 79, 161, 162, 163, 168, 169, 171, 173, 176
potassium channels, 168, 173
power, 47
powers, 102
PP2A, 60, 187, 200
Prader-Willi syndrome, 45
pRB, 133
preconditioning, 121
precursor cells, 80, 120
prednisone, 71
Prednisone, 90
pre-existing, 20, 57, 128, 210
preference, 49, 173, 191

pressure, 168
presynaptic, 43, 162
prevention, 91
probability, x, 103, 161, 163, 166
probe, 19, 27
production, 9, 75, 106, 115, 153, 155, 221
progenitor cells, 42, 104, 105, 120, 122
progenitor-like, 106
progenitors, 120
progesterone, 103, 120
prognosis, 4, 35, 104
prognostic value, 103
program, 51
proinflammatory, 35, 216
proliferation, 1, 2, 3, 6, 7, 10, 11, 20, 23, 27, 28, 29, 30, 33, 81, 106, 109, 114, 123, 124, 144, 149, 181, 182, 189, 190
promote, 201, 204, 205, 210, 212, 216
promoter, 28, 39, 61, 76, 77, 78, 84, 93, 95
promoter region, 93
propagation, x, xi, 161, 162, 163, 165, 166, 167, 169, 172, 175, 176
prophylactic, 120
propionic acid, 221
proposition, 142
prostate, 27, 33, 106, 115, 123
prostate cancer, 27, 33, 115, 123
protease inhibitors, 87
proteases, 4, 75
protein family, 96, 223
protein folding, 123, 168, 172, 175
protein function, 32
protein kinase C, 30, 153, 205, 220, 224
protein kinases, 53, 87, 105, 181, 182, 184, 197, 199, 200, 203, 208, 215, 216
protein sequence, 47
protein synthesis, 43, 57, 61, 68, 71, 90, 194
proteinase, 28
protein-protein interactions, 85, 191, 207, 211
proteolysis, 2, 6, 7, 12, 16, 29, 34, 88, 99, 141
proteome, 28
proteomics, 43
protocol, 112
protocols, 107, 113
protozoa, 4
PSD, 43, 92, 181, 184, 202, 203, 204, 205, 206, 221, 222, 223
pseudo, 89
pseudopodia, 19, 157
pulse, 163

pumps, 152
purification, 32, 87, 218
Purkinje, 76, 93, 162, 172
Purkinje cells, 76, 172

Q

quality of life, 70
quanta, 167
quantum, 111, 124
quantum dot, 111, 124
query, 163

R

race, 16
radial glia, 83
radioresistance, 10
radius, 162
rafts, 171, 174, 175
rain, 38
random, 84, 102, 110, 112, 114, 124, 166
range, 79, 102, 113, 114, 115, 119, 139, 140, 172, 183, 184, 185, 212
rapamycin, 67
rat, 8, 16, 18, 19, 21, 26, 38, 43, 77, 79, 96, 97, 106, 116, 117, 122, 125, 126, 162, 165, 223
rats, 106, 126, 172
reaction rate, 42
reactive oxygen, 144
reactive oxygen species, 144
reading, 77
reagents, 108, 115
reception, 16
receptor-negative, 120
receptor-positive, 120
reciprocal interactions, 107, 115
recognition, 183, 185, 187, 213, 214
recombination, 38, 44, 45, 46, 47, 48, 52, 59, 63
recruiting, 12, 13, 122, 190, 221
recycling, 9, 16, 25, 200
red light, 130
redistribution, 5, 8, 13, 17, 20, 64, 201
reduction, 208
reflection, 98, 117
refractory, 104
regeneration, 9
regular, 109, 112
regulators, 43, 49, 133, 153, 197, 204, 206

reinforcement, 46
relapse, 103
relationship, 2, 8, 19, 20, 22, 31, 35, 151
relationships, 1, 2, 33, 38
relatives, 90
relaxation, 73
relevance, 6, 28, 34, 75, 114, 119
remodeling, 25, 28, 38, 39, 40, 41, 54, 59, 61, 62, 63, 64, 65, 66, 67, 68, 88, 105
remodelling, 41, 49, 186, 224
replication, 48, 79, 127, 128, 130, 131, 133, 134, 135, 136
reporters, 108
repression, 48, 60
reproduction, 129, 221
research, x, 161, 169, 207
researchers, 163
reservoir, 105
residues, 3, 49, 87, 141, 182, 183, 184, 185, 186, 187, 190, 196, 198, 204, 207
resin, 130
resistance, 10, 125, 208
resolution, 165
respiratory, 70
resting potential, 163
restitution, 79
retardation, 45, 90
retention, 70
reticulum, 4, 43, 92, 159, 165, 196
retina, 77, 78, 79, 93, 95
retinoic acid, 125, 168
retroviruses, 79
Reynolds, 99, 220
RFLP, 72
Rho, 40, 59, 82, 143, 147, 182, 187, 188, 189, 190, 200, 201, 204, 205, 207, 208, 210, 211, 215, 219, 224
Rhodophyta, 157
ribosomal, 48
ribosomal RNA, 48
rice, 154
rigidity, 75
rings, 147
RISC, 49
risk, 70
RNA, 37, 39, 42, 43, 44, 47, 48, 49, 52, 53, 57, 59, 60, 63, 64, 65, 66, 67, 73, 185, 186
RNA processing, 185
RNAi, 49, 60, 61, 65
road map, 23
rodent, 93
room temperature, 113
root hair, 150, 153, 158, 159
Russia, 37, 127, 130
Russian Academy of Sciences, 37

S

Saccharomyces cerevisiae, 140, 146, 147, 215
safety, 162, 166
salivary glands, 44, 50, 54
sample, 130
SAP, 193, 203
satellite, 48, 71, 90
satellite cells, 71
scaffold, 79, 81, 140, 144, 146, 181, 187, 191, 192, 193, 194, 195, 196, 198, 200, 201, 204, 206, 208, 209, 212, 213, 214, 215, 216, 217, 218, 221, 223, 224
scaffolding, xi, 43, 87, 179, 180, 181, 182, 187, 188, 189, 190, 191, 192, 194, 196, 199, 200, 202, 204, 205, 206, 209, 212, 215, 216, 217, 220, 221, 223, 224
scaffolds, xi, 30, 94, 179, 181, 190, 194, 206
scatter, 31, 110, 123
scavenger, 15
schizophrenia, 39, 61, 62
Schwann cells, 77, 78, 94
SDF-1, 105
SDH, 6, 29
SE, 33, 91, 92, 93, 99
sea urchin, 140, 143
seals, 23
search, 40, 133, 166
seaweed, 150
secrete, 84
secretion, 109, 146
seeding, 103, 104, 109, 115, 116, 117
segregation, 171
selecting, 119
selective estrogen receptor modulator, 104
selectivity, 146, 188, 212
self-assembly, 175
self-organization, 38
sensing, 26, 35, 157, 207, 224
sensitivity, 18, 26
sensors, 22, 140
separation, 20, 129, 135, 137, 141, 171
sequencing, 50
series, 32, 58, 131, 181, 207

serine, 40, 53, 87, 141, 182, 187, 204
SERMs, 104
serpin, 5, 15, 32
serum, 46, 71, 90, 108, 109, 110, 113, 124, 130
sex, 54, 67
sex chromosome, 54
shape, 14, 15, 17, 18, 19, 25, 100, 102, 159, 170, 198, 199, 203, 212, 219, 222, 224
shares, 10, 147, 210, 214
sharing, 53, 157
shock, 43, 57, 58, 73, 189, 194, 195, 217
shortness of breath, 70
short-term, 120, 121
signal peptide, 3
signal transduction, 25, 27, 29, 40, 53, 74, 98, 157, 183, 184, 185, 195, 196, 200, 202, 203, 208, 212, 213, 214, 216, 217
signaling pathway, 21, 40, 65, 87, 98, 99, 102, 105, 155, 216
signaling pathways, 21, 81, 98, 102, 105, 155, 216
signals, xi, 2, 7, 13, 19, 21, 33, 37, 38, 40, 112, 135, 159, 162, 165, 167, 179, 180, 188, 189, 192, 193, 200, 201, 215
signal-to-noise ratio, 165
signs, 16
similarity, 53, 72, 141, 143, 147, 210
simulation, 168, 172
simulations, 163
siRNA, 49, 63
sites, 3, 4, 27, 38, 39, 44, 46, 47, 54, 66, 76, 78, 82, 84, 92, 99, 101, 102, 103, 104, 105, 122, 140, 165, 167, 180, 182, 188, 189, 191, 192, 196, 197, 198, 200, 201, 204, 205, 207, 209, 211, 214, 216
skeletal muscle, 15, 70, 71, 76, 77, 78, 91, 92, 93, 95, 141, 146
skeleton, 81, 87, 164, 175
skin, 77
smooth muscle, 8, 16, 18, 19, 21, 24, 26, 27, 28, 30, 32, 33, 99, 123
smooth muscle cells, 8, 16, 18, 19, 21, 24, 26, 27, 28, 30, 32, 123
SMS, 45
snake venom, 33
sodium, 117, 168, 169, 171, 220
sodium hydroxide, 117
software, 44, 113, 114, 117, 119
solid tumors, 105
solubility, 172
somatic cells, 50, 62, 129, 150
somatic stem cells, 124

somatostatin, 205
sorbitol, 194, 195
sorting, 50, 108, 124, 168, 169, 209, 219
spatial processing, 45
specialisation, 221
species, 44, 133, 144, 162
specificity, 42, 44, 47, 59, 81, 180, 183, 185, 187, 213, 216, 222
spectroscopy, 31, 174
spectrum, 38
speech, 6, 34
sperm, 194
spermatozoa, 78, 95
S-phase, 128, 129, 130, 134, 135
spinal cord, 162, 168, 170
spindle, 15, 21, 33, 35, 127, 128, 135, 143
spine, 25, 38, 60, 64, 65, 67, 75, 183, 221
spines, 38, 40, 44, 174, 203
spore, 158
sporophyte, 150
St. Petersburg, 37, 130
stability, 39, 49, 61, 73, 84, 94, 167, 171
stabilization, 41, 88, 217
stabilize, 8
stages, 45, 49, 53, 79, 96, 128, 130, 132, 133, 152
standard error, 112
standard model, 162
standards, 189
steady state, 206
stem cells, 41, 59, 70, 78, 95, 101, 102, 106, 113, 115, 120, 121, 122, 123, 124, 125, 126
sterile, 115, 205
stiffness, 15
Stimuli, 65
stimulus, 21, 180, 202
stochastic, 164, 175
stoichiometry, 140, 181
stomach, 210
storage, 13
strain, 46, 51, 58, 84, 85, 151, 209
strains, 46, 48, 54
strategies, 70, 79, 169
strength, 70, 85, 107, 167, 189
stress, 14, 15, 17, 18, 19, 22, 29, 36, 43, 66, 74, 82, 87, 159, 181, 182, 190, 192, 193, 194, 208, 209, 216, 225
stretching, 46
stroma, 103, 104, 105, 120, 122
stromal cells, 101
structural changes, 163, 190

structural characteristics, 72
structural protein, 7, 207
subdomains, 198, 199
substances, 75, 110, 112
substitutes, 33
substrates, 29, 47, 98, 99, 124, 182, 187, 190, 191, 192, 193, 196, 200, 202, 209
summaries, 152
Sun, 200, 217, 219
suppression, 57, 123, 164
suppressor, 187, 216
supramolecular complex, 40, 53
surgery, 94
surprise, 10, 19
survival, 10, 33, 51, 82, 103, 106, 120, 199
surviving, 75
suspensions, 117
Sweden, 26, 130
swelling, 70
switching, 60
symptoms, 70, 75
synapse, 10, 41, 44, 57, 63, 64, 173, 200, 202, 220, 222
synapses, 60, 77, 167, 171, 184, 202, 205
synaptic plasticity, 38, 42, 43, 57, 59, 169, 202
synaptic transmission, 38, 57
synaptic vesicles, 78
synaptogenesis, 40, 70, 80, 88
synaptophysin, 64
synchronization, 134
synchronous, 50
syndrome, 38, 40, 45, 46, 59, 61
synthesis, 4, 13, 25, 42, 43, 44, 46, 57, 61, 68, 71, 90, 97, 130, 133, 155, 163, 168, 169, 194
synthetic, 170
systemic sclerosis, 31
systems, 164, 166, 176

T

T cell, 153, 157, 200
T cells, 153, 200
T lymphocyte, 24, 220
T lymphocytes, 24, 220
tamoxifen, 104, 120
tandem mass spectrometry, 144, 225
targets, 32, 146, 171, 182, 185, 192, 193
teeth, 81, 87
telomere, 45, 46
telophase, 200
temperature, 46, 48, 51, 58, 113, 130
tendons, 117
tension, 22
territory, 62
testis, 189
TGF, 6, 32, 104
theory, 169
therapeutic, 169
therapeutics, 36
therapy, 31, 79, 80, 97, 121, 122
thin film, 169
thin films, 169
thinking, 41
Thomson, 64, 90
threat, 70
threonine, 53, 87, 141, 182, 187, 190, 198, 199, 204
threshold, 215
thrombin, 88
thymidine, 130, 131, 132
thyroglobulin, 13
thyroid, 13, 20, 33, 34
thyroid carcinoma, 34
thyroid gland, 13
time, x, 161, 163, 164, 165, 166, 204, 222
tissue, 10, 28, 71, 72, 73, 75, 77, 79, 80, 97, 101, 103, 105, 115, 116, 118, 125, 126, 164, 184, 210
tissue homeostasis, 10, 184
TNF, 190, 208
TNF-α, 208
tobacco, 158
toxicity, 106
toxin, 18, 26, 142, 147
tracking, 113, 165, 172
traffic, 168, 183, 203
traits, 63, 120
transcript, 50, 72, 76, 77, 78, 93, 94, 106
transcription, xi, 38, 39, 40, 41, 49, 51, 53, 57, 62, 65, 76, 77, 78, 81, 87, 98, 103, 105, 133, 156, 159, 179, 181, 182, 184, 185, 186, 187, 190, 191, 192, 193, 216
transcription factor, xi, 40, 49, 53, 62, 76, 78, 81, 87, 98, 103, 156, 159, 179, 181, 182, 184, 185, 186, 187, 190, 191, 192, 193, 216
transcription factors, xi, 49, 53, 62, 76, 81, 87, 156, 159, 179, 181, 182, 184, 185, 186, 187, 190, 192, 193, 216
transcripts, 44, 49, 68, 75, 76, 79
transducer, 31, 105
transduction, 34, 53, 183, 184, 185, 195, 196, 200, 202, 203, 208, 212, 213, 214, 215, 216, 217

transfection, 108
transfer, xi, 23, 35, 97, 123, 179, 180
transformation, 20, 21, 216
transformations, 110
transforming growth factor, 6
transgenic mice, 84, 120
transgenic mouse, 104
transition, 41, 51, 67, 104, 119, 120, 122, 134, 135, 177
transitions, 41, 64, 110
translation, 38, 39, 41, 42, 43, 49, 57, 59, 63, 67, 68, 76, 87
translocation, 72, 90, 91, 187, 193, 197, 198, 199, 219
translocations, 72
transmembrane, x, 1, 2, 3, 4, 5, 7, 12, 16, 31, 73, 82, 92, 94, 161, 163, 169, 175, 194, 199, 202, 203, 204, 205, 206, 210, 219, 220
transmembrane region, 202
transmission, 14, 38, 39, 57, 180, 192, 202
transmits, 73
transplantation, 103, 104
transport, xi, 34, 39, 40, 43, 58, 63, 65, 66, 164, 179, 180, 185, 199, 211, 212
transposons, 49, 62
transverse section, 151
travel, 110
triggers, 135, 203
tropism, 80, 106, 124
tryptophan, 185
tumo(u)r, 3, 6, 10, 20, 23, 25, 29, 30, 32, 33, 35, 36, 101, 102, 103, 104, 105, 106, 107, 109, 112, 114, 115, 117, 118, 119, 120, 121, 122, 123, 124, 125, 140, 225
tumor cells, 29, 36, 101, 102, 103, 105, 109, 112, 114, 115, 117, 119
tumor growth, 23, 25, 105, 106, 120, 122
tumor necrosis factor, 106, 225
tumor progression, 122
tumorigenesis, 104, 105, 120
tumors, 102, 103, 104, 105, 106, 119, 120, 123
tumour growth, 3
tumours, 119, 120
turnover, 15, 23, 43, 188
tyrosine, 2, 7, 10, 23, 30, 35, 82, 181, 182, 183, 184, 187, 190, 197, 201, 204, 214

U

ultrastructure, 128, 129, 132, 174
ultraviolet, 137
uncertainty, 5
unfolded, 166
uniform, 17, 18, 19, 115, 215
unmasking, 219
urinary, 28
urine, 34
urokinase, 1, 2, 3, 6, 12, 18, 21, 23, 24, 25, 26, 27, 28, 29, 30, 31, 32, 33, 34, 35, 36
UTRs, 59
UV, 136, 137, 189, 194
UV irradiation, 189, 194

V

values, 55, 75
variability, 5, 65, 175
variable, 183, 202
variance, 167
variation, 111, 140
variegation, 48, 68
vascular disease, 16
vascular diseases, 16
vascular endothelial growth factor, 104, 123, 144
vasculature, 103
vasodilator, 185
vector, 79, 113
vehicles, 106, 120, 122
vein, 104
velocity, 163, 170, 175
ventricular zone, 83
versatility, 98
vertebrates, 42, 57
very low density lipoprotein, 36
vesicle, 42, 152, 167, 211
vesicles, 78, 196, 198, 209
vessels, 78
video microscopy, 113, 114, 117
villus, 219
vimentin, 43, 74, 103, 104
viral vectors, 80
viruses, 65
Visa, 39, 41, 65
visible, 18, 132, 133
visual, 162, 175
visual system, 46
visualization, 72, 156
visuospatial, 40
Vitronectin, 6, 25
VLDL, 2, 7

vulnerability, 61

W

water, 115
weak interaction, xi, 179, 180, 212
weakness, 75
Weinberg, 119, 121, 222
wells, 108, 109, 111, 113
western blot, 85
wheelchair, 70
wild type, 50, 51, 54, 55, 57, 78, 85, 86, 87, 88, 209
Wiskott-Aldrich syndrome, 201, 221, 222, 226
Wnt signaling, 81, 87
wound healing, 16, 101, 105, 120, 123
WW domains, 205, 214

X

X chromosome, 46, 49, 53, 56, 66, 72, 89, 90
xenograft, 105, 106

X-linked, 71, 90, 201

Y

Y chromosome, 48
yeast, 32, 41, 49, 139, 140, 141, 142, 143, 146, 147, 153, 158, 181, 191, 194, 213, 216

Z

zinc, 85, 99, 145, 185, 223, 226
zygote, 51
zygotes, 154, 155